Limb Malformations

Stefan Mundlos • Denise Horn

Limb Malformations

An Atlas of Genetic Disorders of Limb Development

Springer

Stefan Mundlos
Institut für Medizinische Genetik
und Humangenetik
Berlin, Germany

Denise Horn
Institut für Medizinische Genetik
und Humangenetik
Berlin, Germany

ISBN 978-3-540-95927-4 ISBN 978-3-540-95928-1 (eBook)
DOI 10.1007/978-3-540-95928-1
Springer Heidelberg New York Dordrecht London
Library of Congress Control Number: 2014956750

Printed on acid-free paper

Springer is part of Springer Science+Business Media (www.springer.com)

Foreword

In this book Stefan Mundlos, Denise Horn, and their associates set out to put more order into a field that Maurice Lamy in his preface to Pierre Maroteaux' 'Maladies osseuses de l'enfant' called 'chaotic' because of the multitude of conditions and their bewildering nomenclature. It focuses on malformations of the limbs – 'dysostoses' in today's nomenclature – and includes a selection of bone dysplasias with prominent limb involvement. Abnormal limbs have been described since the battle in Gath "where there was a man of great stature that had on every hand six fingers and on every foot six toes … also born to the giant" (Old Testament, 2 Sam 21:20). A treasure of malformed limbs can be viewed to this day in the Meckel collection in Halle/Germany that was started in the mid-18th century by Johann Friedrich Meckel, the elder, and brought to blossom by his grandson, Johann Friedrich Meckel, the younger, the very Meckel, who in 1822 recognized a 'defective formation in siblings' that included polydactyly and now is known as the Meckel syndrome, a highly heterogeneous ciliopathy covered in this atlas. Ernst Fischer, in his multivolume "Morphologie der Mißbildungen des Menschen und der Tiere" first published in 1906, a historical 'must' for the scholar of malformations, devoted a large section to developmental limb anomalies. Whereas he and his predecessor pathologists by trade focused on lethal conditions, the study of dysostoses in children and adults was the realm of pediatricians including Eugène Apert, Rudolf Pfeiffer, Walter Fuhrmann, Hans-Rudolf Wiedemann, to name a few. Still, these disorders were too rare to raise wide public interest or concern.

This changed dramatically with the entrance of thalidomide in the drug marked in 1957, and the discovery by another pediatrician-geneticist, Widukind Lenz, of its deleterious effects on early limb development in man. Stefan Mundlos and Denise Horn now come into this tradition with their pioneering work on limb defects.

Major limb malformations are difficult to categorize and to differentiate on clinical and radiological grounds. All of them are individually rare and confusing in their complexity and variability. In these days, the molecular elucidation of many of them helps in their delineation, and determines the spectrum of their expression. This achievement would not have been possible without an intricate relationship between clinical medicine and basic science, personalized by Stefan Mundlos' broad professional background, realized by the fertile intertwining of the Institute of Medical Genetics and the Max Planck Institute for Molecular Biology in Berlin, and documented in this atlas.

The book's main benefit will be in diagnostics. Taxonomy, the art of organizing vast amounts of data, is its indispensable tool. Since Geoffroy Saint-Hilaire, in his 1832 'Traité de Tératologie', differentiated between ectroméliens and syméliens, i.e. reduction and fusion anomalies, numerous classifications have been proposed. The present one offers a coherent system of morphological categories and causally determined subcategories. Similarity between actual and depicted phenotypes will guide the physicians' quest for molecular confirmation of a suspected diagnosis.

Is this old-fashioned? Will computational phenotype/genotype analysis make an atlas a relict of the past? Will we forgo books when digitalized algorhythms have been brought to perfection? Probably not. Both have their own domains. Computers handle fragments to synthesize entities.

Books present entities that reason analyzes. Through analysis we conceive the commonness of conditions, understand their basis and genesis, become experts.

As publications go, this atlas probably will be digitalized. Some students will read it as a book, screen by screen, condition by condition. Others will continue to prefer the compactness of a book, the rustle of paper, the prospect of leafing through pages to pictures on a screen and clicks on a keyboard. They all will enjoy the treasure and clarity of its content and the beauty of its presentation.

Jürgen Spranger
Professor emeritus
Children's Hospital
University of Mainz/Germany

Preface

Congenital malformations are relatively common among newborns. If recognized early, many can be treated, and a complete repair can often be achieved. Our knowledge about this diverse field of medicine has greatly increased over the last decades. We now recognize a myriad of conditions that can be distinguished on clinical grounds as well as by their molecular causes. This book concentrates on a subgroup of skeletal diseases, malformations, and growth defects that predominantly affect the limbs.

Limb malformations are considered a relatively common type of malformation. Because of their bewildering complexity in phenotypes and their frequent association with other malformations and clinical symptoms, they are often difficult to diagnose. Furthermore, abnormalities of the hands are often perceived as stigmatizing, but with adequate and timely surgical and conservative management, many conditions can be improved or even cured. Beyond the clinical interest, skeletal diseases can serve as a paradigm to understand human genetics. The first human disorder recognized to follow the principles of Mendelian inheritance was described by Farabee in 1903. The original pedigree exhibited a classic dominant pattern of segregation over five generations featuring absent or shortened middle phalanges in the hands and feet, a condition now termed brachydactyly type A1 (BDA1). As with many other conditions, the molecular cause of BDA1 has been unraveled, giving us new insights in gene function and basic mechanisms of skeletal development.

For the patient and family members, limb malformations result in various problems, but the extent of these depends on the location and size of the reduction and the functional impairment. Some potential difficulties include questions about the recurrence risk within families; complications with normal development, such as motor skills; the need for assistance with daily activities; limitations in certain movements, sports, or activities; and potential emotional and social issues because of physical appearance. To improve a family's and patient's situation, many medical specialists need to be involved, but communication across disciplines is often hindered by different language and terminology. It is the aim of this book to name, describe, and categorize limb malformations in order to facilitate their correct diagnosis for improved clinical care. This book is therefore addressed to medical geneticists, radiologists, pediatricians, hand surgeons, orthopedic surgeons, and other physicians as well as medical personnel involved in evaluating and treating patients with abnormal limbs.

In contrast to many other genetic conditions that present with rather uniform features, limb malformations are multifaceted in their phenotypic appearances and very heterogenous in their causes. Extreme phenotypic variability and nonpenetrance are common and impose diagnostic challenges on the clinician. In many other genetic disease groups, such as the skeletal dysplasias, a descriptive approach to classify groups and individual conditions has been very successful, even helping to define molecular abnormalities. In limb malformations similar approaches have been taken, and numerous systems for classification of upper-limb anomalies have been proposed. Anatomical classification schemes based on clinical severity can indeed provide useful disease categories that can be used as therapeutic guidelines. However, purely descriptive terminologies cannot account for phenotypic variability, and when true genetic classifications based on etiologies are considered, many systems become outdated as our understanding of genetic and developmental pathology expands. For example, a clinical subdivision of split-hand/foot malformation, polydactyly, or syndactyly based on phenotypic appearance in various subgroups does not withstand the clinical or molecular reality. Studies of large families have shown that so-called distinct phenotypes were part of the phenotypic variability; on the other hand, identical phenotypes were shown to have been caused by different gene defects.

Recent advances in molecular genetics and developmental biology have helped clarify this confusing complexity. Many conditions can now be assigned to certain gene defects, thereby opening the possibility of a molecular diagnosis. However, for many conditions the diagnosed mutation only partially predicts the phenotype with large degrees of variability, even within families. Thus, a diagnosis has to rely on clinical as well as molecular considerations. Only an integration of the two aspects can produce a sufficiently validated disease description, nomenclature, and disease concept that can be used for diagnostic as well as scientific purposes and for the benefit of the patient.

This atlas describes most, but not all, conditions with isolated limb involvement and those syndromes in which abnormalities of the limbs are a consistent and predominant feature. We have concentrated on conditions in which the molecular cause is known. This approach has been facilitated by the enormous increase in knowledge in the field, resulting in a nomenclature and classification that take genetic heterogeneity and clinical variability into account. Whenever possible, we have tried to demonstrate the degrees of clinical variability that are often observed in limb malformations. However, due to limitations of space, this has not been possible in all aspects. The classification used here is clinically oriented and based on phenotypes as well as on genetic/molecular data. This resulted in eight major groups: 1) acromesomelic dysplasias, which are conditions that affect bone formation and/or growth, predominantly in the forearm/leg and hands/feet; 2) brachydactylies, a group of conditions characterized by the shortening or absence of individual bones of the hands and feet; 3) defects of joint formation; 4) contracture deformities, conditions in which connective tissue or muscle problems result in the inability to bend joints; 5) polydactylies, malformations that result in the formation of additional fingers or toes; 6) syndactylies, in which fingers or toes are fused; 7) reduction anomalies, involving the absence of part or all of one or more bones; and 8) conditions with macrodactyly or overgrowth of limbs. In some instances we subdivided groups in those conditions with isolated limb anomalies and those in which limb malformations are associated with other clinical findings. In addition, subdivisions according to anatomical location have been made, and we sorted conditions according to their major clinical problem or involvement. Few limb malformations have isolated defects, and many have features that show overlap among these broad categories. Obviously, these boundaries are artificial and fluid. Nevertheless, we think they are helpful in categorizing these conditions and may be useful in making a correct diagnosis.

The phenotypes of limb malformations and their developmental pathogenicity have been elucidated by many groundbreaking studies on the basic mechanisms of limb development. Based on this work, many malformations can now be understood from their developmental point of view, such as the involvement of the hedgehog pathway in many polydactylies. In the first introductory chapter we give a brief overview of the current concepts of how limbs develop and how the molecular regulatory network that governs limb development is related to certain phenotypes. The clinical evaluation of limbs and the diversity of phenotypes and their interpretation are addressed in the second chapter. In many instances, the clinical evaluation is not sufficient and a radiological examination is necessary, so basic principles of radiology of the limb skeleton are presented in the third chapter. Parents may be dismayed by the appearance of an anomalous hand and may be hoping that surgery can create a "normal" hand. Hand surgery aims at improving function and cosmetic appearance when possible, and includes counseling parents about what is and is not possible with surgery. In the fourth chapter, basic principles of surgery are discussed.

Acknowledgements

Physicians whom we approached to contribute pictures and radiographic films from published and unpublished cases are acknowledged in the figure legends. We wish to express our gratitude to colleagues and friends who contributed to this work:

V. Cormier-Daire, Paris; G. Gillessen-Kaesbach, Lübeck; L. Graul-Neumann, Berlin; R. Habenicht, Hamburg; W. Hülsemann, Hamburg; N. Kantaputra, Chiang Mai; H. Kayserili, Istanbul; R. König, Frankfurt; I. Kurth, Jena; P. Meinecke, Hamburg; J. Opitz, Salt Lake City; A. Rajab, Muscat; J. Spranger, Sinzheim; L. van Maldergem, Besançon; D. Wieczorek, Essen; B. Wollnik, Cologne; B. Zabel, Freiburg.

Our special thanks go to Jürgen Kunze. Many of the clinical figures presented here are from his collection of clinical cases, generated during his time at the Institute for Human Genetics in Berlin. We thank Norbert Brieske for excellent photographic work.

Table of Contents

Part I

Introduction

1 Development of the Limbs

Sigmar Stricker and Stefan Mundlos

Limb Morphology

The limb buds arise from the flank of the embryo and mainly consist of mesoderm originating from the lateral plate covered by a layer of ectoderm. The lateral plate mesoderm (LPM) contains the progenitors for all populations of limb tissues (cartilage, tendon, connective tissue, and so on) with the exception of muscle. Myogenic progenitors originate from the somites and actively migrate into the nascent limb buds. As the limb bud grows distally, the diverse tissue progenitors differentiate and lay down the elaborate pattern of, for instance, skeletal elements. Morphologically the limb can be subdivided into three distinct segments: the proximal stylopod, the medial zeugopod, and the distal autopod. In the stylopod only one skeletal element is found (humerus or femur); in the zeugopod two elements are established (radius and ulna or tibia and fibula); and in the autopod the carpals/tarsals, the metacarpals/metatarsals and five digits arise. Mammalian digits consist of three phalanges with the exception of digit I (thumb or hallux), which possesses only two phalanges.

Limb Initiation

The positions of the limb buds are genetically determined. The *Hox* genes, known as master regulators of embryonic development, are thought to play a key role in generating the morphological diversity along the body axis (Kmita and Duboule 2003). Once the position of the presumptive limbs is set, a series of epithelial-to-mesenchymal interactions between the LPM and the overlying ectoderm leads to the establishment of the limb bud (Capdevila and Izpisua Belmonte 2001). The decisive event in this context is the establishment of a specialized structure from the limb ectoderm, the apical ectodermal ridge (AER). The AER is a thickened epithelial structure that runs along the distal margin of the limb bud from its anterior to its posterior tip. During its establishment, the AER is positioned exactly along the dorsoventral border of the limb bud. Studies performed in the chick have suggested that several molecules expressed in specific domains either in the dorsal or ventral ectoderm are involved in this process, such as Wnt7a, Engrailed-1 (EN-1), and Radical fringe (RFN) (Capdevila and Izpisua Belmonte 2001).

Limb Patterning

Once the limb bud emerges, a complex three-dimensional signaling system is imposed on the undifferentiated mesenchyme to determine the morphology of, for instance, skeletal elements (Fig. 1.1). The AER controls the limb's proximal to distal outgrowth. The zone of polarizing activity (ZPA), a population of mesenchymal cells at the posterior margin of the limb bud, controls anteroposterior (AP) patterning, and the dorsal ectoderm plays a key role in establishing dorsoventral polarity.

The Apical Ectodermal Ridge

The importance of the AER was demonstrated decades ago, when it was shown that chick wings are truncated when the AER is removed (Fig. 1.2). AER removal is quickly followed by cell death in the underlying mesenchyme, which can be rescued by the exogenous application of fibroblast growth factors (FGFs). Consequently, it is widely accepted that the main function of the AER is to provide FGF signaling to the underlying mesoderm. FGFs secreted from the AER keep the mesodermal cells in an undifferentiated state, promote proliferation, and protect from apoptosis. AER-expressed FGFs (FGF4, 8, 9, and 17) thereby induce the expression of FGF10 in the limb mesenchyme, which in turn is required for maintaining FGF8 expression. Thus, FGF8 and FGF10 form an epithelial-mesenchymal positive feedback loop that drives limb outgrowth (Benazet and Zeller 2009) (Fig. 1.1a).

Defects in the establishment or maintenance of the AER in humans lead to truncation syndromes. For example, *Wnt3* is required for AER establishment in the mouse, and human mutations in *WNT3* cause tetra-amelia. Defects in AER maintenance during autopod patterning lead to split-hand/foot syndromes, caused, for example, by mutations in *TP63*, encoding a protein required for AER maintenance.

The Zone of Polarizing Activity

Patterning along the anteroposterior axis has also been elucidated by using the chicken as a model system. Transplantation experiments led to the discovery of a cell population in the posterior limb bud mesenchyme that exhibits posterior-

S. Mundlos, D. Horn, *Limb Malformations*,
DOI 10.1007/978-3-540-95928-1_1, © Springer-Verlag Berlin Heidelberg 2014

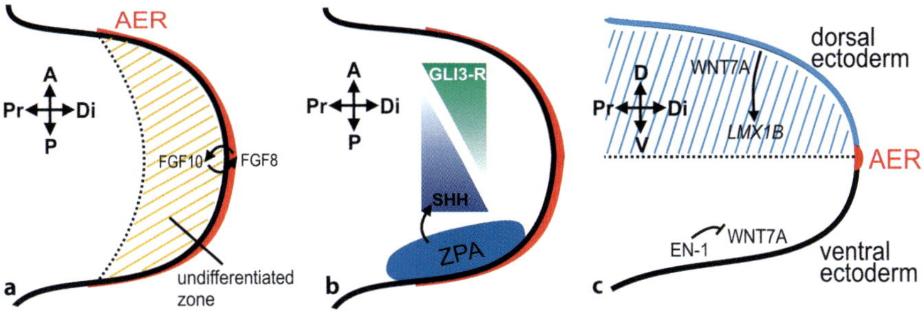

Fig. 1.1 Three-dimensional patterning of the limb bud. **a** Proximal-to-distal outgrowth is under control of the apical ectodermal ridge (AER), a specialized ectodermal structure that runs along the distal rim of the limb bud at the border of the dorsal and ventral half. Fibroblast growth factor 8 (FGF8) from the AER signals to the underlying mesenchyme and keeps cells dividing and undifferentiated and protects from apoptosis (undifferentiated zone). Mesenchymal cells produce FGF10, which signals back to the AER and sustains FGF8 expression (positive feedback). **b** Anteroposterior patterning is controlled by the zone of polarizing activity (ZPA), localized in the posterior mesenchyme of the limb bud. The ZPA produces Sonic hedgehog (SHH), which forms a gradient and acts antagonistically with the repressor form of GLI3 (GLI3-R). **c** Dorsoventral patterning is controlled by the dorsal and ventral ectoderm. The dorsal ectoderm produces the signaling factor WNT7A, which diffuses to the dorsal mesenchyme and induces expression of the transcription factor LMX1B. In the ventral ectoderm, Wnt7a expression is prevented by Engrailed-1 (EN-1). *A* anterior, *D* dorsal, *Di* distal, *P* posterior, *Pr* proximal, *V* ventral

izing activity and was therefore termed the zone of polarizing activity (ZPA). The molecular basis for this was discovered, when Sonic hedgehog (Shh) was proposed to be the diffusible morphogen responsible for polarizing activity (Fig. 1.3). SHH was later proposed to exert its function via antagonism with Glioma-associated oncogene 3 (GLI3). SHH regulates processing of the GLI3 protein: in the absence of hedgehog signaling, GLI3 is constitutively cleaved to a truncated transcriptional repressor (GLI3-R) (Fig. 1.1b). SHH signaling inhibits this cleavage and allows for the accumulation of the full-length activator form of GLI3 in posterior mesenchyme (Zeller et al. 2009). The importance of SHH and GLI3 in mammals has been shown by gene inactivation in the mouse; *Shh* mutant mice lack all digits except for one rudimentary digit in the hind limb; conversely, Gli3 mutants exhibit polydactyly. In humans, mutations leading to misregulated *SHH* expression can cause preaxial or postaxial polydactyly or severe truncation syndromes such as acheiropodia. *GLI3* mutations cause a range of syndromes associated with polydactyly (Anderson et al. 2012).

More recent studies have shed light on the mechanism by which SHH patterns the limb bud. In brief, a timing mechanism was proposed in which ZPA cells measure the time they express SHH. ZPA cells proliferate, so as the limb grows, descendants of the ZPA expand anteriorly. ZPA descendants contribute to digits V and IV and a part of digit III; digits II and partially digit III are subject to paracrine SHH signaling in a classic gradient fashion, while digit I appears to develop independent of SHH. In addition to this, it was recently proposed that SHH has two functions during autopod development: early AP patterning followed by positive regulation of limb bud proliferation to promote expansion of the digit-forming field (Zeller et al. 2009).

Following patterning, the information provided by SHH and GLI3 and other players has to be transmitted into the formation of digit identities. In this context a bone morphogenetic protein (BMP) signaling gradient was proposed as a mediator; however, genetic analysis in the mouse did not support such a role. In the chick it was shown that patterning information is "stored" in the interdigital mesenchyme. Signals from the interdigital mesenchyme are thought to signal to the growing phalanges, providing them with the information necessary for reaching their final length (Zeller et al. 2009).

Dorsoventral Patterning

As outlined above, the AER is established at the dorsoventral (DV) rim of the limb bud, and as would be expected, this process is coordinated with DV patterning of the limb bud mesenchyme. Experiments performed in the chicken showed that the same set of genes that position the AER are involved in DV patterning. The dorsal ectoderm expresses *Wnt7a*, and the ventral ectoderm expresses *EN*-1. Wnt7a is both necessary and sufficient to impose DV patterning (Fig. 1.4). EN-1 inhibits Wnt7a expression in the ventral ectoderm. Wnt7a acts as a morphogen and diffuses to the dorsal mesoderm and induces expression of the transcription factor LMX1B (Fig. 1.1c). LMX1B is considered a major regulator of dorsal patterning in the limb bud mesenchyme. In humans, mutations in LMX1B cause nail–patella syndrome, showing malformations in line with a defect in DV patterning of the limb (Chen et al. 1998).

Integration of Patterning Signals

It is intuitive that these three signaling centers (AER, ZPA, and dorsal ectoderm) must coordinate their function; in other

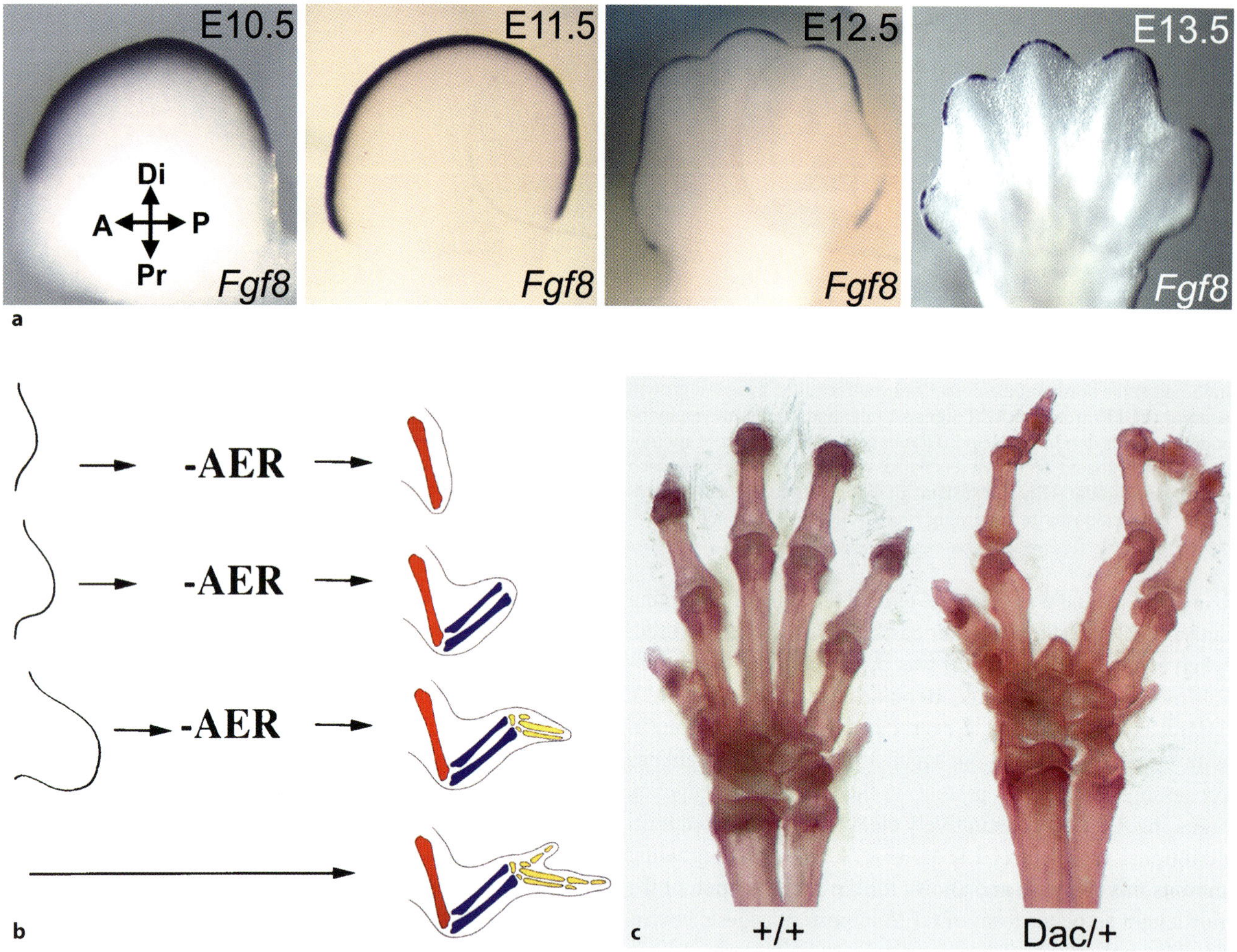

Fig. 1.2 The apical ectodermal ridge (AER). **a** Whole-mount in-situ hybridization for Fgf8 on mouse limb buds from E10.5 to E13.5. Note cessation of Fgf8 expression in regions overlying interdigits versus maintenance of Fgf8 expression overlying the digit condensations. **b** Schematic depiction of AER removal experiments in the chicken. Removal of the AER at sequential time points leads to progressively more distal truncation of the limbs. **c** Degradation of the AER at late time points of limb development leads to ectrodactyly as depicted here for the dactylaplasia mouse mutant, a model for split-hand/foot malformations. *A* anterior, *Di* distal, *P* posterior, *Pr* proximal

words, they require communication (Fig. 1.5). Again, the main concepts of this communication system have been elucidated in the chicken as a model. It was shown that the dorsal mesoderm is required for Shh expression and that Wnt7a was sufficient to replace removed ectoderm. This function is conserved in mammals, since inactivation of *Wnt7a* in the mouse leads to a decrease in Shh expression and loss of posterior digits. Fittingly, mutation of human *Wnt7a* causes limb truncation syndromes (phocomelia) with resemblance to *SHH* mutation. It was noticed early that AER removal not only led to cell death in underlying mesenchyme but also to loss of Shh expression. Interestingly, FGF4 could replace this function of the AER. Likewise, SHH positively regulates *Fgf4* expression in the AER, thus both molecules form a positive feedback loop. This feedback loop is a perfect example of a signal relay in epithelial-to-mesenchymal communication: SHH was shown to positively regulate the expression of Gremlin 1 (*Grem1*), a BMP antagonist. GREM1 inhibits BMP activity, which has a negative influence on the AER (Benazet and Zeller 2009).

Skeletal Condensation

The final output of this concerted effort is the establishment of a correctly patterned limb skeleton together with other tissue types such as tendons and muscles. The skeleton of the limb arises via the process of endochondral ossification. Endochondral ossification is a process that involves the formation of a cartilaginous template of the future skeleton, which subsequently becomes replaced by bone. This process starts with the formation of a cartilaginous condensation consisting of osteochondroprogenitor cells that will give rise to chondrocytes and perichondral cells. The chondrocytes form the actual cartilaginous condensation, which is surrounded by flattened cells, the perichondrium (Fig. 1.7a).

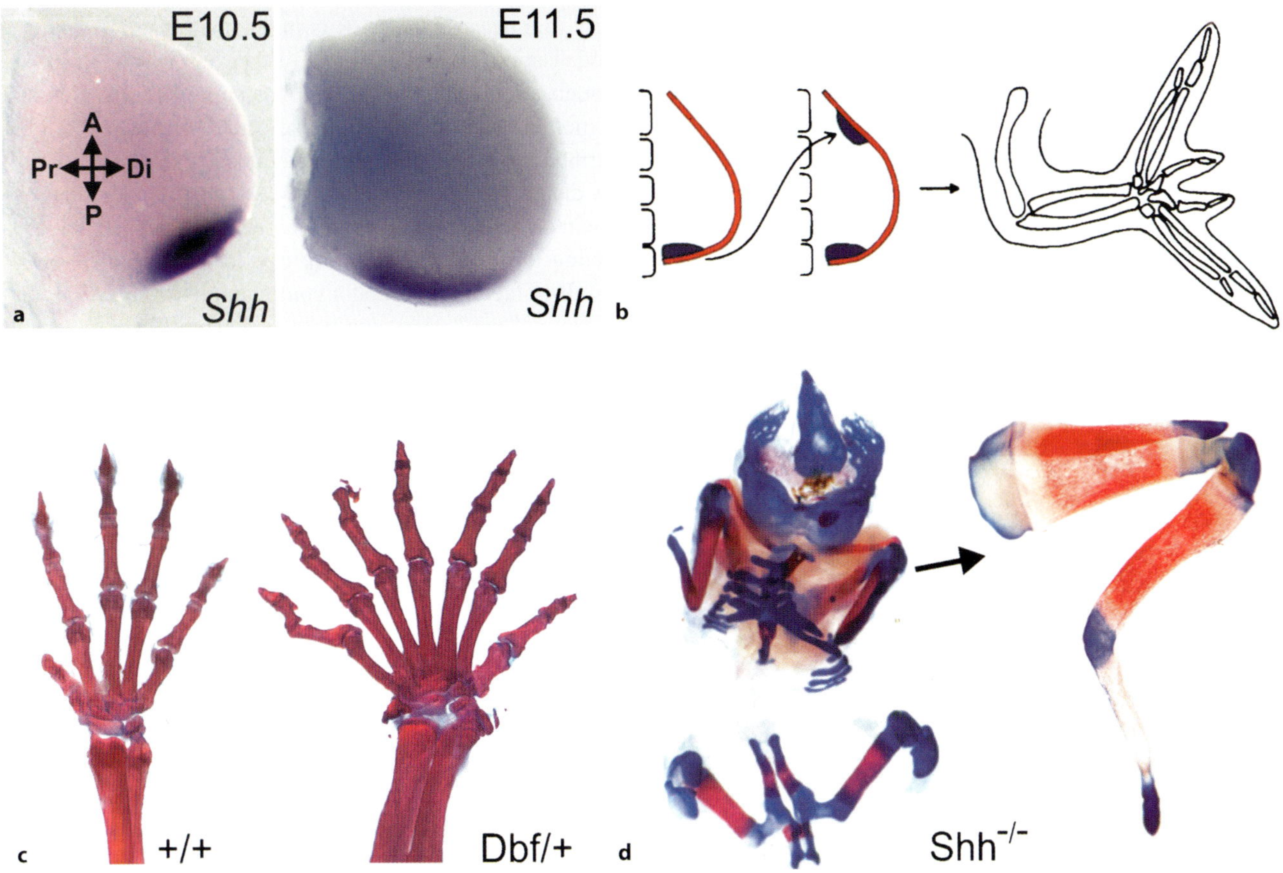

Fig. 1.3 The zone of polarizing activity (ZPA). **a** Whole-mount in-situ hybridization for Sonic hedgehog (*Shh*) at E10.5 and E11.5. **b** Ectopic ZPA activity at the anterior end of the limb bud (here by transplantation of ZPA cells from a posterior chicken wing bud to an anterior wing bud) leads to mirror-image duplication of skeletal elements. **c** Ectopic activation of *Ihh* expression (a paralog of Shh) in anterior limb bud mesenchyme leads to preaxial polydactyly in the Doublefoot (Dbf) mouse. **d** Shh loss of function leads to limb truncation and loss of distal skeletal elements. *A* anterior, *Di* distal, *P* posterior, *Pr* proximal

Chondrogenic condensations express the transcription factor SOX9, which is required for chondrogenesis. In humans, haploinsufficiency of *SOX9* causes campomelic dysplasia, a condition in which endochondral ossification is severely impaired, and a hypoplastic trunk and limb skeleton forms. Therefore, *Sox9* can be considered a master regulator of chondrogenesis. SOX9 performs this role by inducing the expression of chondrocyte-specific genes such as collagen type 2 alpha 1 (*Col2a1*) and by inducing other prochondrogenic transcription factors such as SOX5 and SOX6 (Kawakami et al. 2006). A plethora of evidence highlights the importance of signaling molecules belonging to the transforming growth factor beta (TGFβ) family in the regulation of chondrogenesis (Stricker and Mundlos 2011b). Among this family, the so-called BMPs are of pivotal importance for chondrogenesis. BMPs stimulate chondrogenesis in vitro and in vivo, and expression of dominant-negative receptors in the chick leads to disrupted chondrogenesis. BMPs are able to induce *Sox9* expression in vitro and in vivo, and combined inactivation of BmpR1b and BmpR1a leads to severe hypoplasia of the limb skeleton (Kawakami et al. 2006).

Growth of Skeletal Elements

After establishment of the condensation, the cartilage further differentiates by forming the growth plate (Fig. 1.7b). Here, small roundish cells start to strongly proliferate and concomitantly polarize to form clonal stacks of cells. The cells further differentiate to prehypertrophic and hypertrophic chondrocytes, which finally become apoptotic and make way for the bone marrow cavity. In parallel, cells in the perichondrium differentiate to osteoblasts and start to form the cortical bone. In addition, osteoblasts follow blood vessels invading the cavity formed by the removal of hypertrophic cartilage and form the trabecular bone. The growth plate carries out the longitudinal expansion of the skeletal element after the condensation phase. This is accomplished by the interplay of proliferation, columnar organization, and hypertrophy, which altogether drive longitudinal growth of skeletal elements.

Recent evidence suggests that signaling via the WNT/planar cell polarity pathway is essential for chondrocyte polarization (Romereim and Dudley 2011). Proliferation is mainly controlled by FGF signaling. Growth plate cells express FGF

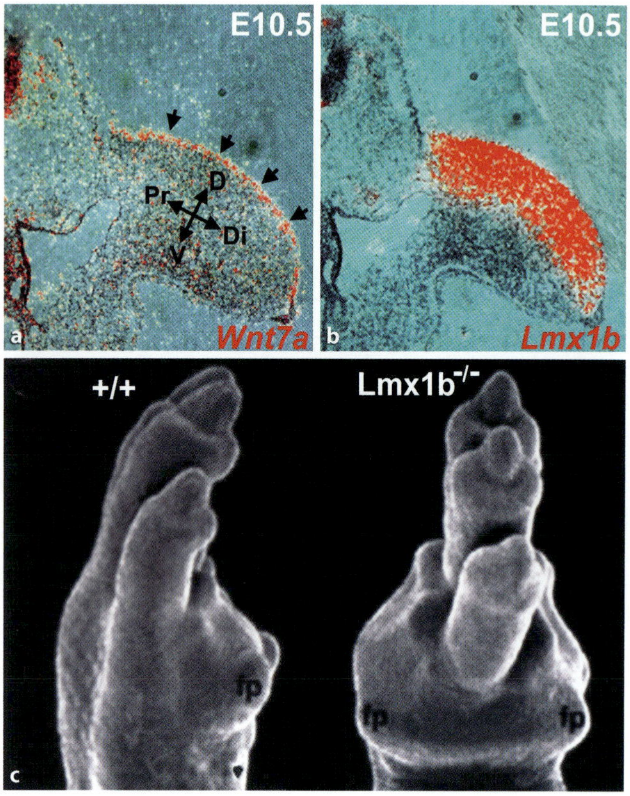

Fig. 1.4 The dorsal ectoderm and dorsoventral patterning. **a,b** In-situ hybridization for Wnt7a and Lmx1b in E10.5 mouse forelimb buds. **c** Development of double-ventral limbs in Lmx1b-deficient mice. *D* dorsal, *Di* distal, *Pr* proximal, *V* ventral, *fp* foot pads (From Chen et al. 1998)

receptor type 3 (FGFR3), which negatively regulates proliferation of chondrocytes. In humans, activating mutations in FGFR3 lead to the most common short stature syndrome, achondroplasia (Kronenberg 2003). Prehypertrophic chondrocytes express a member of the hedgehog family called Indian hedgehog (IHH). IHH is thought to diffuse across the growth plate and induce the expression of parathyroid hormone-like hormone (PTHLH) in periarticular chondrocytes. PTHLH in turn diffuses into the growth plate and signals to its receptor PTHR1, which is expressed slightly proximal to IHH. Signaling by PTHR1 prevents cells from differentiating to IHH-expressing prehypertrophic chondrocytes, thereby closing a negative feedback loop. This loop is considered one of the main signaling relays that controls the pace of chondrocyte differentiation and thus bone growth, together with several other mechanisms. IHH is also necessary for osteoblast differentiation in the perichondrium (Kronenberg 2003).

Digit Elongation

AER activity is described to cease around E12 in the mouse concomitant with the shutdown of the ZPA. This is not entirely true because the AER is maintained distal to the digit condensations, where it drives further outgrowth. However, condensation of the phalanges has some peculiarities that are not shared with the other skeletal elements of the limb. During limb growth, the skeletal condensations basically follow distal outgrowth. Current models of patterning along the proximodistal axis (Tabin and Wolpert 2007) predict that cells leaving the AER influence are free to undergo differentiation. It in fact appears that a combination of AER–FGF and ectodermal WNT signaling keeps cells undifferentiated, and once this repressive function is relieved, cells differentiate to, for instance, chondrocytes (Zeller et al. 2009). Digits, on the other hand, actively contribute to their elongation. Examination of digit growth in the chicken showed that a population of cells exists anterior to the digit condensation that is required for outgrowth. This signaling center, which has been termed the phalanx-forming region (PFR), shows strong activity of the BMP signaling pathway, and intensity of pathway activity was correlated to digit elongation and identity. Via the PFR, undifferentiated distal cells are recruited to the condensation, thus elongating it distally (Fig. 1.4a). The activity of the PFR depends on the presence of the AER but also on IHH signaling emanating from the condensation itself, which means that the digit condensation promotes its own outgrowth via the PFR. This additional level of complexity is expected to render the digit condensations more prone to mutation-induced malformation, which is indeed the case. At least two syndromes of the brachydactyly disease family of digit-shortening syndromes are caused by a defective PFR. Mouse models for both brachydactyly type A1 (BDA1), caused by mutation in IHH, and brachydactyly type B1 (BDB1), caused by mutation in ROR2, showed decreased BMP pathway activity, causing a decreased rate of progenitor incorporation into the digit condensation. As it turns out, most members of the brachydactyly disease family are caused by mutations in members of the BMP signaling pathway, further strengthening the importance of this mechanism pathway (Stricker and Mundlos 2011b).

Digit Separation

Elongation of the digits is intimately coupled with their separation. As digits grow out, the tissue in between the condensations regresses and becomes removed by apoptosis (Fig. 1.6a,d). A key role in distinguishing regions subject to further growth (that is, digit regions) versus interdigit regions prone to degeneration is played by the AER. As mentioned, the AER is maintained overlying the digit condensations and promotes proliferation and survival of subjacent mesenchyme. FGF signaling has a protective role against interdigital apoptosis (Montero and Hurle 2010). Activated FGF signaling is observed in Apert and Pfeiffer syndromes that are caused by mutations in FGF receptor genes and exhibit

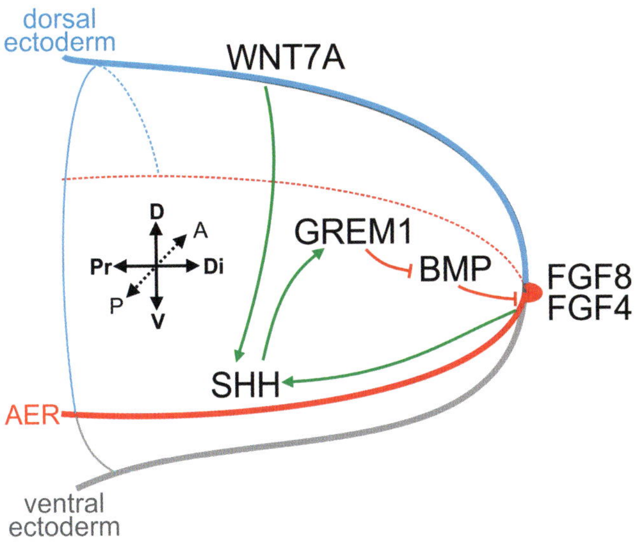

Fig. 1.5 Interaction of patterning centers during limb development. WNT7A produced by the dorsal ectoderm is required for the maintenance of SHH expression in the zone of polarizing activity (ZPA) coupling dorsoventral to anteroposterior patterning. Distal outgrowth is linked to ZPA activity via a complex epithelial-mesenchymal feedback loop. SHH produced by the ZPA diffuses to the limb mesenchyme and induces expression of Gremlin1, encoding GREM1, a secreted antagonist of bone morphogenetic proteins (BMPs). BMPs negatively regulate the function of the apical ectodermal ridge (AER). GREMLIN1 relieves the AER of this inhibition, thus sustaining AER activity. FGF4 from the AER in turn maintains Shh expression in the ZPA, closing the loop. *A* anterior, *D* dorsal, *Di* distal, *P* posterior, *Pr* proximal, *V* ventral

(among other features) syndactyly (Stricker and Mundlos 2011a). There is long-standing evidence that BMP signaling is involved in interdigital apoptosis. Applying high doses of BMP to interdigital mesenchyme in the chick induces apoptosis. In the mouse, combined inactivation of several mesenchymal BMPs has provided genetic evidence for a requirement of BMP signaling for interdigital apoptosis. However, this can also be interpreted to be secondary to inhibition of *Fgf8* expression in the AER. Several other factors have been involved in interdigit regression, including retinoic acid (RA). It is noteworthy that RA synthesis in interdigital spaces is defective in mouse models for human synpolydactyly that show reduced interdigital apoptosis and ectopic cartilage condensations (Montero and Hurle 2010).

Joint Development

The limb skeletal elements grow distally as a continuous condensation, which concomitantly becomes subdivided by the insertion of synovial joints (Fig. 1.6a–c). One of the best marker genes expressed in joint cells is Gdf5 encoding a member of the Tgfβ superfamily (Fig. 1.6c). Genetic lineage studies have shown that Gdf5-positive cells give rise to the joint surface as well as the joint capsule and ligaments. This expression pattern would suggest a role of GDF5 in

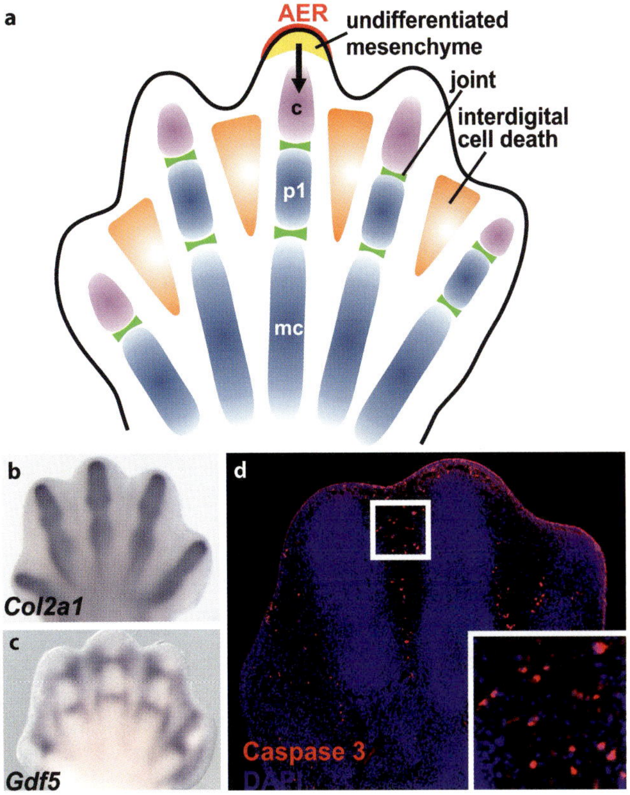

Fig. 1.6 Elongation and separation of digits. **a** Schematic depiction of a developing autopod. Metacarpals (*mc*) and proximal phalanges (*p1*) have already formed, while distal structures are still undergoing condensation (*c*). The apical ectodermal ridge (*AER*) is maintained anterior to the growing condensations and keeps underlying cells undifferentiated (depicted only for the middle finger). From this pool, cells are continuously recruited to the growing condensation (*arrow*). Concomitant with digit elongation, synovial joints are inserted in a proximal-to-distal order, and interdigital mesenchyme regresses by apoptosis. **b,c** Whole-mount in-situ hybridization on mouse E13.5 forelimb autopods for Col2a1 (marking digit condensations) and Gdf5 (marking joints). **d** Detection of interdigital cell death via immunolabeling for activated caspase 3 on section of mouse E13.5 forelimb autopod

joint induction; however, GDF5 appears to have an opposing function. Exogenous application of GDF5 inhibits joint formation and induces cartilage differentiation and proliferation (Archer et al. 2003). In agreement, homozygous loss of function mutations in *GDF5* cause recessive generalized acromesomelic chondrodysplasia of the Grebe (MIM 200 700), Hunter–Thomson (MIM 201 250), and Du Pan (MIM 228 900) types. This predicts that inhibition of GDF5 and putatively other members of the TGFβ family is necessary for joint formation, which is indeed the case. Mutations in the BMP antagonist NOGGIN cause symphalangism (MIM 185800) and multiple synostosis syndrome (MIM 186500). Strikingly, gain-of-functions in GDF5 either by increased receptor binding or insensitivity to NOGGIN cause joint fusions. GDF5 binds to its high-affinity receptor BMPR1B, and a subset of BMPR1B mutations can also cause a symphalangism phenotype. This suggests that tight

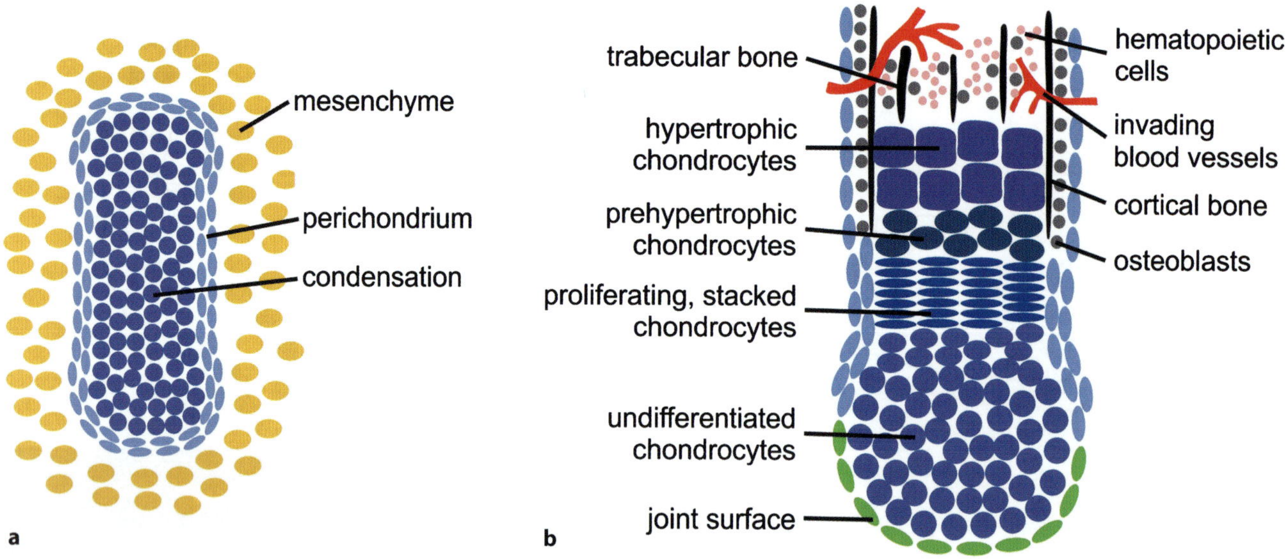

Fig. 1.7 Cartilage condensation and growth. **a** The initial cartilaginous anlagen are formed from undifferentiated mesenchyme. Cells condense and undergo chondrogenic differentiation. The condensation is surrounded by a perichondrium consisting of specialized flattened cells. **b** In the cartilage, growth plate chondrocytes undergo differentiation from rounded undifferentiated cells ("resting" chondrocytes) to proliferative chondrocytes that polarize and form characteristic clonal stacks of cells. The chondrocytes further differentiate to prehypertrophic and hypertrophic chondrocytes that enlarge and are finally removed by apoptosis. In parallel, cells in the perichondrium differentiate to bone-forming osteoblasts that start to form the cortical bone (bone collar). Osteoblasts invade alongside blood vessels. Osteoblasts form trabecular bone, and hematopoietic cells colonize the bone marrow cavity

control of BMP signaling is required for joint formation, but that BMP ligands expressed in the presumptive joint area (such as GDF5) signal back to the condensation. This might have a dual function: promoting condensation maintenance and growth as well as spacing distances between two joints. In agreement, brachydactyly type C (BDC) caused by GDF5 mutations can exhibit hypersegmentation of digits (Stricker and Mundlos 2011b).

Apart from BMP antagonism, other factors and pathways have been implicated in joint formation. It was shown that the WNT/β-catenin pathway can induce the formation of synovial joints, while loss of β-catenin results in joint fusions. IHH was also involved in joint formation, since Ihh mutant mice show fused phalanges. It was suggested that IHH acts synergistically with Wnt/β-catenin signaling in this process (Stricker and Mundlos 2011b).

Limb Identity

As outlined above, the limbs are thought to be positioned along the body flank by the pattern of HOX gene expression. Subsequently, current models hold that this information is promoted to other local signaling mechanisms that then specify the identity of the forelimbs and hind limbs. Forelimbs conspicuously express the T-Box gene *Tbx5*, while the hind limb exclusively expresses a paralogous gene, Tbx4 (Duboc and Logan 2011). Experiments in the chick had indicated an instructive role of both genes in determining limb identities. However, this view was not supported by genetic analysis in the mouse, highlighting that information obtained from model systems has to be treated with care (Duboc and Logan 2011). TBX4 induced expression of *Pitx1*, and misexpression of Pitx1 in chick forelimbs led to the development of hind limb characteristics. Moreover, misexpression of *Pitx1* in mouse forelimbs also led to hind-limb-like morphological alterations, while inactivation of *Pitx1* caused changes in some features that are characteristic for hind limbs, such as the patella, that were in line with a partial conversion to a forelimb morphology. In humans, PITX1 mutations were detected in two syndromes that, fittingly, are either hind-limb-specific or lead to morphological changes in forelimbs toward hind limb-like features. Homozygous putative loss of function mutations in PITX1 were detected in "clubfoot and various other lower extremity anomalies" (MIM 119800) and in patients exhibiting polydactyly and/or tibial hemimelia but normal upper extremities. Conversely, genomic rearrangements upstream of PITX1 were associated with autosomal-dominant Liebenberg syndrome (MIM 186550), which exhibits upper limb deformities indicative of a hind-limb-like morphology such as a loss of the olecranon. It was suggested that the rearrangements might lead to a misexpression of PITX1 in the forelimb, thus causing arm-to-leg conversion (Spielmann et al. 2012 and references therein).

References

Anderson E, Peluso S, Lettice LA, Hill RE (2012) Human limb abnormalities caused by disruption of hedgehog signaling. Trends in Genetics 28:364–373

Archer CW, Dowthwaite GP, Francis-West P (2003) Development of synovial joints. Birth Defects Res C Embryo Today 69:144–155

Benazet JD, Zeller R (2009) Vertebrate limb development: moving from classical morphogen gradients to an integrated 4-dimensional patterning system. Cold Spring Harb Perspect Biol 1:a001339

Capdevila J, Izpisua Belmonte JC (2001) Patterning mechanisms controlling vertebrate limb development. Annu Rev Cell Dev Biol 17:87–132

Chen H, Lun Y, Ovchinnikov D, Kokubo H, Oberg KC et al (1998) Limb and kidney defects in Lmx1b mutant mice suggest an involvement of LMX1B in human nail patella syndrome. Nat Genet 19:51–55

Duboc V, Logan MP (2011) Regulation of limb bud initiation and limb-type morphology. Dev Dyn 240:1017–1027

Kawakami Y, Rodriguez-Leon J, Izpisua Belmonte JC (2006) The role of TGFbetas and Sox9 during limb chondrogenesis. Curr Opin Cell Biol 18:723–729

Kmita M, Duboule D (2003) Organizing axes in time and space; 25 years of colinear tinkering. Science 301:331–333

Kronenberg HM (2003) Developmental regulation of the growth plate. Nature 423:332–336

Montero JA, Hurle JM (2010) Sculpturing digit shape by cell death. Apoptosis 15:365–375

Romereim SM, Dudley AT (2011) Cell polarity: the missing link in skeletal morphogenesis? Organogenesis 7:217–228

Spielmann M, Brancati F, Krawitz PM, Robinson PN, Ibrahim DM, Franke M et al (2012) Homeotic arm-to-leg transformation associated with genomic rearrangements at the PITX1 locus. Am J Hum Genet 91:629–635

Stricker S, Mundlos S (2011a) FGF and ROR2 receptor tyrosine kinase signaling in human skeletal development. Curr Top Dev Biol 97:179–206

Stricker S, Mundlos S (2011b) Mechanisms of digit formation: human malformation syndromes tell the story. Dev Dyn 240:990–1004

Tabin C, Wolpert L (2007) Rethinking the proximodistal axis of the vertebrate limb in the molecular era. Genes Dev 21:1433–1442

Zeller R, Lopez-Rios J, Zuniga A (2009) Vertebrate limb bud development: moving towards integrative analysis of organogenesis. Nat Rev Genet 10:845–858

2 Clinical Assessment and Anthropometry of the Limbs

Denise Horn

General Background of Terminology

The developmental axes of the limb are specified as distal versus proximal (digit tip to shoulder/hip), anterior versus posterior (thumb/hallux to digit V), and dorsal versus ventral (back of hand/foot to palm/sole). The latter two terms are based on embryological terminology. Joints are specified by their adjacent bones; for instance, the metacarpophalangeal joint II specifies the joint connecting the distal metacarpal with the proximal phalanx of digit II.

The individual segments of the limbs can be defined based on embryological terms such as zeugopod (humerus/femur), stylopod (radius/ulna; tibia/fibula), and autopod (hand/foot including carpals/tarsals). Here we use the specific descriptions of the affected bone (humerus or femur) and use the term zeugopod to describe a more general abnormality that affects both bones. Figure 2.1 illustrates the skeletal anatomy and general terms.

The terms "finger" and "toe" generally refer to digits II–V in the hands and feet, respectively, thus excluding the thumb and the great toe (hallux). The term "digit" is a more general term to describe any finger/toe including the thumb/hallux. Here we prefer to use the term "digit" to describe general anomalies, and we refer to "finger" or "toe" to distinguish from "thumb" or "hallux" or hand versus foot, respectively. The term "ray" refers to skeletal elements on either the radial or the ulnar side of the limb, thus potentially including the corresponding long bone, carpal bones, metacarpals, and phalanges.

The digits are numbered I–V (or VI and more in polydactyly) from the radial/tibial side of the limb starting with the thumb/hallux. Polydactyly is described as preaxial (thumb/hallux side), postaxial (5th finger/toe side), or central or interaxial (between digits I and V). Additional digits may represent a complete duplication of a digit that is separated or partially fused with other digits. Incomplete duplications may arise from the metacarpals or any of the phalanges. In this case the description includes the point(s) of fusion.

Inspection of the Limbs

Inspection of the hands and feet includes information concerning their proportion in relation to the limbs and the whole body, the length and proportion of the digits and toes, the position of the digits, the contours of the hand and foot muscles, and the presence of syndactyly. Inspection of palmar and digital creases gives information about joint location and mobility. By making a fist by flexing the fingers, the relative length of the metacarpals can be assessed. Mild skin syndactyly can be discovered by spreading out the fingers. At the feet, the height of the plantar arch should be judged with the patient standing.

Measurement of the limbs, hands, or feet is recommended if abnormalities are suspected, such as abnormal lengths of digits and/or palms, as well as abnormal length of hands or feet. Palm length refers to the length from the distal wrist crease to the flexion crease at the base of the middle finger. The middle fin-

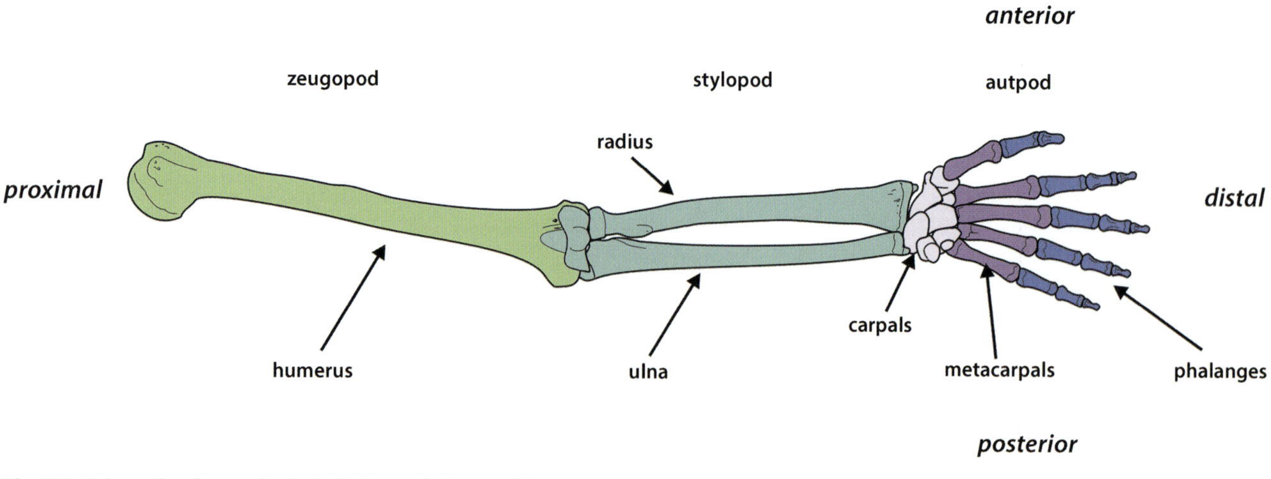

Fig. 2.1 Schematic of upper limb skeletal morphology and terms

S. Mundlos, D. Horn, *Limb Malformations*,
DOI 10.1007/978-3-540-95928-1_2, © Springer-Verlag Berlin Heidelberg 2014

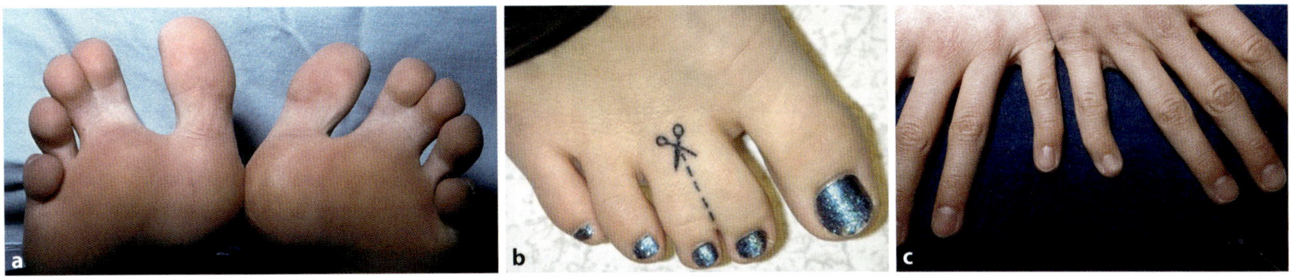

Fig. 2.2 Minor abnormalities and normal variations. **a** II/III toe syndactyly. **b** Toe syndactyly and problem to solution Berlin style. **c** Clinodactyly of the 5th finger

ger length is defined as the distance from the flexion crease at the base of this finger to the distal end. To assess limb shortening, the arm span has to be evaluated, which has a normal range of about ±5 % of the body length. The reader is referred to Hall et al. (2007) for detailed descriptions of several methods of measurements and for the corresponding data.

Palpation of the Extremities

Each joint should be extended passively to its full extent. Limitation of joint mobility means that joint contractures or camptodactyly are present. Hyperextension of joints corresponds to joint laxity. With the patient seated or lying down, the range of motion of the foot joints is evaluated.

Normal Variations and Minor Abnormalities

A spectrum of normal variations of hand and feet features can be observed; for instance, the palmar crease shows a broad variability of normal variations. A single transverse palmar crease can be observed in 4 % of the normal population. Mild syndactyly of toes II/III is a minor anomaly with no significance. However, it may occur together with other conditions, such as Smith–Lemli–Opitz syndrome and other syndactyly-associated limb malformations. Kirner deformity refers to an angulation within the distal phalanx of the 5th finger with thickening of the epiphysis. Clinodactyly is curving of a finger to the radial or ulnar side. Most frequently the 5th finger is affected in terms of radial clinodactyly. A short and broad distal phalanx of the thumb is a relatively frequent minor abnormality, also referred to as brachydactyly type D. It is often an accompanying feature of brachydactyly type E. Figure 2.2 shows normal variations of the hands and feet.

Disruptions

Disruptions due to amniotic bands are frequently associated with abnormalities of the limbs, especially the hands and feet. Disrupted embryonic or fetal development of the limbs can occur due to vascular disruption. Normal embryonic development may also be disrupted by external factors that act on a genetically normal embryo, such as thalidomide embryopathy.

Dysplasias

Bony changes of the limbs (short metacarpals, for example) are part of the spectrum of many skeletal dysplasias; in particular, the 3rd, 4th, and 5th metacarpals can be associated with diverse skeletal dysplasias such as Albright hereditary osteodystrophy or acrodysostosis. The term dysplasia refers to abnormalities of bone and/or cartilage as a tissue. As such, they usually affect bone growth and/or stability. The overall pattern of the skeleton (that is, the number and the type of bones) remains intact.

Dysostosis

The term dysostosis refers to the absence, duplication, or other type of malformation that is caused by early developmental defects. Thus, in contrast to dysplasias, dysostoses are defects of patterning, and their pathology is not active at the time of inspection.

Types of Limb Malformations and General Classification

One of the first classifications of limb anomalies was published by Frantz and O'Rahilly (1961). Temtamy and McKusick divided the limb anomalies into several categories and subdivided them into syndromic and nonsyndromic types (1969, 1978). The classification of genetic skeletal disorders also includes forms of dysostoses and syndromic disorders with involvement of the extremities (Warman et al. 2011). Standard terms for anomalies of the hands and feet were suggested by Biesecker et al. (2009) with the goal of reaching consensus regarding the definitions. Early classification attempts were based purely on descriptive terms. However, with the increasing success of molecular genetics and the identification of the molecular causes in the majority of

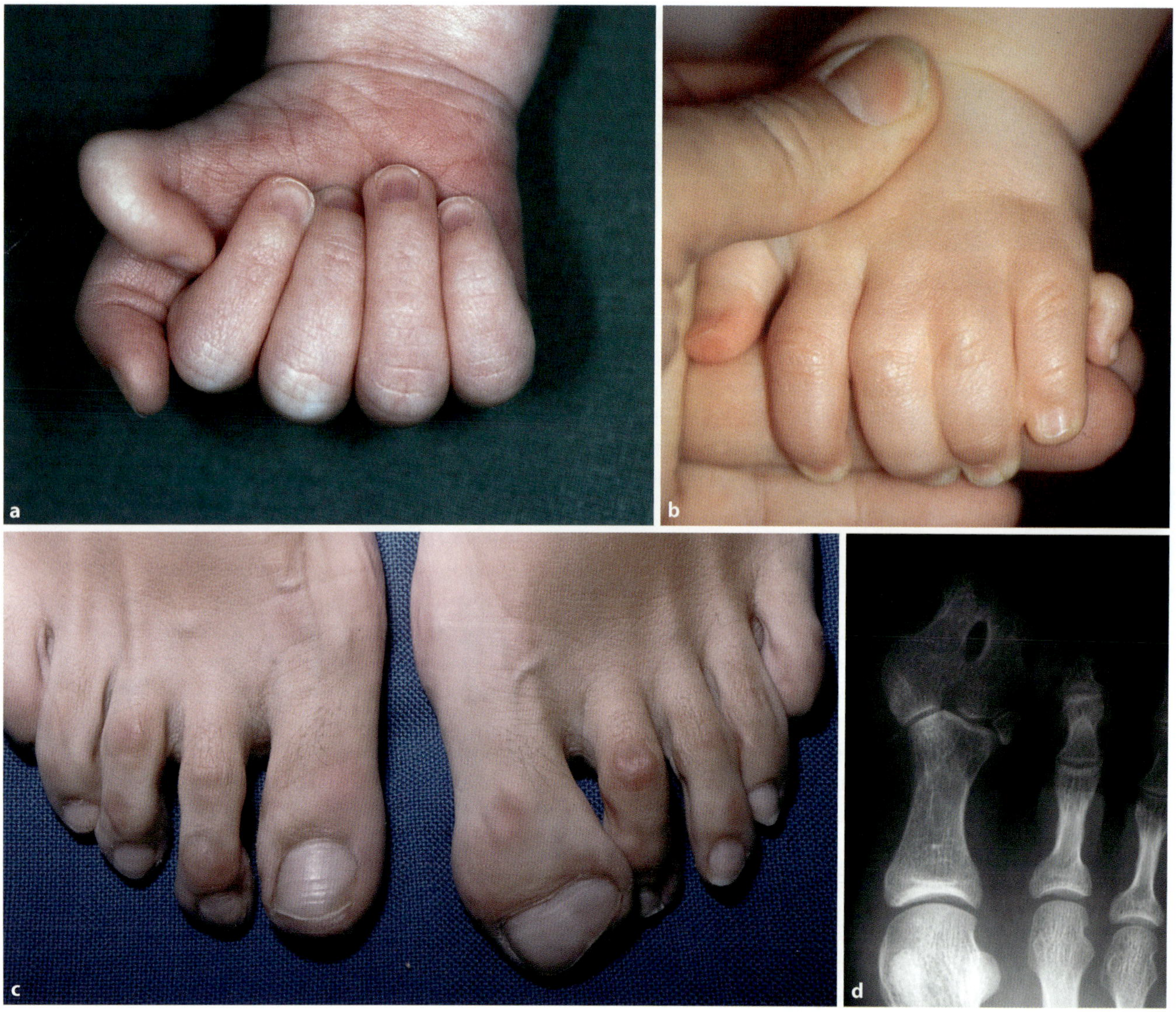

Fig. 2.3 Polydactyly. **a** Preaxial; duplication of thumb. **b** Postaxial; additional finger at ulnar side. In addition, note cutaneus syndactyly III–IV. **c** Broad hallux on the left. **d** Corresponding radiograph showing duplication of distal phalanx

known and defined conditions, it became clear that disease descriptions needed to be developed that were more than purely descriptive.

In this book we predominantly follow the Temtamy and McKusick (1969, 1978) classification with modifications and extensions of some groups. We also took over the subdivision of isolated and associated forms of particular limb anomalies, but integrated dysplasias that predominantly affect the limbs, including acromesomelic dysplasias and syndromic disorders with involvement of the extremities. Most of these follow the classification of genetic skeletal disorders, 2010 revision (Warman et al. 2011). In general, we attempt to combine phenotypic and molecular descriptions and, whenever possible, aim at fusing the molecular and clinical nomenclature. The primary approach, however, remains clinical and is centered on the patient and his or her phenotype. The following major limb malformations can be distinguished clinically. In many cases the clinical categories will overlap, resulting in complex pictures that need to be described in detail in order to make a diagnosis.

Polydactyly

Polydactyly is defined as the occurrence of supernumerary digits or portions thereof. These conditions are further classified as postaxial polydactyly, preaxial polydactyly, and central polydactyly. Polydactyly is often accompanied by syndactyly, in particular (but not exclusively) affecting the additional digit(s) and their next neighbor. Postaxial polydactyly (PAP), defined as an additional digit on the ulnar side of the hand, is a relatively frequent malformation. It can be further subclassified into two types: In type A, a well-formed extra digit articulates with the 5th or a 6th metacarpal, and

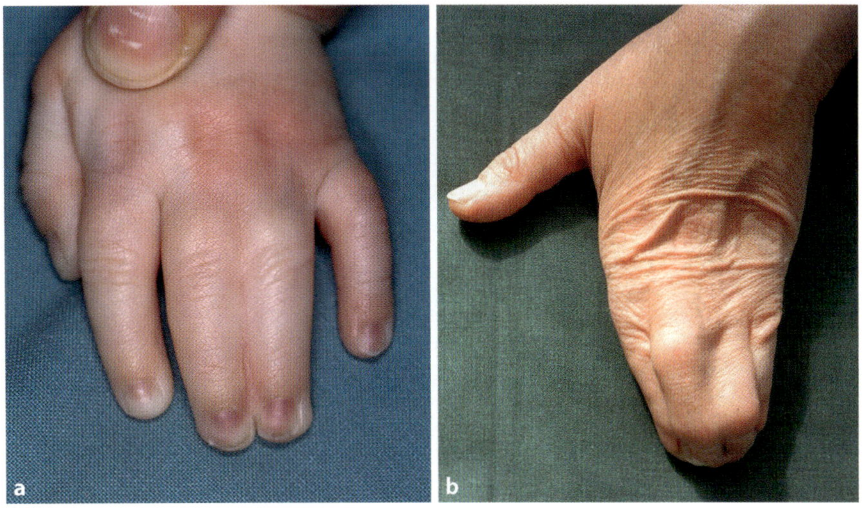

Fig. 2.4 Syndactyly. **a** Cutaneous syndactyly III/IV, also called type I syndactyly. **b** Complete syndactyly II–V with bony fusion of the distal phalanges

in type B, a rudimentary, poorly developed extra digit (also known as pedunculated postminimus) is present. It is a frequent form of polydactyly in certain populations. Preaxial polydactyly (PPD) refers to additional digits on the radial/tibial side of the hand/foot. The simplest form involves duplication of one or more of the skeletal components of a biphalangeal thumb/hallux. This may range from mere broadening of the distal phalanx with slight bifurcation at the tip to full duplication including the metacarpals. Thenar hypoplasia may be associated or the only minor sign. PPD can be associated with a digitized or triphalangeal thumb. In this case, the thumb has three instead of two phalanges and has the appearance of a finger. Triphalangeal thumbs may or may not occur as part of a duplication. The most common type of central polydactyly is synpolydactyly, in which an additional finger arises between digits III and IV. Usually, these three fingers are combined in a syndactylous web, and there can be bony fusion at various levels. An extreme form of polydactyly is mirror-image polydactyly. Here, the entire hand/foot is duplicated around the 1st digit. Mirror-image polydactyly can be accompanied by complete syndactyly. Examples of polydactyly phenotypes are shown in Fig. 2.3.

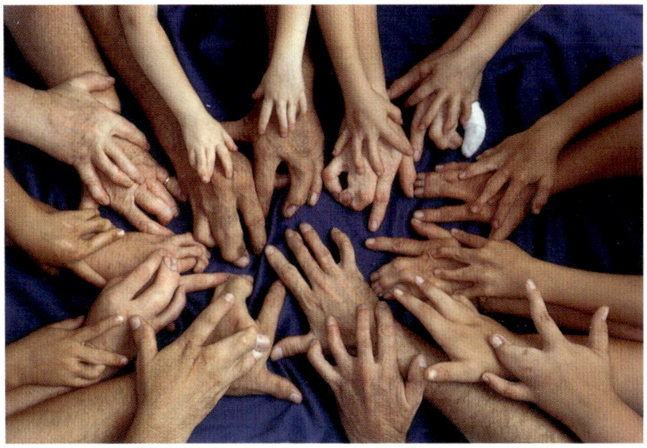

Fig. 2.5 Family with synpolydactyly, *HOXD13* associated

Syndactyly

Syndactyly means a cutaneous or bony fusion of one or more digits. The severity of cutaneous syndactyly varies from mild expression to severe involvement with joined digits to the level of the corresponding nails. In bony fusions between one or more phalanges of adjacent digits, abnormally broad digits are formed. Historically, syndactyly has been subdivided into the following forms: syndactyly type I, fusion of the 3rd and 4th fingers and/or the 2nd and 3rd toes; syndactyly type II, fusion of the 3rd and 4th fingers with partial or complete duplication of a digit within the syndactylous web; syndactyly type III, fusion of the 4th and 5th fingers or the 3rd, 4th, and 5th fingers; syndactyly type IV (Haas type), complete cutaneous fusion of all fingers with additional preaxial and/or postaxial digits; and syndactyly type V, fusion of the 4th and 5th metacarpal and/or metatarsal bones. In some instances this nomenclature correlates with specific disease entities; in others, it does not. This is mainly due to the extensive variation in phenotypes within a genetically defined condition, resulting in considerable overlap among the different types. These categories may therefore serve as a phenotypic description but should not be used as diagnostic terms. Examples of syndactyly phenotypes are shown in Fig. 2.4. Figure 2.5 shows a family with *HOXD13*-related synpolydactyly (fusion of the 3rd and 4th fingers with an additional digit in the syndactylous web).

Brachydactyly

Brachydactyly means shortening of digits due to anomalies of any of the phalanges, metacarpals, or/and metatarsals. We use a modified version of Bell's original 1951 classification

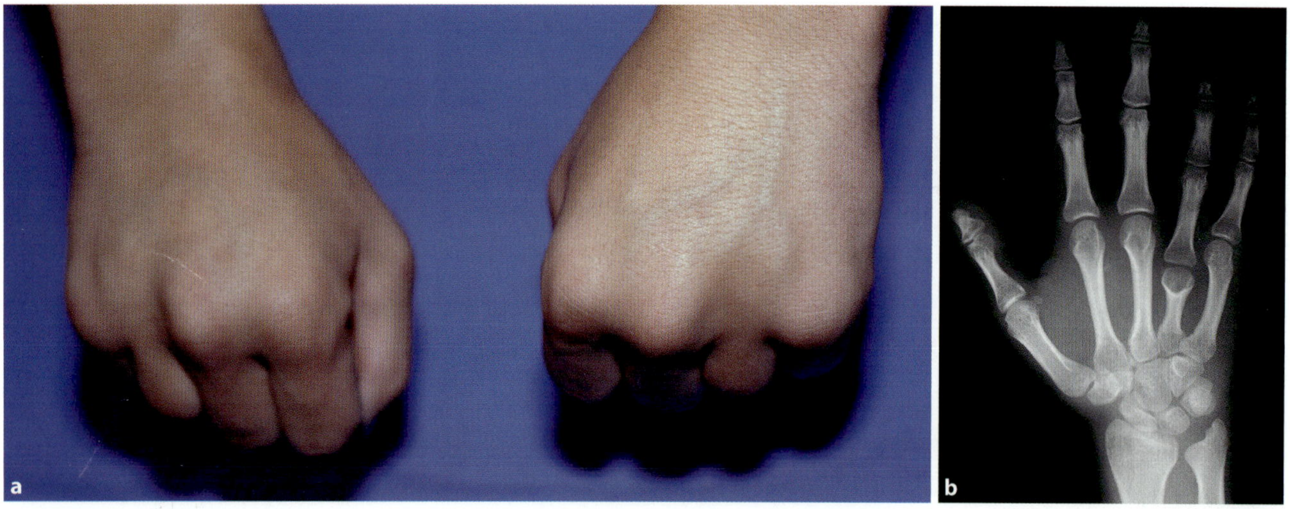

Fig. 2.6 **a** Knuckle sign in brachydactyly type E. Note retraction of the 4th knuckle due to a short metacarpal IV. **b** Corresponding radiograph

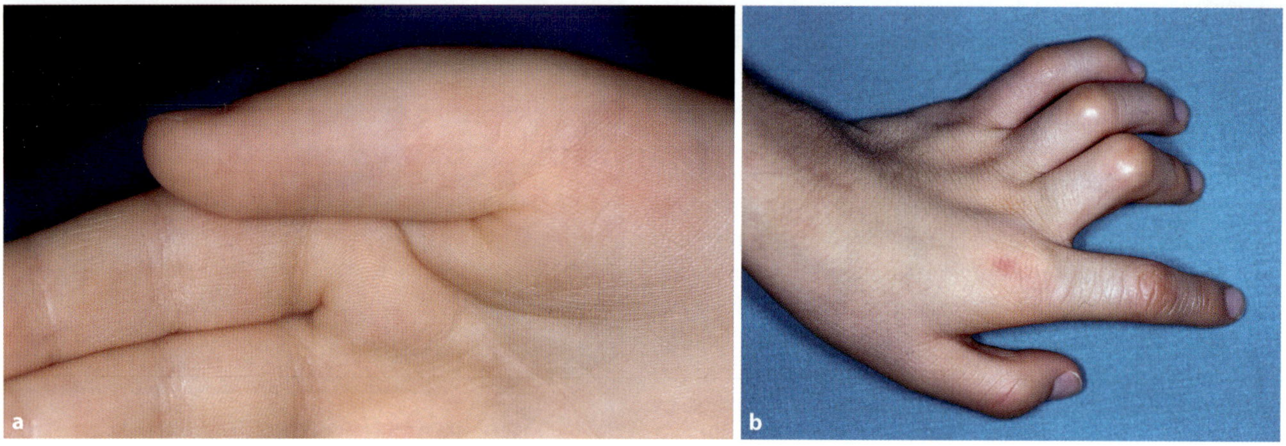

Fig. 2.7 Abnormal joint formation in symphalangism. **a** Symphalangism of interphalangeal joint of thumb. Note absence of flexion crease. **b** Camptodactyly and inability to extend fingers

(Mundlos 2009). For a detailed assessment, a radiological examination is necessary. Type A refers to shortening of the middle phalanges. Subtype A1 is defined by shortening of all middle phalanges, whereas in A2, shortening is confined to the middle phalanges of the 2nd and 5th fingers. Subtype A3, which is shortening of the middle phalanx of the 5th finger, is a frequent minor anomaly or part of more complex phenotypes. All other described subtypes are variants of the above. Type B refers to shortening and/or absence of the terminal and sometimes middle phalanges of digits II–V. It has been subdivided into types B1 and B2; the latter is accompanied by syndactyly. Type C brachydactyly is the most complex type. Finger IV is the least affected and thus the longest. The first metacarpal can be very short; the phalanges of fingers II, III, and V are hypoplastic; and on radiographic films often four instead of three phalangeal ossification centers can be seen (hyperphalangism). Type D brachydactyly refers to a short and broad terminal phalanx of the thumb. Type E is shortening of one or more metacarpals and/or metatarsals, often accompanied by short phalanges. Short metacarpals can be examined by the presence or absence of the "knuckle sign" (Fig. 2.6a).

Abnormalities of Joint Formation and Mobility

The joints are frequently affected in limb malformations. Examination of all joints for full or limited range of motion is therefore mandatory. Syndactylies frequently result in restricted joint mobility because of differences in length between digits. This may result in contractures that need to be released surgically. Contracture deformities are characterized by displacement anomalies without osseous primary changes in the skeletal structures. Typical examples of isolated contractures deformities are camptodactyly, Dupuytren contracture, and congenital clasped thumb. Camptodactyly is a term used to describe the inability to extend the proximal or distal interphalangeal joint of digits. These conditions have to be distinguished from abnormalities of joint formation, which

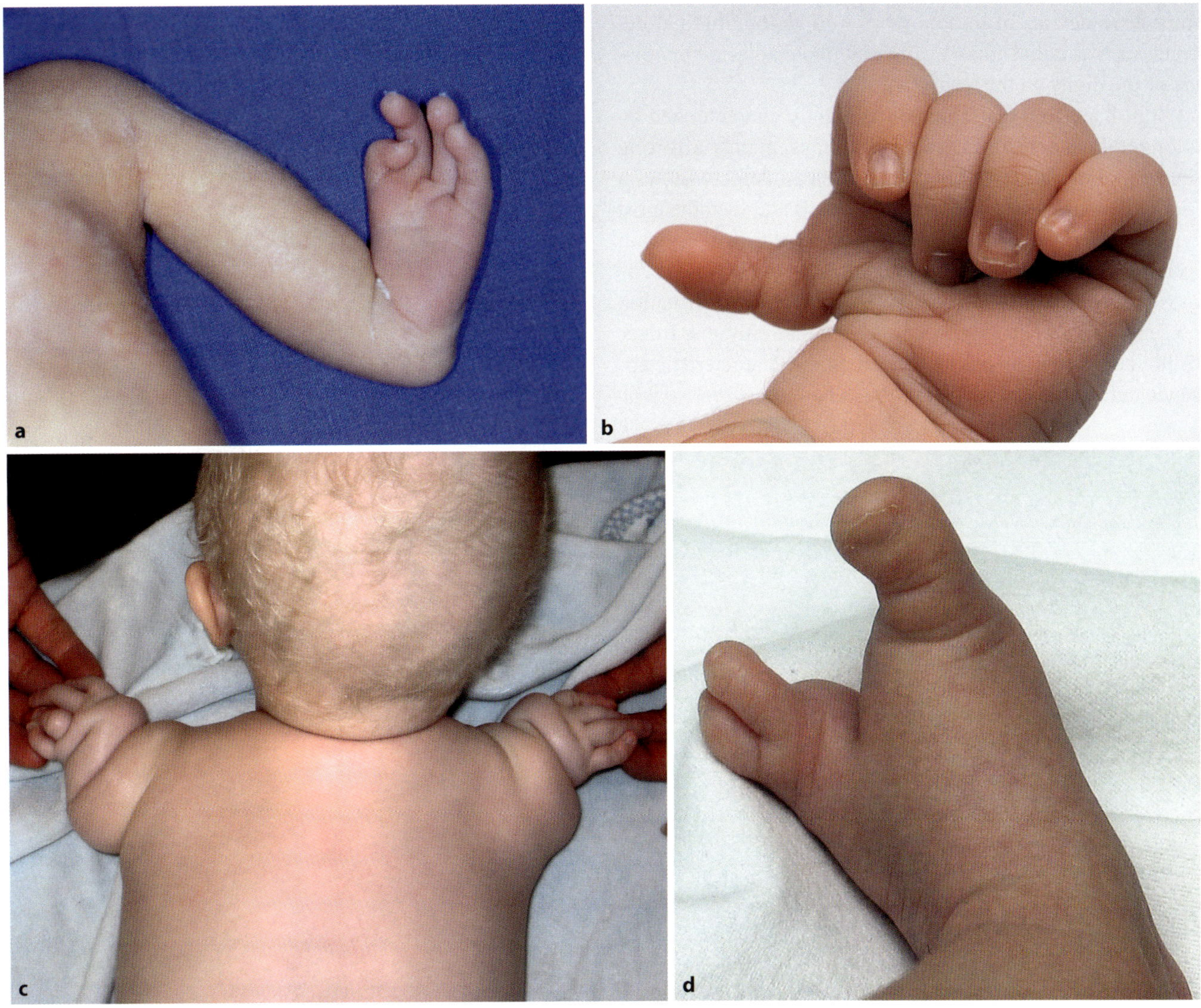

Fig. 2.8 Absence deformities. **a** Absence of radius, resulting in angulation of hand. **b** Hypoplastic and deformed thumb as minimal manifestation of radial ray deficiency. **c** Phokomelia in TAR syndrome. **d** Typical ectrodactyly of the foot

involve the separation of cartilaginous anlagen of the skeletal elements from each other early in development. In this case the radiograph shows a true fusion of skeletal elements with a bony bridge or a reduced interphalangeal joint space in the case of a cartilaginous fusion. This is not the case in contracture deformities. Reduced mobility in the phalangeal joints during fetal development results in reduced or absent phalangeal creases, a reliable clinical sign that should be further validated by radiology. Fusion of the interphalangeal joints is referred to as symphalangism. In the large joints (elbow, knee, or shoulder), a reduction in mobility often results in the formation of pterygiae. Carpal or tarsal synostosis refers to a fusion of two or more carpal or tarsal bones, which can occur in isolation or in association with other bony changes such as a dysplastic elbow joint and brachydactyly. Camptodactyly due to limited joint movement and the absence of flexion creases in symphalangism are shown in Fig. 2.7.

Absence Deformities

Absence deformities consist of the absence or hypoplasia of skeletal structures of the limbs. They can be subdivided according to anatomical location. Peromelia refers to distally missing structures, whereas amelia is the lack of all limb structures. "Terminal transverse" describes the (unilateral) absence or hypoplasia of distal structures of the limbs with more or less normal proximal structures. Examples of terminal transverse defects of the hands and feet include absence of one or more phalanges, absence of one or more digits, or absence of the entire hand or foot. A more severe manifestation of this type of defect includes an absence deformity of the forearm, including the hands. Phocomelia, in contrast, describes an intercalary deficiency of limbs in which a normal or almost normal hand or foot appears to emerge directly from the shoulder or hip. Radial and ulnar defects include transverse defects of these rays as well as longitudinal defects, such as radial aplasia, with or without aplasia/hypoplasia of the digits on the respective side.

Split-hand/foot malformation is mainly characterized by a longitudinal defect of hand and foot rays, mainly affecting the central digital ray. This type of skeletal defects shows a markedly variable phenotype. In the hands and feet, the most typical abnormality is the absence of the 3rd digital ray with a cleft extending to the level of the carpal or tarsal bones. The most severe manifestation of split-hand/foot malformation presents as monodactyly, which means that only one (ulnar or fibular) digital ray has developed. Some characteristic absence deformities are shown in Fig. 2.8.

References

Biesecker LG, Aase JM, Clericuzio C, Gurrieri F, Temple IK, Toriello H (2009) Elements of morphology: standard terminology for the hands and feet. Am J Med Genet A 149A(1):93–127

Frantz CH, O'Rahilly R (1961) Congenital skeletal limb deficiencies. J Bone Joint Surg 43A:1202

Hall JG, Allanson JE, Gripp KW, Slavotinek AM (2007) Handbook of Physical Measurements, 2nd edn. Oxford University Press, New York

Mundlos S (2009) The brachydactylies: a molecular disease family. Clin Genet 76(2):123–136

Temtamy S and McKusick VA. Synopsis of hand malformations with particular emphasis on genetic factors. In: Limb malformations BD:OAS. White Plains: The National Foundation 1969 V(3):125.

Temtamy S, McKusick VA (1978) The genetics of hand malformations. The National Foundation March of Dimes. Birth Defects: Original Article Series XIV:3

Warman ML, Cormier-Daire V, Hall C, Krakow D, Lachman R, LeMerrer M et al (2011) Nosology and classification of genetic skeletal disorders: 2010 revision. Am J Med Genet A 155A(5):943–968

Radiology of the Limb

Ralph Lachman

3

Long Bone Radiologic Anthropometry

Assessment of the extremities needs to be approached methodically. One must be familiar with certain terminology:

- Rhizomelia, or proximal bone shortening (humerus, femur)
- Mesomelia, or middle bone shortening (radius/ulna, tibia/fibula)
- Acromelia, or hand and foot shortening
- Brachydactyly, or finger and toe shortening
- Parts of the growing bone (epiphysis, metaphysis, diaphysis)

Unlike the situation when dealing with most skeletal dysplasias, in many dysostoses there can be absence of entire bone segments. This may occur symmetrically or asymmetrically. Hypoplastic long bone segments also can be present either unilaterally or bilaterally. It is important to ascertain whether the hypoplasia is proximal, distal, or generalized and whether the bone has maintained its normal caliber. A transverse cutoff can also occur, or there can be a drop-out of singular and/or combined bone segments (radius and ulna) with intact normal proximal/distal bones, as in phocomelia (thalidomide embryopathy). Are the epiphyses involved as well as the combined metaphyseal and diaphyseal portions? Another consideration is possible osseous fusion (synostosis) between two bones across a joint space or between adjacent bones. All other bones must be looked at because there may be clues regarding contiguous involvement of the extremities (for instance, acetabular changes in femoral-facial syndrome). The foot is an important structure, but it contains an enormous amount of normal variation, especially in the young individual; therefore, it is often much more difficult to interpret as to abnormal findings.

In this newer imaging era, magnetic resonance imaging (MRI) can help in ascertaining muscular involvement, vascular abnormalities, and so on. Computed tomography (CT) can also be helpful in some cases. As a general rule, the nonenhanced MRI delineates the soft tissues, noncalcified cartilage, and marrow, while bone is a "black hole." A contrast MRI can reveal vascular changes. On the other hand, CT delineates the osseous elements quite well. It is important to realize that bypassing the plain film not uncommonly leads to major, preventable miscalculations. Most diagnoses of dysostoses of the extremities need only plain film examination.

To accurately evaluate the extremities in a patient with abnormal limb development, one must recognize the normal size and bony configuration of the extremities. This is complicated by age-related changes. Earlier in this text, limb development was discussed. We are now going to look at each of the long bones separately as to how they appear on radiographs normally so that one will be able to ascertain whether they manifest hypoplasia, missing portions, or other anomalous development. Long and short tubular bones have four basic portions that contribute to growth and development: the epiphyses, the growth plate, the metaphysis, and the diaphysis. They are recognized and delineated in the growing fetus (ultrasound, MRI, fast CT) and in the child (radiograph) until the growth plate has fused (Fig. 3.1).

We begin with the *upper extremity long bones*:

The *humerus*, as with other long bones, has epiphyses at both ends. The proximal humeral epiphysis ossifies postnatally and normally will be present just after term. At the elbow, the distal humeral growth centers ossify much later. The growth plate proximally is much more active and contributes to most of the humeral growth in length. The diaphysis is narrowed in the midshaft region, and the metaphyseal regions are widened at both ends (Fig. 3.2a, b, d). The *radius* and *ulna* have anatomy similar to the humerus, except their more rapid-growing centers are distal rather than proximal. The radius has significant widening at the distal end, while both ends of the ulna and the proximal end of the radius are only mildly widened. Central diaphyseal modeling (narrowing) is minimal for both bones (Fig. 3.2a, c, e).

Next let us look at the *lower extremity long bones*:

The *femur* has epiphyses at both ends. Proximally it also contains two apophyseal centers, the greater and lesser trochanters (by definition these do not contribute to growth in length). The distal femoral epiphysis ossifies at 38±2 weeks of gestation (it is the fastest growing epiphyseal/growth-plate center in the body), while the proximal center (capital femoral epiphysis) normally ossifies at about 6 weeks to 3 months of age. The neck of the femur is almost like a separate diaphysis from the intratrochanteric groove region up to the proximal femoral growth plate. There is very significant widening of the femur distally but not proximally. Modeling (periosteal bone development) of the diaphysis, as with most other long bones, results in some mild central narrowing (Fig. 3.2f–h, j). The *tibia* and *fibula* are typical long bones with fairly symmetrical widening at both ends and

S. Mundlos, D. Horn, *Limb Malformations*,
DOI 10.1007/978-3-540-95928-1_3, © Springer-Verlag Berlin Heidelberg 2014

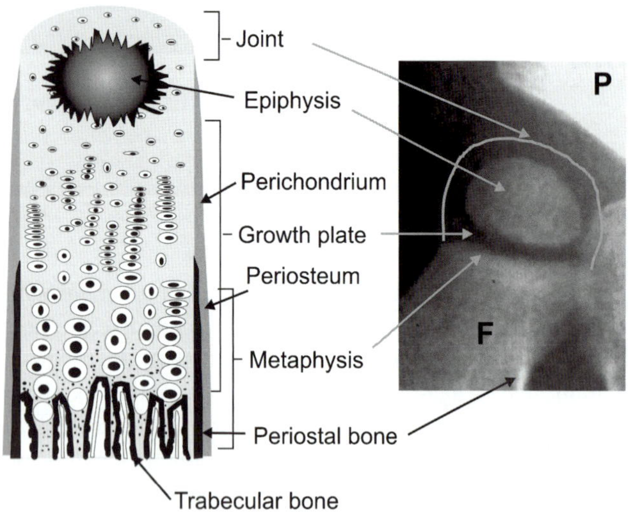

Fig. 3.1 The growth plate and its appearance in plain film radiology. *P* pelvis, *F* femur

epiphyseal centers at each end (the proximal tibial epiphysis ossifies at 40±2 weeks of gestation and is the second fastest growing growth plate). Tibial midshaft diaphyseal narrowing is present but is hardly noticeable in the fibula (Fig. 3.2f, g, i, k).

Hand Anthropometry

The human hand is a very complex structure. It consists of 19 short tubular bones and eight carpal bones. It also contains a significant amount of normal variation. This variability and complexity are related to the developmental function of the hand as a working unit. The radiographic appearance of the hand bones (rather than just clinical hand assessment) is often the best way to evaluate abnormalities. The short tubular bones of the hand are formed by epiphyses, metaphyses, and diaphyses similar to the other extremity bones, but true metacarpals proximally can also contain pseudoepiphyses that may have clinical significance.

The size of the bones as well as their timing of ossification is an important consideration and can be broken down as follows:

- Length of the metacarpals and phalanges
- Relative slenderness of these short tubular bones
- Size, configuration, and developmental ossification of the carpal bones

The normal radiographic appearance of hands during development/bone growth is shown in Fig. 3.2l–p.

The short tubular bones of the hand (metacarpals and phalanges)

Most commonly the assessment can be made by simply viewing the hand and wrist radiograph. Small incremental changes in length can be difficult to gauge. Direct age-related measurements have been created with appropriate tables (Garn et al. 1972; Gefferth 1972). However, because the actual single bone reduction may not be significant without a relationship to the other bones, relative bone length tables were created. Because the absolute numbers are so variable relative to radiographic technique, a relative bone length pattern profile analysis (MCPP) was created (Poznanski et al. 1972). Subsequently an adjustment was suggested for the MCPP to a "total length" measurement valuable for certain syndrome analysis; also, possible errors can be produced by different population usage (Dijkstra 1983; Arias-Cazorla and Rodriguez-Larraide 1983). Another addition to pattern profile analysis is the use of *Q*-scores rather than *Z*-scores for younger individuals (birth to 7 years) (Dijkstra and Venema 1991). IBM-compatible software for MCPP is available (Hosenfeld et al. 1991). It is important to point out that many of these entities do not have characteristic, much less diagnostic, pattern profiles. Also, with the advent of molecular/gene analysis of these disorders, perhaps the MCPP plays a less important role.

The short tubular bones and carpal centers of the hand are divided into the 1st/radial ray and ulnar ray for developmental purposes, yet for polydactyly considerations into preaxial (thumb side), postaxial (5th finger side) and interaxial (central) divisions. Radiologically, I feel it is best to separately analyze the thumb from the rest of the digits. The thumb has only two phalanges (exception: triphalangeal thumb). The 1st metacarpal notably has its epiphysis proximally appearing like a phalanx. Phylogenetically it suggests that the "true metacarpal" of the thumb was later incorporated into the carpus.

The metacarpals II–V have their epiphyses on the distal end of bone. On the proximal end of these metacarpals, pseudoepiphyses and pseudoepiphyseal notches can occur normally (most prevalent on metacarpals II and V), while

Fig. 3.2 Radiographs of normal limbs at various ages. Humerus and radius/ulna in **a–e**, hands in **l–p**, and femur and tibia/fibula in **f–k**. **a** Newborn. Normal upper extremity; humerus is longer than radius/ulna. **b** An 8-year-old. Normal humerus radiograph. **c** An 11.5-year-old. Normal radius/ulna radiograph. **d** A 16-year-old female. Normal humerus; almost completely fused growth plates. **e** A 16-year-old female. Normal radius/ulna; almost completely fused growth plates. **f** Newborn. Normal lower extremity; femur longer than tibia/fibula; not quite term infant (no ossified epiphyses at the knees). **g** A 1-year-old. Normal lower extremity; proximal fibula is shorter than tibia. Note epiphyses at proximal, distal femur, proximal tibia. **h** A 3-year-old. Normal femur. **i** A 3-year-old. Normal tibia/fibula. **j** A 14-year-old. Normal proximal femur/hip. **k** A 14-year-old. Normal knee-tibia/fibula; proximal fibula is shorter than tibia. **l** Newborn. Normal anteroposterior hand radiograph; no carpal/epiphyseal ossification. **m** A 3-year-old male. Normal hand radiograph. **n** A 3-year-old female. Normal hand radiograph. **o** A 12-year-old female. Normal hand radiograph. **p** An 11-year-old male. Normal hand radiograph; note decreased skeletal maturation in the male

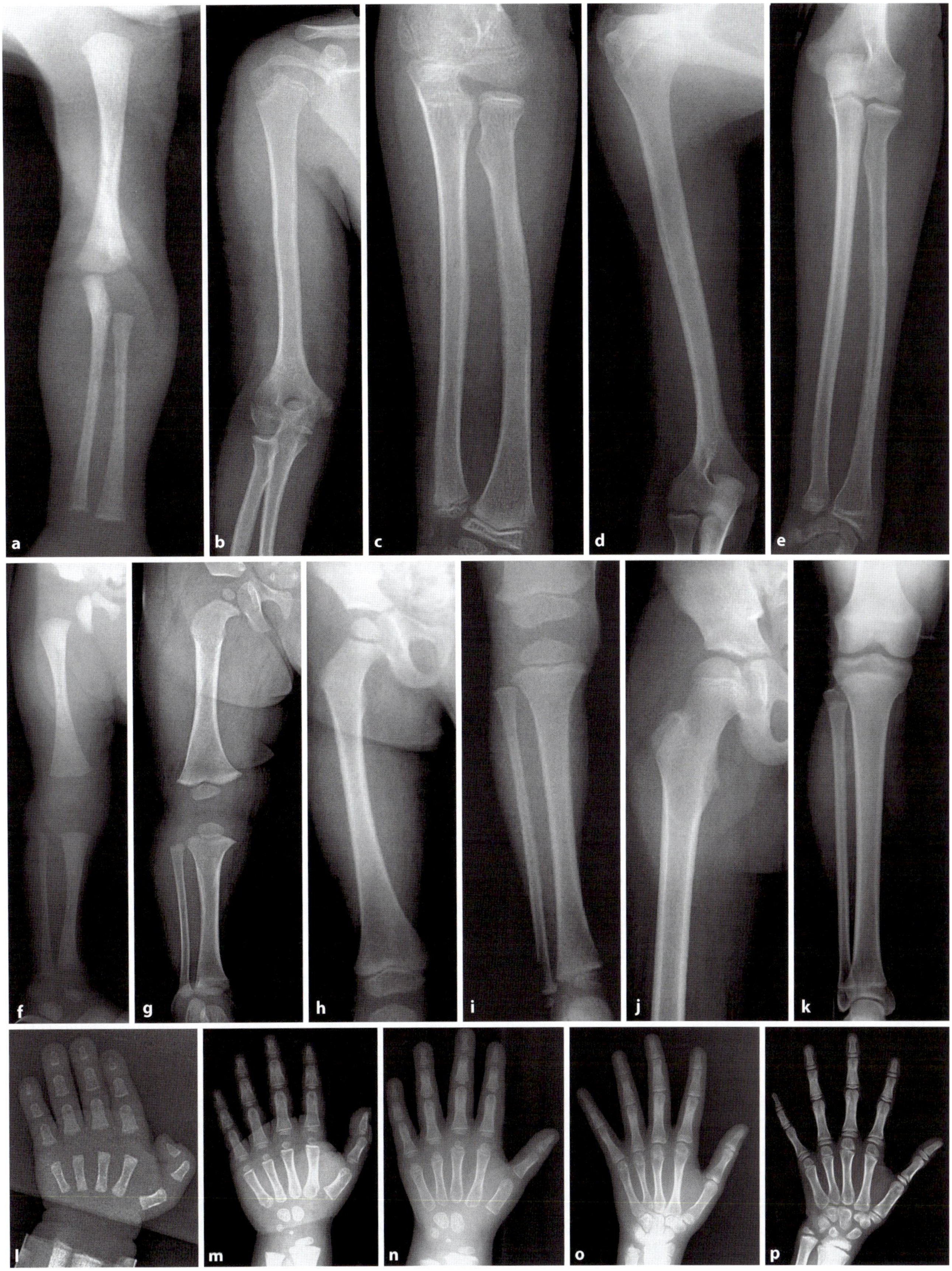
a
b
c
d
e
f
g
h
i
j
k
l
m
n
o
p

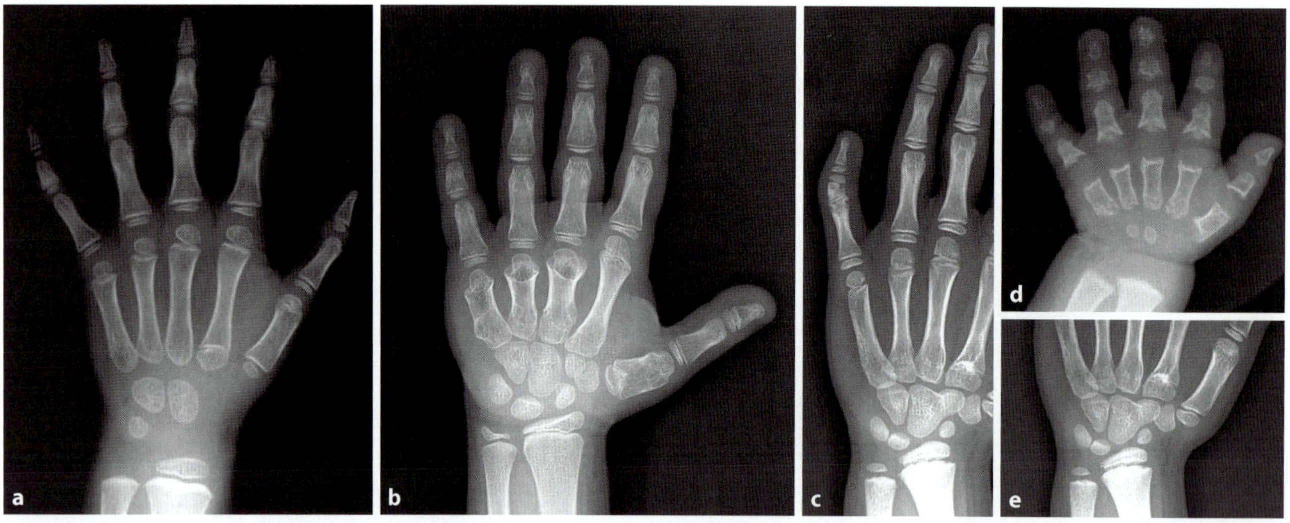

Fig. 3.3 **a** Hand of an individual with cleidocranial dysplasia. Note pseudoepiphyses at distal metacarpal I and proximal metacarpal II. **b** Brachydactyly type E. Very short metacarpals III–V; metacarpal II is the longest. **c** Symphalangism (fusion of joints) of the interphalangeal joint of digit V. **d** Multiple cone-shaped epiphyses in Ellis–van Creveld syndrome. **e** Fusion of carpal bones (capitate and trapezoid)

multiple pseudoepiphyses can be syndromic (cleidocranial dysplasia; Fig. 3.3a). These short tubular bones have a similar shape to the previously discussed long bones, with mild narrowing of/near their central diaphysis. The length of metacarpals is quite important. The longest metacarpal is the 3rd, followed by II, IV, and then V (Fig. 3.2n–p). The metacarpal index is a measure of relative slenderness (Sinclaire et al. 1960; Joseph and Meadow 1969; Parish 1966). For radiographic evaluation of the isolated brachydactyly syndromes, one measurement is the metacarpal sign, which is similar to the clinical evaluation of the length of the 4th metacarpal in relation to the 3rd and 5th metacarpals. This is, of course, helpful for evaluating brachydactyly type E (Fig. 3.3b). The remaining isolated brachydactyly syndromes usually do not require a special system of radiographic analysis . The 1st metacarpal is by far the shortest. It has a slightly different shape (more rectangular with less central narrowing). Pseudoepiphyses are fairly common on the distal end.

Digits II–V each have three phalanges. The more proximal digital phalanges are longer, with a progressive decrease in size as one goes distally. Their epiphyses are on the proximal end of these short tubular bones. Their metaphyseal ends are all normally wider than the distal portions. The two phalanges of the thumb (proximal and distal) are shaped similarly to the other phalanges and are sized like the middle and distal phalanges of the rest of the hand. The distal, also called terminal, phalanges contain the nail bed and have a specific radiological appearance. The so-called tuft normally has a chess-pawn shape.

Phalanges and metacarpals are connected by joints. Radiologically these joint spaces are, of course, not ossified and can best be seen by MRI, but joint space narrowing is appreciated by a decreased distance between the ends of bones, which can lead to complete obliteration or fusion (Kosowicz 1965; Fig. 3.3c).

Cone-shaped epiphyses involve both metacarpals and phalanges and have a different frequency in varying populations. They can be found in a number of syndromes and usually lead to precocious fusion and bone shortening (Giedion 1967; Fig. 3.3d). Another interesting abnormal finding in the phalanges (and metacarpals) are “angels.” They consist of wing-shaped lateral excrescences and are associated with several syndromes and skeletal dysplasias (Giedion et al. 1993; Merrill et al. 2012). The embryological/fetal development of hand ossification is rather interesting. The tufts (distal phalanges) are the first to ossify, followed by the metacarpals and the proximal and middle phalanges, in that order (O’Rahilly and Gardner 1972). The 5th middle phalanx ossification can be delayed until term.

The Carpus

The carpal centers in humans number eight and were often named by their shape and size (Fig. 3.2p). They are varied in size, configuration, and time of appearance. The navicular (scaphoid) and the greater multiangular trapezium are part of the 1st ray. The carpal bones normally begin to ossify after birth (±3 months). The first to ossify are the capitate and hamate, and ossification is completed with the pisiform. The shape of the carpal bones can vary greatly. Phylogenetically the very “primitive hand” has three rows of carpal centers. In higher species (most modern reptiles and mammals), there is retention of the 3rd row, but some have one or two os centrale carpal centers instead of a middle row of four ossifications. Developmentally, an os centrale is present at 6 weeks of human gestation and later fuses with the scaphoid and is rarely seen as a normal variant (Kivell and Begun 2007, 2009). An os centrale can be found in humans as a feature of certain syndromes (hand-foot–uterus syndrome, Holt–Oram syndrome, otopalatodigital syndrome, Larsen syndrome). Carpal fusions appear either as isolated anomalies, as part of congenital malformation syndromes, or secondary to severe inflammatory processes such as rheumatoid arthritis (Fig. 3.3e).

Radiological / Imaging Evaluation

Anthropometry (the study of the sizes and proportions of the skeletal system) is very important not only in the evaluation of limb development (dysostoses) but in skeletal dysplasia and syndrome diagnoses as well. In doing a genetic skeletal survey, one begins the examination with the ascertainment of possible shortening of the rhizomelic (proximal) portions of the extremities, followed by the mesomelic (middle) portions of the limbs, and finally the acro (distal) elements (hands/feet) (Lachman 2007).

Skeletal Maturation (Bone Age)

The assessment of skeletal maturation is performed radiologically by obtaining a film of the left hand and wrist. There are ossification differences between each hand that are related to the handedness of the individual, but these differences are minor. The atlas of skeletal development by Gruelich and Pyle is the most commonly used and practical methodology (Gruelich and Pyle 1971). Pediatric radiologists have long been aware that disharmonious epiphyseal-carpal ossification exists even in the normal individual. Not uncommonly there is a significant delay of carpal ossification compared with the epiphyseal ossification of the metacarpals and phalanges. As a result, bone age readings (if such disharmonious ossification is present) should have a slight reduction of the bone age reached with the epiphyseal ossification assessment. The epiphyseal ossification of the distal radius and ulna is usually in line with the hand epiphyseal ascertainment. Bone age assessment is not really that important when dealing with dysostoses. It is also not very valuable in most skeletal dysplasias or in syndrome evaluations, where there is often marked nonspecific carpal-epiphyseal disharmonious ossification.

Normal Variants

Variations of the norm in the skeletal system are extremely numerous but play a very important role in radiography, especially in pediatric radiology (the assessment of radiographic developmental abnormalities). For dysostosis evaluation in particular, normal variation in the hands plays a key role. Many normal variants exist in the short tubular bones and carpal bones of the hand and wrist. For help with this important evaluation of deciding what is normal and what is pathological, physicians can consult Keats and Anderson's atlas of normal variants (Keats and Anderson 2013) and Freyschmidt's *Borderlands of Normal and Early Pathological Findings in Skeletal Radiography* (Freyschmidt et al 2001).

References

Arias-Cazorla S, Rodríguez-Larralde A (1983) Metacarpophalangeal pattern profiles in Venezuelan and northern Caucasoid samples compared. Am J Phys Anthropol 73(1):71–80

Dijkstra PF (1983) Analysis of metacarpophalangeal pattern profiles. Rofo 139(2):158–159

Dijkstra PF, Venema HW (1991) Metacarpophalangeal pattern profiles: Q-score for ages from birth to 7 years. Am J Med Genet 40(1):107–114

Freyschmidt J, Brossmann J, Sternberg A, Wiens J (2001) Köhler/Zimmer's Borderlands of Normal and Early Pathological Findings in Skeletal Radiography, 5th edn. Thieme, Stuttgart

Garn SM, Hertzog K et al (1972) Metacarpophalangeal length in the evaluation of skeletal malformations. Radiology 105:375–381

Gefferth K (1972) Metrische Auswertung der kurzen Röhrenknochen der Hand von der Geburt bis zum Ende der Pubertät: Längenmasse. Acta Paediat Acad Sci Hung 13:117–124

Giedion A (1967) Cone-shaped epiphyses of the hands and their diagnostic value. The tricho-rhino-phalangeal syndrome. Ann Radiol (Paris) 10(3):322–329

Giedion A, Prader A et al (1993) Angel-shaped phalango-epiphyseal dysplasia (ASPED): identification of a new genetic bone marker. Am J Med Genet 47(5):765–771

Greulich WW, Pyle SI (eds) (1971) Radiographic Atlas of Skeletal Development of the Hand and Wrist, 2nd edn. Stanford University Press, Stanford, CA

Hosenfeld D, Hosenfeld F et al (1991) IBM-PC compatible software for establishing metacarpophalangeal pattern profiles. Clin Genet 39(5):396–400

Joseph MC, Meadow SR (1969) The Metacarpal Index of Infants. Arch Dis Child 44:515–516

Keats TE, Anderson MW (2013) Atlas of Normal Roentgen Variants That May Simulate Disease, 8th edn. Saunders/Elsevier, Philadelphia

Kivell TL, Begun DR (2007) Frequency and timing of scaphoid-centrale fusion in hominoids. J Hum Evol 52(3):321–340

Kivell TL, Begun DR (2009) New primate carpal bones from Rudabánya (late Miocene, Hungary): taxonomic and functional implications. L Hum Evol 57(6):697–709

Kosowicz J (1965) The roetgen appearance of the hand and wrist in gonadal dysgenesis. Am J Roetgenol 94:354–361

Lachman RS (2007) Radiology of Syndromes, Metabolic disorders, and Skeletal Dysplasias, 5th edn. Mosby/Elsevier, Philadelphia

Merrill AE, Sarukhanov A et al (2012) Bent bone dysplasia-FGFR2 type, a distinct skeletal disorder, has deficient canonical FGF signaling. Am J Hum Genet 90(3):550–557

O'Rahilly R, Gardner E (1972) The initial appearance of ossification in staged human embryos. Am J Anat 134:291–308

Parish JG (1966) Radiographic measurements of the skeletal structure of the normal hand. Brit J Radiol 39:52–62

Poznanski AK, Garn SM et al (1972) Metacarpophalangeal pattern profiles in the evaluation of skeletal malformation. Radiology 104:1–11

Sinclaire RJG, Kitchin AH et al (1960) The Marfan syndrome. Quart J Med 53:19–46

4 Surgical Management Principles for Congenital Upper Limb Malformations

Ulrich Mennen

It takes a professional lifetime to get a feel for managing congenital upper limb malformations. This is because each deformity is unique – even the two sides in bilateral cases differ. Furthermore, the special investigations to evaluate more deeply than the obvious phenotype are in fact no more than a shadow; for example, radiographs only cast a shadow of calcified tissue (bone), and therefore the full picture cannot be appreciated. Cartilaginous parts and soft tissues that are also always involved cannot be visualized by radiographs. In other words, all tissues must be assessed and dealt with simultaneously.

The overriding principle when planning or suggesting a management protocol is to always test it against the two fundamental rules: First, and most important, will the treatment improve function? Second, will it improve the cosmetic appearance? Special investigations are essential, especially in the more complex deformities. Apart from the gold-standard radiographic image, computed tomography (CT) and three-dimensional (3D) imaging, high-definition sonar (static and video), and nuclear magnetic resonance imaging (MRI) prove to be very informative, particularly regarding the soft tissue aberrations and extent of soft tissue masses. Recently, 3D printing or additive manufacturing has been a major development to create a 3D model of the anatomical variation, which helps to visualize the deformity. This technique is also used to manufacture implants, build missing anatomical parts, and design orthotics and prosthetics.

It is advisable for the management strategy to be planned by a team of experts, which may include the surgeon, occupational therapist, orthotist, prosthetist, physiotherapist, biokineticist, and geneticist, as well as on occasion the psychologist. In general, persons with congenital anomalies adapt remarkably well to their deformities. They are innovative in developing the skills to perform activities of daily living, sport, work, and social interaction (Fig. 4.1).

Conservative Management

Conservative (nonsurgical) management includes hand therapy, manipulation, and the application of splints.

The main aim of **hand therapy** is to help optimize the individual's ability to cope with activities of daily living (ADL) and work. Hand therapists visit the homes and workplaces of patients to advise on structural changes and ergonomic adaptions (bathroom, kitchen, tools, instruments, machinery, car, and so on) to assist and optimize their ability to perform ADL and work. Many helpful gargets and devices are available to assist with all kinds of deformities. Hand therapists also have an important educational role to play toward parents, teachers, and employers.

Manipulation can be used to correct contractures, provided the therapy is started soon after birth. The newborn still has the hormone relaxin in his body (from his or mother; it assists in softening the ligaments during the birth process). A typical example is camptodactyly. In more than 90 % of cases, this congenital flexion contracture of the finger can be fully or near fully rectified if manipulation is done regularly soon after birth.

Manipulation can also be used to improve a deformity to facilitate surgery. Examples include radial dysplasia (radial club hand) and arthrogryposis multiplex congenita (AMC). In radial club hand, the radially dislocated hand is gently manipulated by distal distraction and ulnar "bending" at the wrist level. This will stretch the short tissues on the radial side. The improved position can then be held by a well-molded splint. In AMC, the upper limb typically has, among other deformities, the elbow fixed in extension, the wrist in fixed flexion, the thumb in the palm, and fixed flexion contractures of the fingers. Gentile manipulation to reverse these contractures will decrease the severity of the deformities. This will make the surgery less extensive.

Splints can be either static (passive) or dynamic (active). They can be made from many kinds of material. Choosing the correct material and type of splint is crucial to maximize the efficacy of this treatment modality. Manufacturing of splints is a highly specialized process done by occupational therapists. Splints have to be user friendly, effective, and easy to fit. Unfortunately, one often sees splints and orthoses that are uncomfortable and annoying to wear, and they achieve less than intended. It is extremely difficult to make well-fitting splints for babies, and much experience is needed! Before deciding to provide a splint for a baby, the surgeon and therapist have to be absolutely convinced that the device will be effective and lead to improved function and cosmetic appearance, and that it will not be used primarily to satisfy the parents or the attendant (surgeon or hand therapist).

Unfortunately, terms such as "trick movements" are used, which have negative connotations. Each person will develop adaptive skills to cope with his or her deficiency. These should never be ridiculed but should be nurtured and augmented. After all, the patient has a unique anatomical aberration, and he or

S. Mundlos, D. Horn, *Limb Malformations*,
DOI 10.1007/978-3-540-95928-1_4, © Springer-Verlag Berlin Heidelberg 2014

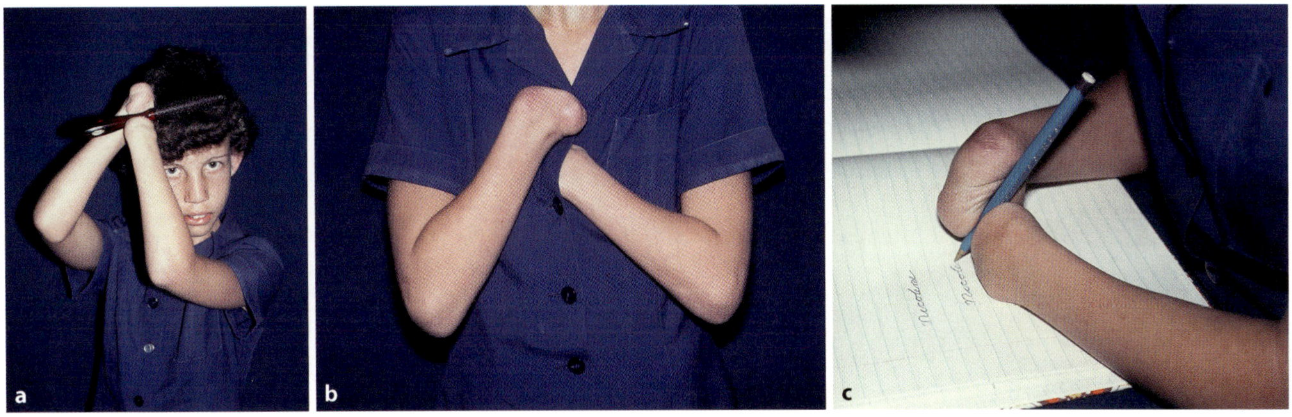

Fig. 4.1a–c Bilateral absence of hands (severe form of symbrachydactyly). This girl is able to do all activities of daily living and won her school's "neat writing" competition

she will know best how to cope with ADL. In small children, spontaneous play is more effective than specific exercises. In older children the emphasis is on developing and coping with skilled activities, including writing, typing, and other ADL.

Surgery

When planning surgery the following principles should guide decision making:

First surgery The first surgical procedure is the most important. This has to be definitive and comprehensive. Subsequent procedures should be reserved for further smaller corrections, such as dealing with scar contractures or deviant growth. Staged surgery may be indicated when, for instance, blood supply becomes compromised, such as in a three-web syndactyly. Stage one would release webs 1 and 3, and at stage two, after 6 months, web 2 would be released. Some conditions, however, need not be done in stages. Circumferential removal and resuturing of the skin of an amniotic band in one sitting is widely accepted as the method of choice.

Timing of surgery. it is generally agreed that if surgery is contemplated, early surgery (that is, between 3 and 12 months of age) is significantly better than later. Scar tissue formation is less, adaption to the new anatomy/position is better, and the altered anatomy becomes part of the natural body image. In the infant, grasp and pinch coordination are integrated by the age of 1 year. By 3 years of age, the child has a full awareness of prehension and spatial perception. This underlines the necessity for early surgery. The survival rate of free toe phalangeal transfers to lengthen fingers, such as in symbrachydactyly, is markedly better if done before 9–12 months of age.

Another time to perform early surgery is when a deformity interferes with function and development. Examples include complete syndactyly between fingers of unequal length. The longer finger is tethered by the shorter one, preventing full extension of, especially, the proximal interphalangeal joint, causing permanent abnormal joint development.

Combined procedures. In patients with multiple deformities such as AMC, combining surgical procedures under one general anesthetic is advisable to reduce the number of operating room visits. In such a case, the upper limb surgeon would address the elbow and wrist on one side (carpectomy to improve wrist extension, and muscle transfer at the elbow to restore elbow flexion), while at the same sitting the lower limb surgeon would correct the clubfoot on the contralateral side. At the second session, the plaster changes can be done and the other wrist/elbow and foot can be operated on.

Comprehensive surgery. Congenital malformations seldom involve only one type of tissue. The abnormal anatomy is a combination of various tissues that are either underdeveloped, overdeveloped, malpositioned, or absent. Therefore, surgery must address all the different tissues at the same time (skin, tendons, ligaments, bone, joints, nerves, and vessels as necessary). For example, in thumb duplication all of the above forms part of the surgical procedure; simple amputation of one of the two thumbs is not always indicated. More complex procedures may need to be performed; for example, Bilhaut-Cloquet resection–fusion or reconstruction of joints and ligaments after amputation of the less "dominant" thumb.

In radial club hand deformities, skin flaps, bone osteotomies, joint reconstruction, and tendon transfers are essential to correct the malformation and rebalance the affected joints. Deforming tissue (such as short tendons) is often transferred to act as correcting structures.

Normal tissue versus scar tissue. Scar tissue consists of longitudinally arranged collagen fibers forming bands of hard tissue. Scars usually develop after an injury of some kind, which leads to inflammation, the healing process, and eventually scar formation. These collagen bands tend to shorten when they mature, causing contractures. These contractures can have deforming effects on tissues and joints. Also, scars do not grow as fast as normal, unscarred tissue. Surgical incisions should be designed and placed in such a position that the possible development of scar contractures is reduced to a minimum. Scar formation can be normal, hypertrophic, or

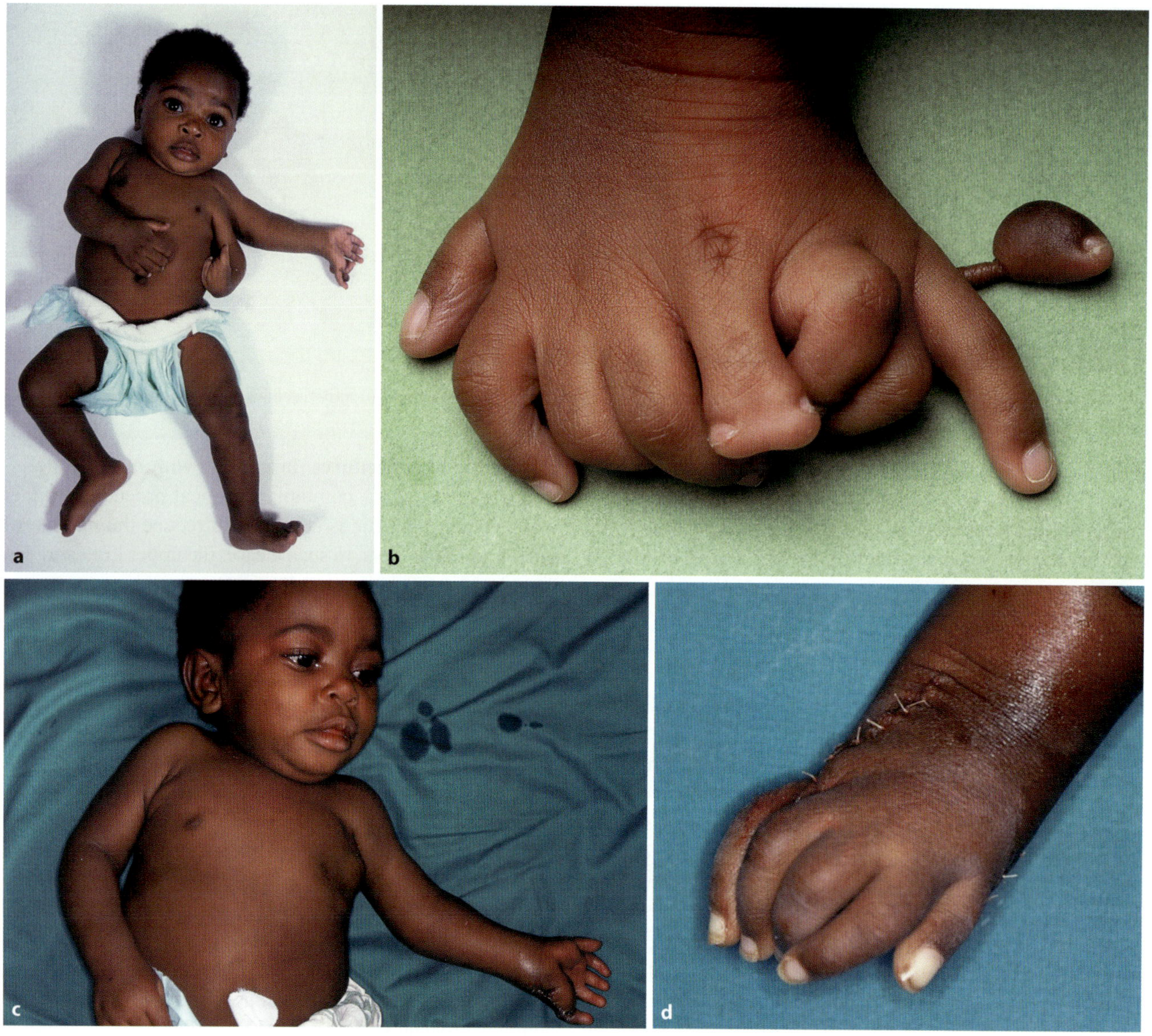

Fig. 4.2 **a** Upper limb triplication with radial dimelia and mirror-image duplication (**b**) on left side. The third arm was amputated, which included a scapula and brachial plexus (**c**). The 10 fingers were reduced to five (**d**)

very severe, with the formation of unsightly keloids. In some congenital conditions, particularly in patients with macrodactyly combined with syndactyly, severe scarring can occur to such an extent that the common measures to treat scars (scar massage, cortisone injection, pressure garments, silicone dressing) are ineffective. Methotrexate has been proposed to combat excessive scar formation.

Surgical Options

Surgical decision making involves a few basic options:

(1) **Reduction** of tissue, as in macrodactyly, polydactyly, "floating thumb," duplicated or excessive tissue (Fig. 4.2), and "mirror hand" (Fig. 4.3)

(2) **Addition** of tissue, as in skin grafts in syndactyly and camptodactyly, skin flaps used in creating a 1st web space (Figs. 4.4, 4.5), and pollicization of an index finger

(3) **Stabilization** of joints, as in arthrodesis of a dysplastic metacarpophalangeal joint of the thumb, ligament reconstruction after resection of a Wassel IV thumb polydactyly, and muscle transfer to stabilize the thumb (such as Huber abductor digiti minimi muscle opponensplasty)

(4) **Correction** of deformities, as in radial dysplasia, ulnar dysplasia, cleft hand, and congenital dislocated radial head (Figs. 4.4, 4.6)

(5) **Increased movement**, as in carpectomy and elbow arthrolysis in AMC, as well as muscle transfer for active elbow flexion; another example is tendon repositioning in distal arthrogryposis

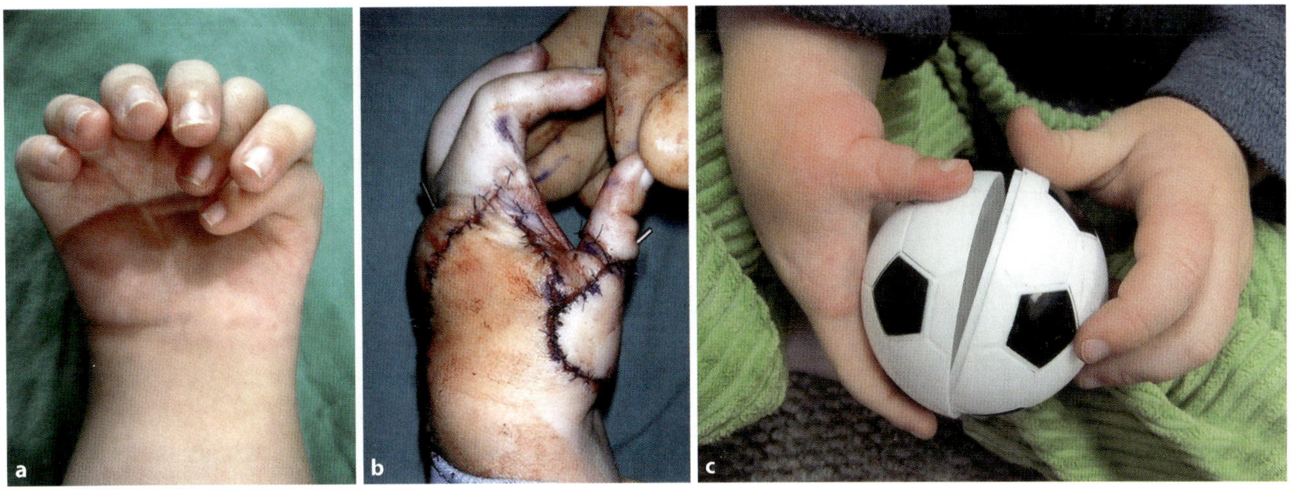

Fig. 4.3 **a** Mirror-image duplication with no radius but with two ulnas and seven symmetrical fingers. **b** Tendon transfers at the wrist, amputation of the excess fingers, and pollicization of the dominant radial finger were done. **c** The result is a functional hand with a thumb

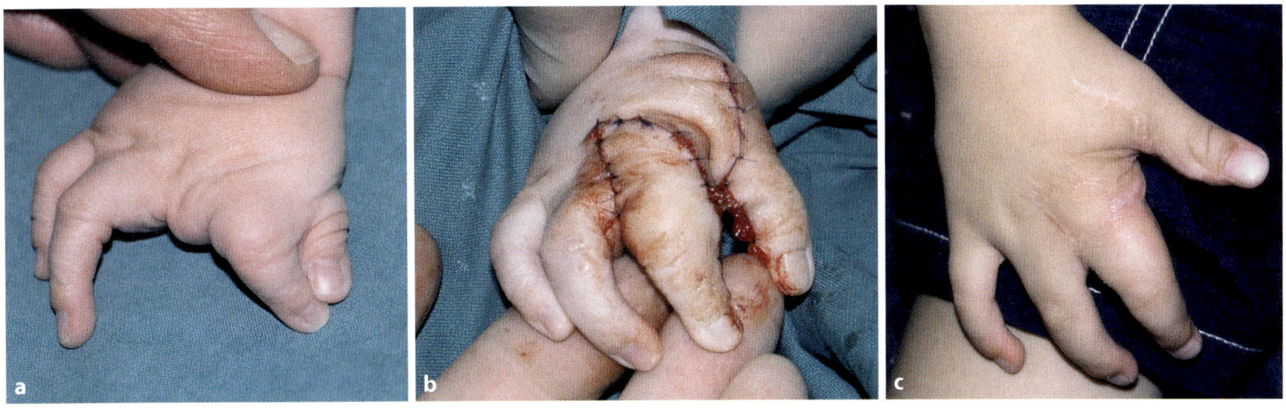

Fig. 4.4 "Cleft hand." **a** Preoperative appearance. **b** After reconstruction and transfer of the abnormal web to the 1st web area. **c** Result

(6) A **combination** of the above (Fig. 4.7)

The following examples illustrate these basic principles.

Polydactyly

This deformity can take many forms. The principle is to reduce the number of digits to five (four fingers and one thumb). It is important to make sure that the retained digits are the best in terms of function and appearance as well as the favored ones being used. A finger will not be used normally if the cortical representation is inadequate.

If the extra finger is on the ulnar side, the most common procedure if the finger is rudimentary is to tie a tight knot at the base, at birth. This will cause ischemia to the digit and result in dry gangrene, and the finger will fall off in due course. Alternatively, a formal amputation needs to be done to remove the extra finger.

Polydactyly of the thumb is more complex. The ulnar thumb is, fortunately, usually the "dominant" one of the two. The radial extra thumb is amputated, and the radial collateral ligament of the metacarpophalangeal joint, if involved, needs to be reconstructed. In some thumb polydactyly cases, two smaller but equal-size thumbs are found. These could be combined by resecting a wedge (one-half or one-third of each thumb) and then closing the remaining outer parts into one thumb.

Central polydactyly is even more complex. One commonly finds an extra metacarpal or phalanx, or both, that lies transverse. This bone needs to either be removed by resection (*reduction*) to correct the deformity (*correction*) or be used to augment incomplete digits (*addition*). The resected bone can be interposed in a short digit to lengthen the finger, or it can be turned from its abnormal transverse position into a normal position to support a digit lacking some of its bones. The web space then needs to be reconstructed. Various flaps have been designed to create a normal-looking web space.

The **triphalangeal thumb** often looks like a finger rather than a thumb because of the three phalanges. The length of the thumb needs to be reduced by either removing one of the extra phalanxes or, more commonly, performing arthrodesis to remove one of the joints, at the same time destroying (re-

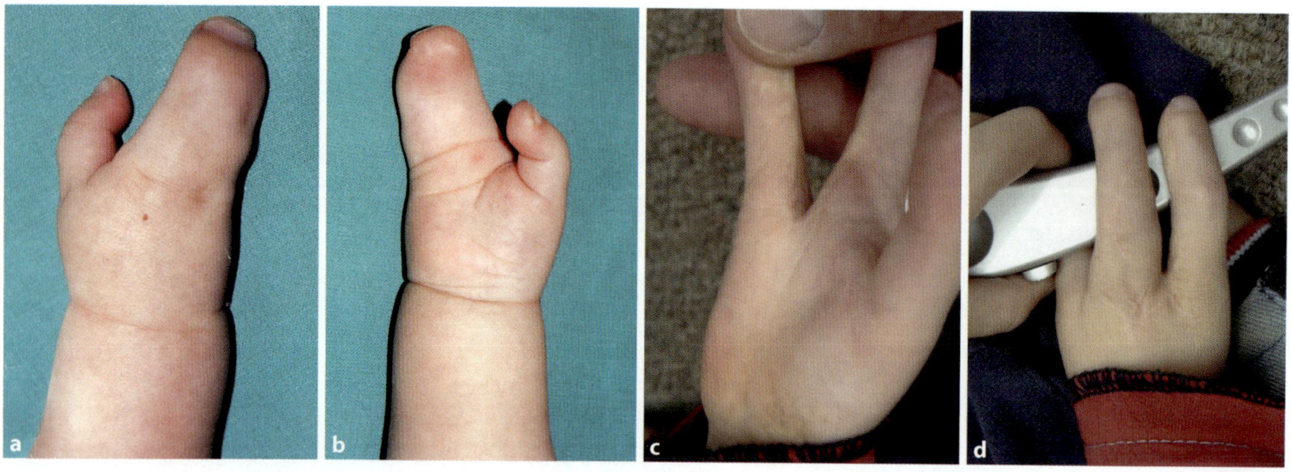

Fig. 4.5 Syndactyly of two fingers of unequal length, dorsal (**a**) and palmar (**b**) views. **c, d** Early release is indicated to allow free movement of the joints, which is essential for normal development

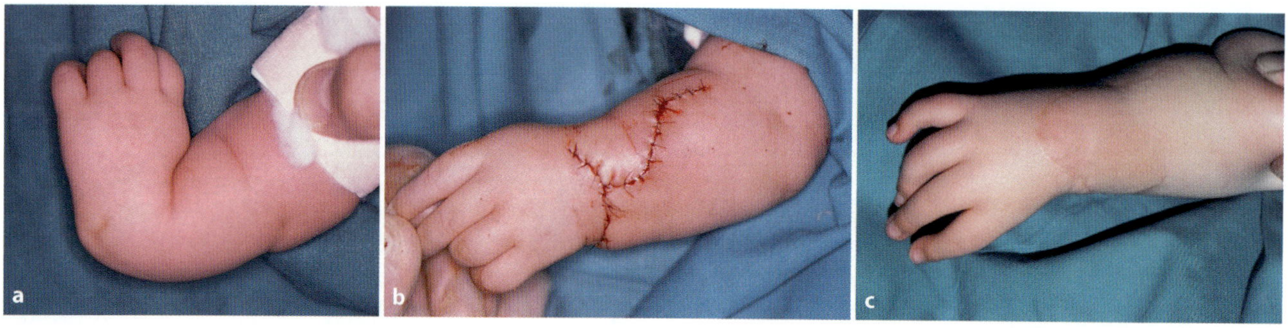

Fig. 4.6 **a** Radial dysplasia ("radial club hand"). **b** The curved ulna was osteotomized at multiple levels; the hand was repositioned on the distal end of the ulna; and tendon transfers were essential to rebalance the wrist. Note the dorsal skin flaps, which transfer excess ulnar skin to the radial side. **c** Result

moving) the near growth plate (physis), thus further reducing the potential growth of the thumb.

Syndactyly

Syndactyly, or "fused fingers," can be either simple (soft tissue fusion) or complex (bone and soft tissue fusion). The nails can also be fused in either of these two types. The treatment to release the fused fingers (*increased movement*) can take many forms. The timing of the separation should be around 6 months of age to prevent tethering of fingers of unequal length and to allow the digital joints to develop normally.

Cutaneous syndactyly. This is the simplest type and involves only the skin. However, in some cases the normal neurovascular separation, which occurs at the level of the normal web, may split more distally. When releasing the skin, it is imperative to start distally and carefully follow the digital nerve and artery proximally. If the spit occurs more distal than the intended new web, the nerve can be gently teased apart (split) to the desired level. The artery poses a challenging problem. In general, the dominant branch is kept, and the lesser artery is tied off. It is assumed that the digit with the lesser artery has a "dominant" arterial contribution on the contralateral side. For this reason, adjacent syndactylies are never released at the same time; if the contralateral artery is compromised in any way, the finger may be lost to ischemia. The second syndactyly release is usually only done after 6 months to encourage restoration of optimal blood supply to the finger.

Creation of an expandable web. Numerous flaps to create a "normal" web have been described. The author prefers to use a palmar flap, gives a more natural web and leaves minimal scarring on the dorsum of the hand.

Skin incision. A zig-zag skin incision between the fingers is made to reduce the chance of scar contracture. Closure of the skin may leave areas without skin. These areas are covered by a full-thickness skin graft, taken from, for instance, the volar aspect of the wrist.

Complex syndactyly. The above principles hold true for the complex type, which additionally involves fused phalanges. This bony fusion needs to be osteotomized. The raw bony area is smoothed down and trimmed to resemble a normal-looking phalanx, and it is usually covered with "bone wax" to prevent adhesions from forming on the raw bony surface.

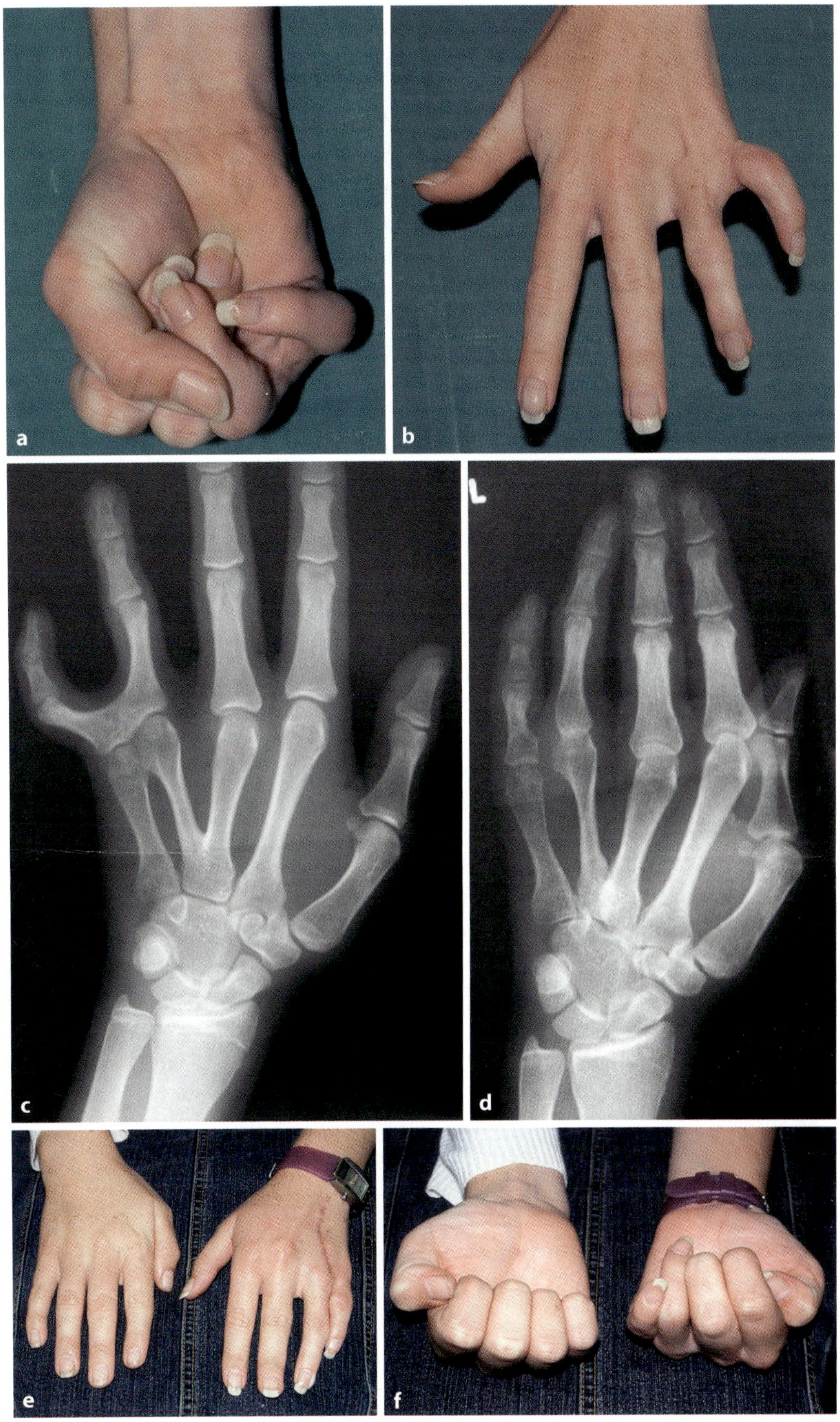

Fig. 4.7 Dysplastic metacarpals and phalanges resulting in unacceptable appearance and poor function. **a** Fist. **b** Open hand. **c** Corresponding radiograph shows multiple bony fusions involving the carpals, as well as metacarpals III/IV and proximal phalanges IV and V. **d** Postoperative radiograph. **e, f** Corrective osteotomies, joint and ligament reconstructions, and tendon transfers resulted in good function and a pleasing cosmetic appearance

Nail syndactyly. In many syndactylies the nails are also fused together. The aim is to create nail folds on the adjoining sides. Again, many flaps have been designed. The author prefers the one described by Buck-Gramcko, which uses long and relatively narrow fingertip skin flaps that are rotated to produce almost normal-looking nail folds after the nails have been separated.

Symbrachydactyly

Symbrachydactyly presents with various degrees of finger development, from missing fingers to short fingers. The treatment will depend on the potential functionality of the hand. The standard classification recognizes the following types:

Short finger type. The fingers are smaller than on the contralateral side, but they are fully functional and therefore need no surgical intervention

Oligodactylic type. The thumb and small finger are usually present, whereas the other fingers are small nubbins (rudimentary finger remnants). The digits are mostly unstable and small. Stability and elongation can be achieved by joint arthrodesis, free toe phalangeal interposition transfer, or distraction with an external distractor and subsequent bone interposition graft (*addition*). Any add-on, on-top bone graft may lengthen a digit initially, but almost all of the transplanted bone will be resorbed after a few years. The digits can also be relatively lengthened by deepening the web spaces between the fingers (*increased movement*). The useless nubbins are removed because they have no function and often tear, causing pain and infection (*reduction*).

Monodactylic type. Only the thumb is present, with or without any nubbins. The thumb may be unstable and short and can be treated the same way as above. To give the thumb a pillar to pinch against, free neurovascular toe transfer may be done to replace the absent small finger (*addition*).

Peromelic type. No digits are present, with or without nubbins. Presently the only possible option is a double toe-to-hand neurovascular transplant. Toe-to-hand transfer may have become routine in some centers, but this is a major procedure that leaves an undesirable cosmetic defect in the foot. It is remarkable to see how functional these children become without any fingers (Fig. 4.1), thus begging the question of whether major surgery such as toe-to-hand transfer is warranted.

Cleft Hand

The surgical principle is to transfer the large "cleft" in the hand to the 1st web space to increase the span between the thumb and index finger. This is done by variously described rotation flaps.

At the same time, the index finger metacarpal is transferred toward the ulnar side and fixed into the place of the absent middle finger metacarpal. This will then obliterate the "cleft" (*combination procedure*).

Absent or Hypoplastic Thumb

In cases of an absent thumb, or the rudimentary thumb ("floating thumb") often seen in radial club hand, the index finger (if fully functional) may be transferred to the thumb position (pollicization; *addition*). This involves removing the index finger metacarpal; preserving the nerves, arteries, and as many veins as possible; creating a 1st web with skin flaps; transferring muscles (for example, the 1st dorsal interosseus muscle becomes the new abductor pollicis brevis muscle, and the 1st palmar interosseus muscle becomes the new adductor pollicis muscle); transferring tendons (for example, the extensor digitorum communis tendon becomes the new abductor pollicis longus tendon); and shortening tendons (for instance, the extensor indicis proprius tendon becomes the new extensor pollicis longus tendon).

This "ultimate procedure" in hand surgery should be done only if the child has a well-functioning index finger and uses it to pick up objects. Another indication that this pollicization will be functional is a rotational "attitude" of the index finger, as if it wants to be a thumb.

These pollicized index fingers become stronger and sturdier as the child grows. Some are so realistic in function and appearance that only careful examination of the hand will reveal previous surgery.

Prostheses and Orthoses

Although very sophisticated artificial replacement parts for the hand and arm are available that perfectly mimic the appearance of the hand, they are very rarely worn permanently because these gadgets have no feeling (sensation) or proprioception. A common complaint is that "they are always in the way." Even a cosmetic device to disguise an abnormal-looking hand is often used only temporarily because the artificial hand has an obvious "dead" look. However, in some cases a device can be applied to assist function, such as a strapped-on pillar to act as a post against which a one-fingered hand can pick up and hold objects. In the lower limb, prostheses for defects are very successful. Stability to carry the body weight is of prime importance. As opposed to the upper limb, sensation and proprioception do not matter in the lower limb.

Conclusion

Consider surgical correction only if the outcome is certain to be better than the preoperative state. Some congenital deformities perform perfectly well regardless of appearance, contractures, or anatomical deficits. Be careful about amputating an "odd" finger, for instance; such a finger may be used as a very important support in ADL and work.

References

Green DP, Hotchkiss RN, Pederson WC, Wollfe SW (eds) (2005) Green's Operative Hand Surgery, 5th edn. vol. 2. Elsevier Churchill Livingstone, Philadelphia, pp 1375–1528 (part VI)

Gupta A, Kay SPJ, Scheker LR (eds) (2000) The Growing Hand. Mosby, London, p 1156

Part II

Disorders: Polydactyly Isolated

5 Preaxial Polydactyly

MIM 174400

Synonyms
Thumb polydactyly

Major Clinical Findings
Preaxial polydactyly (PPD) refers to additional digits on the radial/tibial side of the hand/foot. The simplest form involves duplication of one or more of the skeletal components of a biphalangeal thumb/hallux. This may range from mere broadening of the distal phalanx with slight bifurcation at the tip to full duplication including the metacarpals. It is a frequent form of polydactyly in certain populations. Thenar hypoplasia may be associated or may be the only minor sign.

Genetic Transmission
Autosomal dominant, autosomal recessive, reduced penetrance, polygenic.

Differential Diagnosis
PPD is a common finding in many limb malformation syndromes. Isolated PPD should be differentiated from PPD with triphalangeal thumb. In many conditions, PPD, hypoplasia of the thumb, and triphalangeal thumb can be part of a phenotypic spectrum and thus the manifestation of one condition.

References

Bingle GJ, Niswander JD (1975) Polydactyly in the American Indian. Am J Hum Genet 27:91–99

Graham JM Jr., Brown FE, Hall BD (1987) Thumb polydactyly as a part of the range of genetic expression for thenar hypoplasia. Clin Pediat 26:142–148

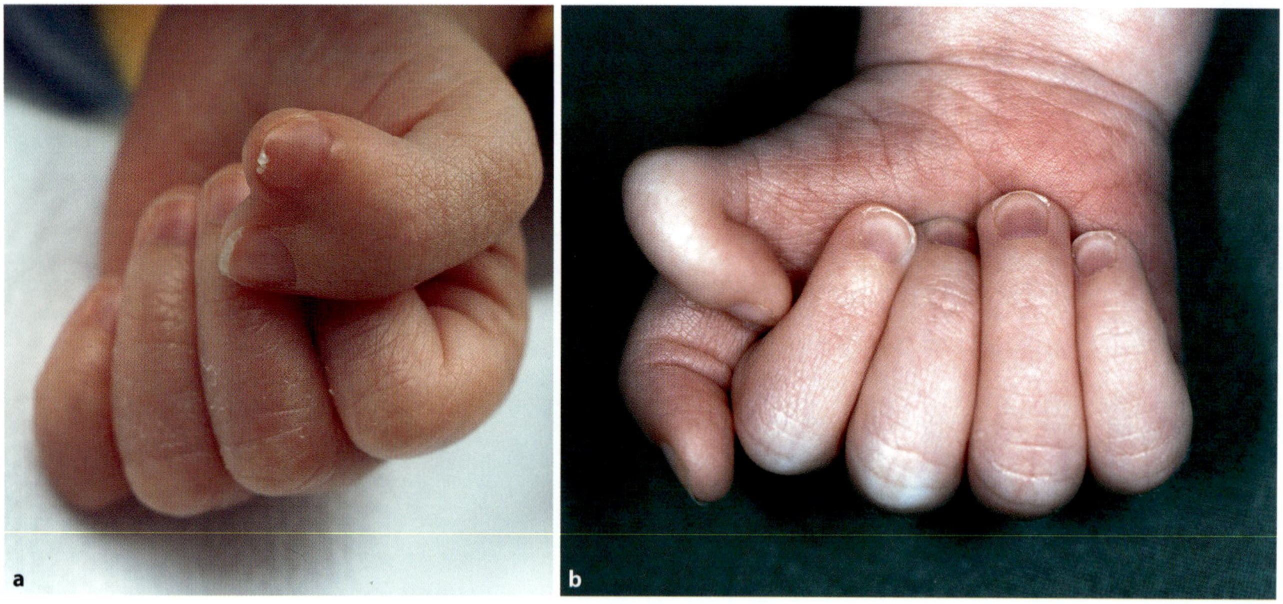

Fig. 5.1 **a** Partial duplication of thumb. **b** Preaxial polydactyly with nonfunctional thumb

S. Mundlos, D. Horn, *Limb Malformations*,
DOI 10.1007/978-3-540-95928-1_5, © Springer-Verlag Berlin Heidelberg 2014

Postaxial Polydactyly

MIM 174200

6

Major Clinical Findings

Postaxial polydactyly (PAP), defined as an additional digit on the ulnar side of the hand/foot, is a relatively frequent malformation. There are distinct population differences. PAP is about 10 times more frequent in blacks than in whites (~ 20 per 1,000 in blacks). PAP can be further subclassified into two types. In type A, a well-formed extra digit articulates with metacarpal V or VI. This type appears to be inherited in an autosomal dominant fashion with high penetrance. In type B, also known as pedunculated postminimi, a rudimentary, poorly developed extra finger is present. In this type, variable expressivity and reduced penetrance are common, suggesting more complex types of inheritance. However, both types have been observed in one family.

Genetic Transmission

Autosomal dominant, autosomal recessive, reduced penetrance, polygenic.

Differential Diagnosis

PAP is a common finding in many limb malformation syndromes. Among the chromosomal syndromes, PAP occurs almost exclusively with trisomy 13, in which about 75 % of cases show this feature.

Molecular Pathology

PAP has been linked to mutations in *GLI3*. Evidence exists for several other loci, in particular duplications on 13q21.

Remarks

PAP deserves a special place in the history of genetics. In 1756 Maupertuis (1698–1759), who was at the time director of the Academy of Sciences in Berlin and who has been considered a predecessor of Mendel, published the pedigree of Jacob Ruhe, a surgeon in Berlin. Ruhe, his mother, grandmother, and two sons (out of six children) had PAP. Maupertuis concluded that the disorder could be transmitted by either males or females, thereby refuting the preformationist theories generally accepted at the time.

References

Emery AEH (1988) Pierre Louis Moreau de Maupertuis (1698–1759). J Med Genet 25:561–564

Orioli IM (1995) Segregation distortion in the offspring of Afro-American fathers with postaxial polydactyly. Am J Hum Genet 56:1207–1211

Radhakrishna U, Bornholdt D, Scott HS, Patel UC, Rossier C, Engel H et al (1999) The phenotypic spectrum of GLI3 morphopathies includes autosomal dominant preaxial polydactyly type-IV and postaxial polydactyly type-A/B; no phenotype prediction from the position of GLI3 mutations. Am J Hum Genet 65:645–655

Scott-Emuakpor AB, Madueke EDN (1976) The study of genetic variation in Nigeria. II. The genetics of polydactyly. Hum Hered 26:198–202

Ventruto V, Theo G, Celona A, Fioretti G, Pagano L, Stabile M et al (1980) A and B postaxial polydactyly in two members of the same family. Clin Genet 18:342–347

S. Mundlos, D. Horn, *Limb Malformations*,
DOI 10.1007/978-3-540-95928-1_6, © Springer-Verlag Berlin Heidelberg 2014

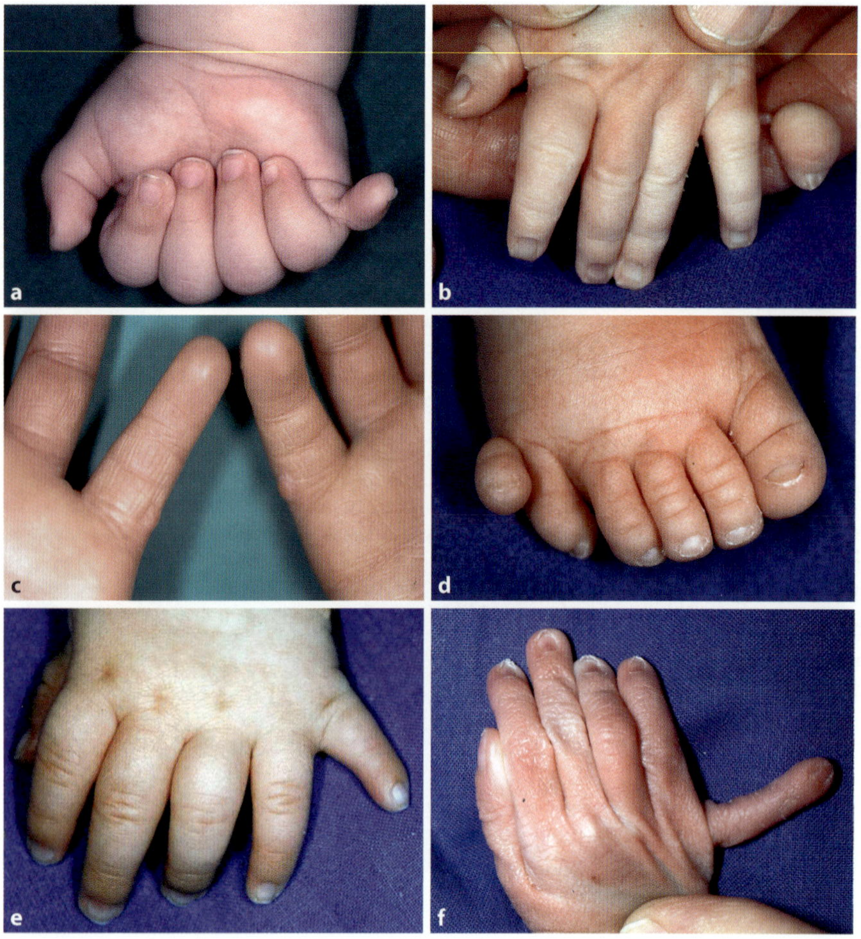

Fig. 6.1 a–d Postaxial polydactyly (PAP) type B. **a** Minimally developed extra finger (postminimus). **b** Extra finger is attached to finger V by a thin skin tag. **c** Small skin protrusion as a minimal version of PAP type B. **d** Postaxial polydactyly of foot. **e, f** Postaxial polydactyly type A. **e** Full extra digit with fusion at distal metacarpal V. **f** Fully developed extra digit with unstable articulation

Greig Cephalopolysyndactyly Syndrome

MIM 175700

7

Major Clinical Findings

Greig cephalopolysyndactyly syndrome is characterized by macrocephaly with a broad and prominent forehead and polysyndactyly. Typical findings in the limbs are postaxial polydactyly of the hands (postaxial polydactyly type B, such as a small digit attached by a skin tag to the medial border of digit V) and preaxial polydactyly of the feet (duplication of the hallux). However, other combinations are possible with variable expressivity. The thumbs/halluces may be broad or partially duplicated. Postaxial polydactyly may be complete or more subtle, consisting of only a vestigial digit along the lateral aspect of the limb. Syndactyly primarily affects fingers III and IV but is variable, ranging from near complete webbing to fully separated digits. In the feet, toes I–III are most often affected. Syndactyly is usually cutaneous but may also be osseous. Craniofacial anomalies include high forehead and frontal bossing, macrocephaly, hypertelorism, and downward slanting palpebral fissures. Learning disabilities and absence or hypoplasia of the corpus callosum may be present. Mild degrees of hydrocephalus occur at low frequency.

Genetic Transmission

Autosomal dominant.

Differential Diagnosis

There is substantial overlap with Pallister–Hall syndrome, which is also caused by mutations in *GLI3*. But in addition to synpolydactyly, Pallister–Hall syndrome features imperforate anus; epiglottic, laryngeal, and other airway abnormalities; and hypothalamic hamartoblastoma. Furthermore, the hand phenotype appears to be distinct, mainly featuring central (poly)syndactyly. The conditions are generally considered to be clinically distinct entities. Acrocallosal syndrome also shows similar features, and distinguishing between the two conditions may be difficult. Agenesis of the corpus callosum and large intracranial cysts may serve in differentiating acrocallosal syndrome from Greig cephalopolysyndactyly syndrome.

Molecular Pathology

Greig cephalopolysyndactyly syndrome is caused by loss of function mutations in *GLI3*. The GLI family of zinc finger transcription factors is related to the *Drosophila cubitus interruptus* (*ci*) gene. Ci was shown to be primarily located in the cytoplasm bound to a multiprotein complex consisting of the proteins fused, costal, suppressor of fused, and protein kinase A. Upon exposure to hedgehog signaling, ci is freed from the cytoplasmic complex and is transferred into the nucleus, where it activates target genes. Under another stimulus in the absence of hedgehog signal, ci is cleaved just after the zinc finger domain and is translocated into the nucleus. In this case, however, it serves as a suppressor. In vertebrates the system works in a very similar manner. In the limb, this results in a gradient of Gli3 across the anterior–posterior axis based on the asymmetry of hedgehog signal from the zone of polarizing activity. Gli3 activator is present close to the hedgehog signal, whereas gli3 repressor is more active distant to the signal and thus in the posterior part of the bud. In Greig cephalopolysyndactyly, one allele is inactivated, resulting in a reduction of both the repressive and the activating signals.

References

Ausems MG, Ippel PF, Renardel de Lavalette PA (1994) Greig cephalopolysyndactyly syndrome in a large family: a comparison of the clinical signs with those described in the literature. Clin Dysmorphol 3(1):21–30

Balk K, Biesecker LG (2008) The clinical atlas of Greig cephalopolysyndactyly syndrome. Am J Med Genet A 146A(5):548–557

Johnston JJ, Olivos-Glander I, Killoran C, Elson E, Turner JT, Peters KF et al (2005) Molecular and clinical analyses of Greig cephalopolysyndactyly and Pallister–Hall syndromes: robust phenotype prediction from the type and position of GLI3 mutations. Am J Hum Genet 76(4):609–622

Kalff-Suske M, Wild A, Topp J, Wessling M, Jacobsen EM, Bornholdt D et al (1999) Point mutations throughout the GLI3 gene cause Greig cephalopolysyndactyly syndrome. Hum Mol Genet 8(9):1769–1777

Litingtung Y, Dahn RD, Li Y, Fallon JF, Chiang C (2002) Shh and Gli3 are dispensable for limb skeleton formation but regulate digit number and identity. Nature 418(6901):979–983

Vortkamp A, Gessler M, Grzeschik KH (1991) GLI3 zinc-finger gene interrupted by translocations in Greig syndrome families. Nature 352(6335):539–540

S. Mundlos, D. Horn, *Limb Malformations*,
DOI 10.1007/978-3-540-95928-1_7,

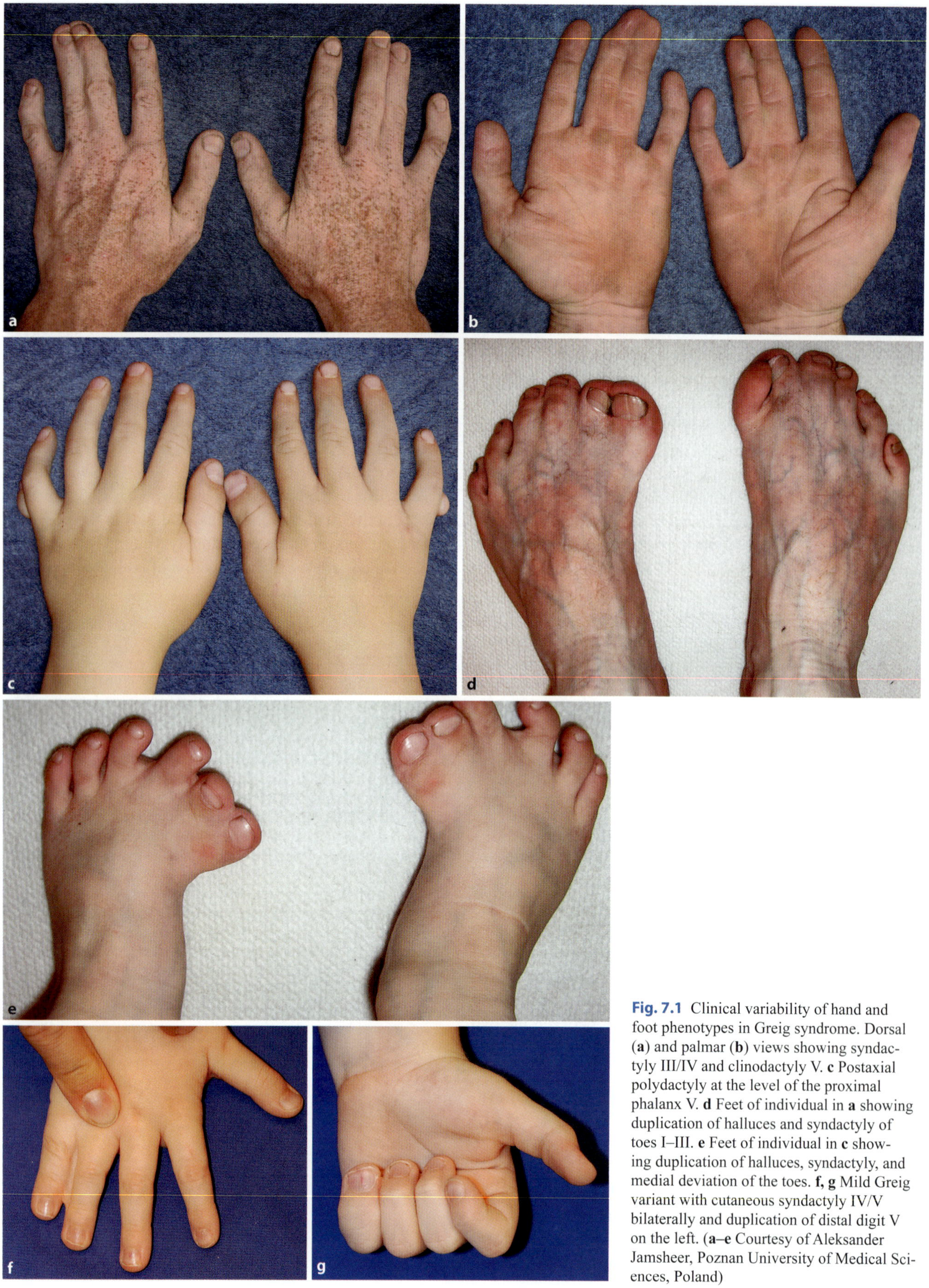

Fig. 7.1 Clinical variability of hand and foot phenotypes in Greig syndrome. Dorsal (**a**) and palmar (**b**) views showing syndactyly III/IV and clinodactyly V. **c** Postaxial polydactyly at the level of the proximal phalanx V. **d** Feet of individual in **a** showing duplication of halluces and syndactyly of toes I–III. **e** Feet of individual in **c** showing duplication of halluces, syndactyly, and medial deviation of the toes. **f, g** Mild Greig variant with cutaneous syndactyly IV/V bilaterally and duplication of distal digit V on the left. (**a–e** Courtesy of Aleksander Jamsheer, Poznan University of Medical Sciences, Poland)

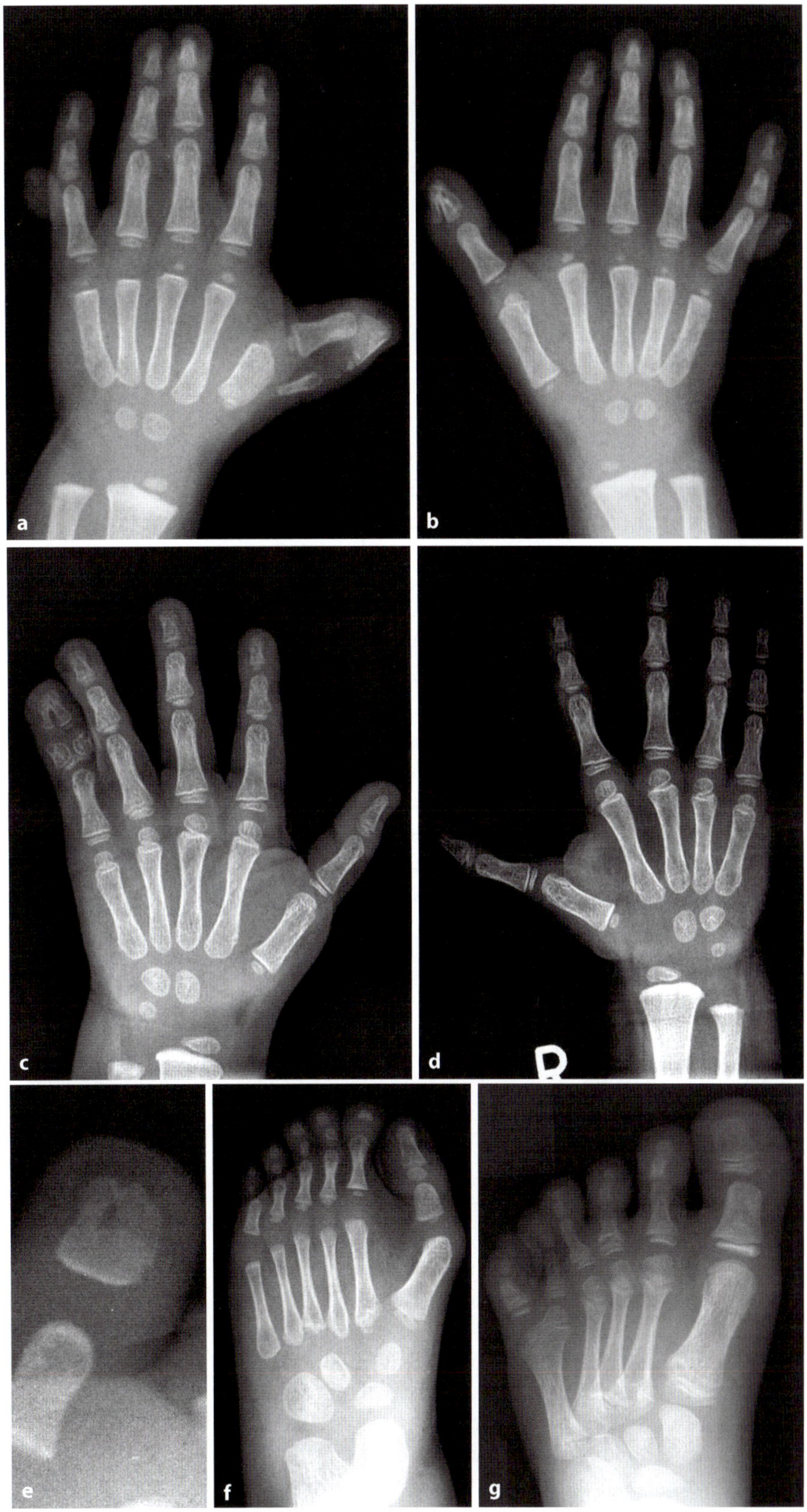

Fig. 7.2 Variability in radiographic findings. **a** Short and broad metacarpal I, partial duplication of thumb with broad, fused distal phalanx. Cutaneous syndactyly III–IV and postaxial polydactyly at the level of the proximal phalanx. **b** Other hand of same individual, showing postaxial polydactyly and distal duplication of the thumb as well as mild II/III and III/IV soft tissue syndactyly. **c, d** Corresponding radiographs for Fig. 7.1f, g: soft tissue syndactyly, otherwise normal radiograph on the right side. Duplication of middle and distal phalanges of digit V with distal bony fusion on the left. **e** Minimal phenotype with duplication of the distal phalanx. **f, g** Foot phenotypes: **f** Enlarged/angulated hallux, postaxial duplication, and hypoplastic middle/distal phalanges of digits I–VI. **g** Broad hallux and postaxial polydactyly arising from the distal portion of broad/fused metacarpal V

8 Triphalangeal Thumb-Polydactyly Syndrome

MIM 174500

Synonyms
Polydactyly of triphalangeal thumb
Preaxial polydactyly with triphalangeal thumb
Polydactyly of triphalangeal thumb

Major Clinical Findings
Triphalangeal thumb-polydactyly syndrome comprises variable forms of thumb malformation with or without syndactyly of other digits. The thumbs may be triphalangeal, duplicated, or both. The triphalangeal thumb consists of three phalanges instead of the normal two and may thus look like an index finger instead of a thumb. The phenotype is highly variable and can range from an apparently normal thumb with a small delta phalanx to a fully formed digit. Polydactyly may consist of two normal thumbs or triphalangeal thumbs or a combination. Without duplication, isolated triphalangeal thumbs are usually well formed and fully functional. Syndactyly may occur between the 3rd, 4th, and 5th fingers and is sometimes associated with bony synostosis in the distal phalanges of the same fingers. In the most severe cases, a complete syndactyly of all fingers is observed, giving a cuplike appearance to the hands.

Preaxial and postaxial polysyndactyly of the feet is a common feature. No other organ manifestations or dysmorphic features are present.

Genetic Transmission
Autosomal dominant.

Differential Diagnosis
Triphalangeal thumbs may occur in practically all conditions with abnormalities of the radial ray, such as Holt–Oram syndrome. Duane–radial ray syndrome, also known as Okihiro syndrome, shows similar anomalies of the upper limb but can be differentiated by the presence of ocular and renal anomalies and the absence of severe congenital heart defects. Preaxial polydactyly with or without triphalangeal thumb is a feature of Townes–Brooks syndrome. Lacrimo-auriculo-dento-digital (LADD) syndrome features duplication of the distal phalanx of the thumb, triphalangeal thumb, and syndactyly in addition to obstruction of the nasal lacrimal ducts and cup-shaped pinnas with mixed hearing deficit. Other conditions with triphalangeal thumb include Nager acrofacial dysostosis, VATER association, and Diamond–Blackfan anemia.

Molecular Pathology
Triphalangeal thumb is caused by missense mutations in the zone of polarizing activity regulatory sequence (ZRS), a regulatory element involved in *SHH* gene regulation in the limb. The identical phenotype was described in families with tandem duplications of the ZRS. As shown in mice, mutations, insertions, or deletions of the ZRS result in ectopic expression of Shh in the anterior margin of the limb bud in addition to its normal posterior expression domain. This "double dose" results in duplications, as previously shown by transplantation experiments of the zone of polarizing activity in chick embryos.

References

Furniss D, Lettice LA, Taylor IB, Critchley PS, Giele H, Hill RE et al (2008) A variant in the sonic hedgehog regulatory sequence (ZRS) is associated with triphalangeal thumb and deregulates expression in the developing limb. Hum Mol Genet 17(16):2417–2423

Hill RE (2007) How to make a zone of polarizing activity: insights into limb development via the abnormality preaxial polydactyly. Dev Growth Differ 49(6):439–448

Klopocki E, Ott CE, Benatar N, Ullmann R, Mundlos S, Lehmann K (2008) A microduplication of the long-range SHH limb regulator (ZRS) is associated with triphalangeal thumb-polysyndactyly syndrome. J Med Genet 45(6):370–375

Lettice LA, Heaney SJ, Purdie LA, Li L, de Beer P, Oostra BA et al (2003) A long-range Shh enhancer regulates expression in the developing limb and fin and is associated with preaxial polydactyly. Hum Mol Genet 12(14):1725–1735

Zguricas J, Snijders PJ, Hovius SE, Heutink P, Oostra BA, Lindhout D (1994) Phenotypic analysis of triphalangeal thumb and associated hand malformations. J Med Genet 31(6):462–467

S. Mundlos, D. Horn, *Limb Malformations*,
DOI 10.1007/978-3-540-95928-1_8, © Springer-Verlag Berlin Heidelberg 2014

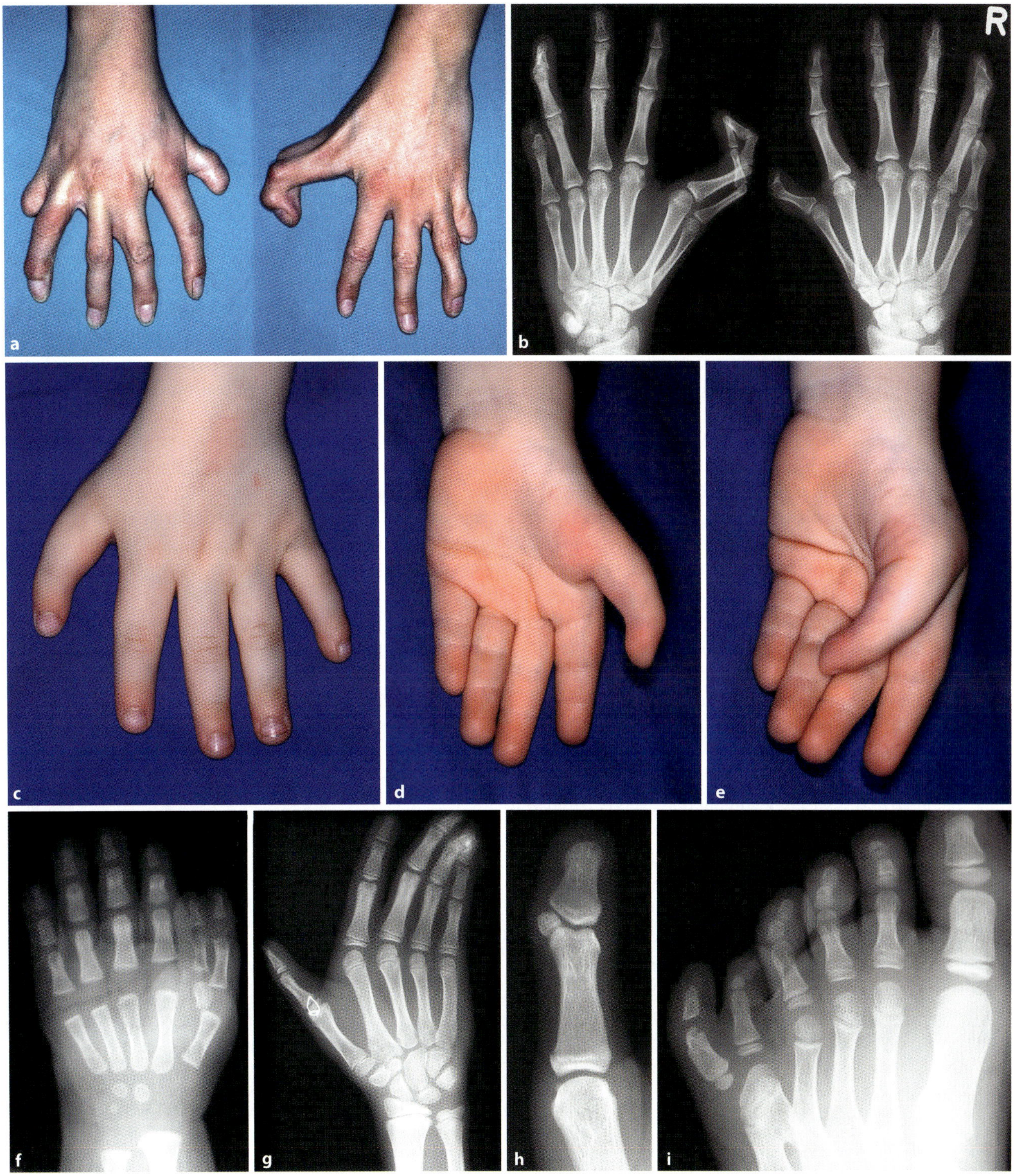

Fig. 8.1 **a** Dorsal view of hands with triphalangeal thumb. **b** Corresponding radiograph showing preaxial hypoplastic digit, a fingerlike triphalangeal thumb, and hypoplastic 5th digit on the right hand. On the left, preaxial duplication of the triphalangeal thumb, hypoplastic middle phalanx, and almost absent distal phalanx of digits IV and V, respectively. **c–e** Triphalangeal thumb, partially opposable. **f–i** Radiographic findings. **f** Duplication of thumb with smaller interaxial component. **g** Surgical correction of the thumb. Soft tissue syndactyly III–V with terminal bony fusion. **h** Small additional ossification center on the lateral side of the distal interphalangeal joint (mimicking a sesamoid bone) as minor manifestation of triphalangeal thumb. **i** Foot phenotype showing postaxial polysyndactyly

9 Synpolydactyly

MIM 186000

Synonyms
Syndactyly, type I
Synpolydactyly with foot anomalies

Major Clinical Findings
Synpolydactyly (SPD) is characterized by syndactyly of fingers III and IV with an additional finger in the syndactylous web. Syndactyly may also involve finger V. The supernumerary digit may branch from metacarpal IV, giving it a Y-shaped appearance, or from one of the proximal or middle phalanges, or it may appear as a completely duplicated digit. Syndactyly may be cutaneous or involve bony bridges between phalanges. Also seen are fusion of nails within the syndactyly, abnormal growth and/or bending of the finger in the web, agenesis and/or hypoplasia of phalanges in the web, and hypoplasia of the middle phalanges of finger V. Delta phalanx, true double epiphyses, pseudoepiphyses, and cone-shaped epiphyses occur. The feet most frequently show postaxial polydactyly with variable syndactyly of toes II–VI. The middle phalanges of toes II–V are often hypoplastic. Preaxial polydactyly is rare. Reduced penetrance is observed, even within one individual. The condition is phenotypically variable. Other manifestations include III/IV syndactyly without polydactyly (syndactyly type I, or zygodactyly), postaxial polydactyly without syndactyly, and distal hypoplasia of the digits.

Homozygous individuals have been described. In one person there was pentadactyly, syndactyly III/IV/V, and brachydactyly of all fingers, with the metacarpals having a round, carpal-like shape. In more severe cases, polydactyly together with complete syndactyly III–VI and duplication of the thumbs has been observed. Extreme brachydactyly has resulted in very short hands in which the index finger was the only separate, identifiable digit. Delayed bone age and osteopenia have been observed in all affected individuals. The feet are characterized by a relatively large great toe and severely hypoplastic syndactylous toes. Radiologically, the metatarsals and phalanges are largely fused and round. In another case, oligodactyly with only three toes was observed.

Genetic Transmission
Autosomal dominant.

Differential Diagnosis
Central polydactyly is also observed in Pallister–Hall syndrome.

Molecular Pathology
SPD was originally described in association with an expansion of the polyalanine stretch located in the N-terminal in *HOXD13*. Normally, this stretch codes for 15 alanines. In SPD an expansion of this repeat by an additional 7–14 alanines is present. The length of the repeat correlates with the severity and penetrance of the malformations. Individuals with a +7 alanine expansion show a high degree of interfamilial as well as interindividual variability and reduced penetrance. With increasing length of the repeat, variability is reduced, and penetrance increases. The expansion of the alanine repeat has been shown to result in Hoxd13 protein degradation and cytoplasmic aggregation. In a mouse model recapitulating SPD, mutant Hoxd13 was shown to induce extra digits by decreasing retinoic acid synthesis. This results in a reduction of chondrocytic differentiation in the interdigital mesenchyme and, as a consequence, formation of additional cartilage anlagen, which subsequently develops into additional digits. The polyalanine expansion appears to function as a combination of loss of function and gain of function. SPD-like phenotypes have also been observed with a variety of missense and frameshift mutations in *HOXD13*.

References

Albrecht AN, Kornak U, Böddrich A, Süring K, Robinson PN, Stiege AC et al (2004) A molecular pathogenesis for transcription factor associated poly-alanine tract expansions. Hum Mol Genet 13(20):2351–2359

Goodman FR (2002) Limb malformations and the human HOX genes. Am J Med Genet 112(3):256–265

Goodman FR, Mundlos S, Muragaki Y, Donnai D, Giovannucci-Uzielli ML, Lapi E et al (1997) Synpolydactyly phenotypes correlate with size of expansions in HOXD13 polyalanine tract. Proc Natl Acad Sci U S A 94(14):7458–7463

Kuss P, Villavicencio-Lorini P, Witte F, Klose J, Albrecht AN, Seemann P et al (2009) Mutant Hoxd13 induces extra digits in a mouse model of synpolydactyly directly and by decreasing retinoic acid synthesis. J Clin Invest 119(1):146–156

Muragaki Y, Mundlos S, Upton J, Olsen BR (1996) Altered growth and branching patterns in synpolydactyly caused by mutations in HOXD13. Science 272(5261):548–551

Yucel A, Kuru I, Bozan ME, Acar M, Solak M (2005) Radiographic evaluation and unusual bone formations in different genetic patterns in synpolydactyly. Skeletal Radiol 34(8):468–476

S. Mundlos, D. Horn, *Limb Malformations*,
DOI 10.1007/978-3-540-95928-1_9,

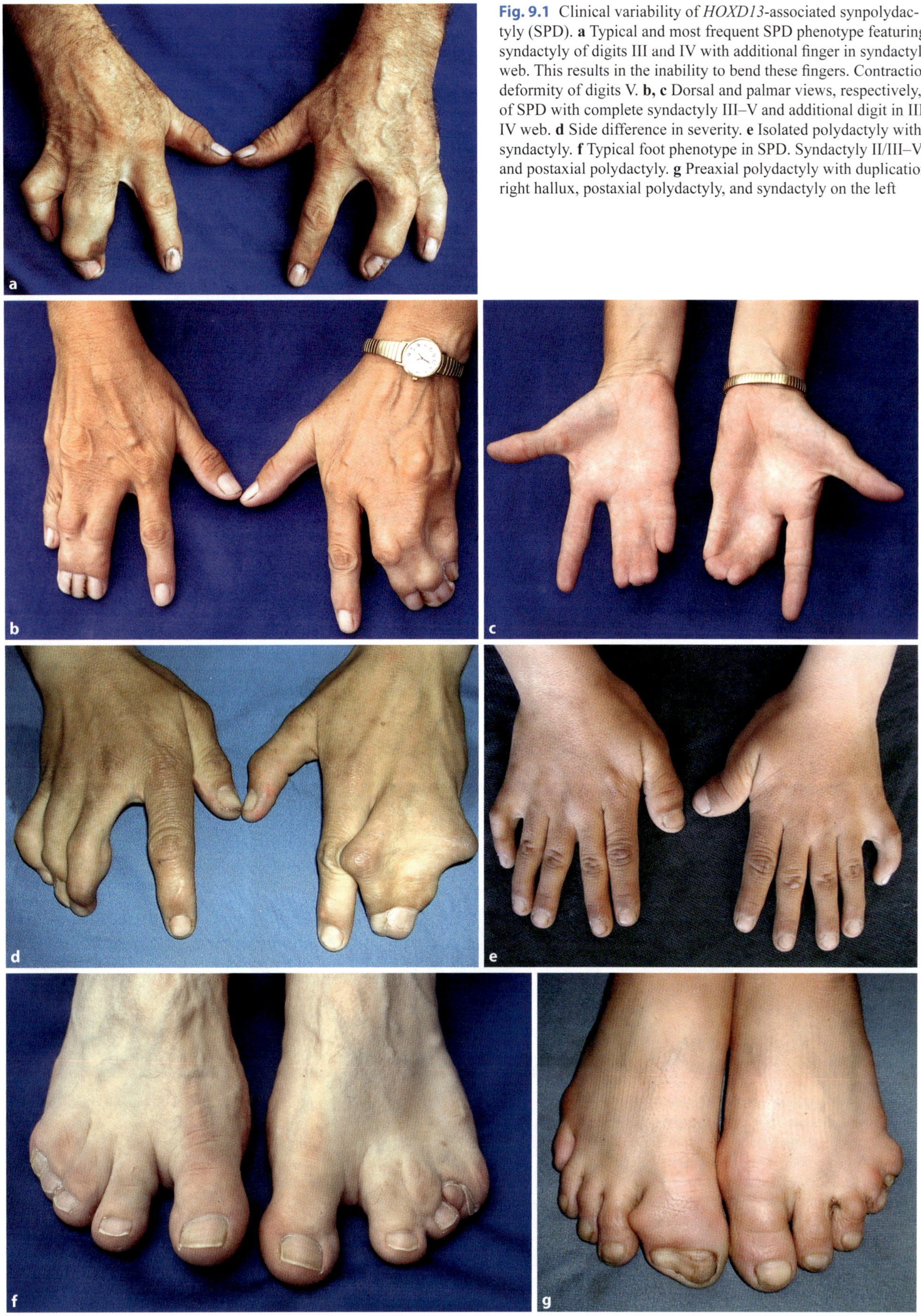

Fig. 9.1 Clinical variability of *HOXD13*-associated synpolydactyly (SPD). **a** Typical and most frequent SPD phenotype featuring syndactyly of digits III and IV with additional finger in syndactylous web. This results in the inability to bend these fingers. Contraction deformity of digits V. **b, c** Dorsal and palmar views, respectively, of SPD with complete syndactyly III–V and additional digit in III/IV web. **d** Side difference in severity. **e** Isolated polydactyly without syndactyly. **f** Typical foot phenotype in SPD. Syndactyly II/III–V and postaxial polydactyly. **g** Preaxial polydactyly with duplication of right hallux, postaxial polydactyly, and syndactyly on the left

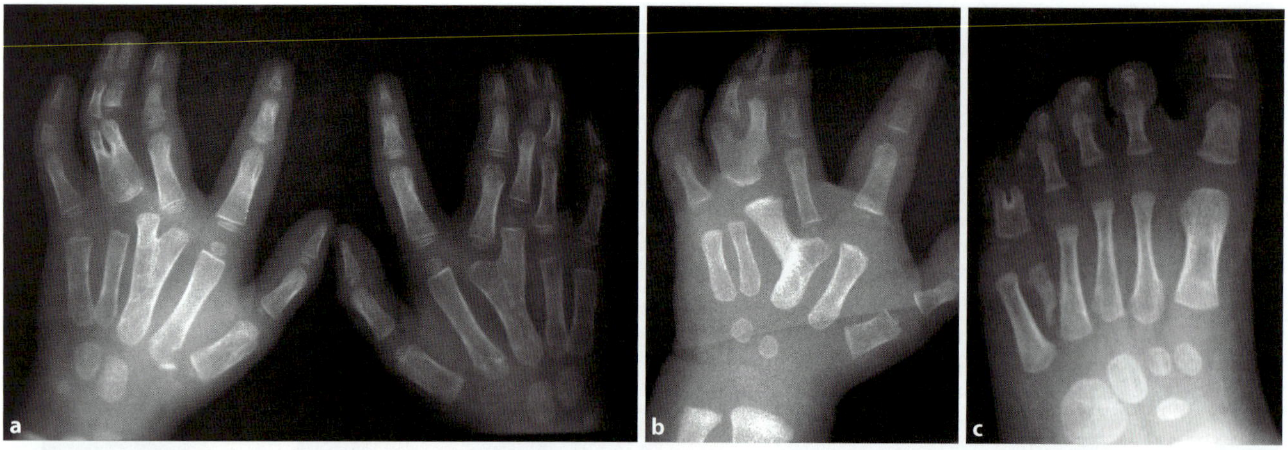

Fig. 9.2 Radiographic findings in *HOXD13*-associated synpolydactyly (SPD). **a** Radiograph corresponding to Fig. 9.1a showing bifurcation of metacarpal III. An additional digit arises from the ulnar side. Partial fusion of phalanges with phalanges of digit IV. Hypoplasia/dysplasia of middle phalanges of digits V. **b** Complex interaxial synpolydactyly. Branching of short 3rd metacarpal producing interaxial duplication of the proximal phalanx of digit IV with separate fusion and clinodactyly of digit V. Soft tissue syndactyly of III–IV/V. **c** SPD foot phenotype showing a small additional metatarsal between digits IV and V and proximal phalangeal synostosis. Soft tissue syndactyly involving all digits

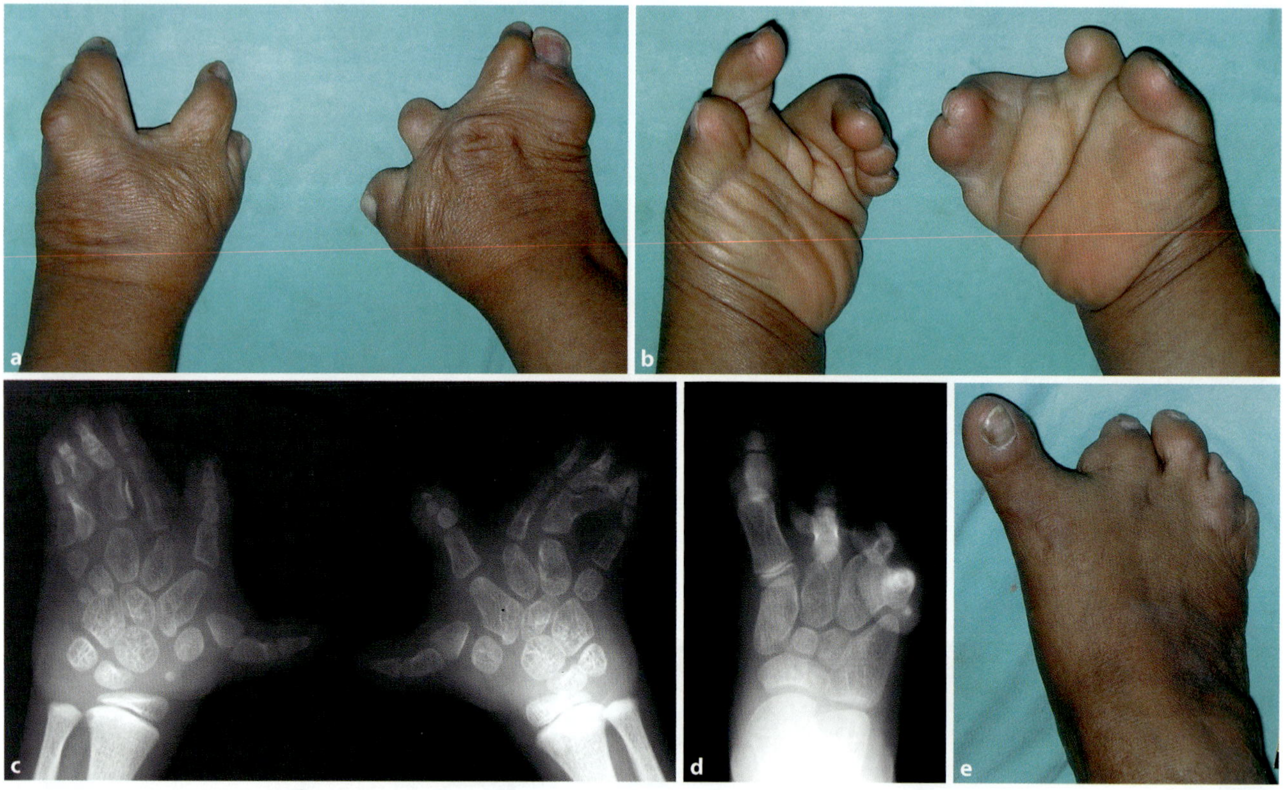

Fig. 9.3 Homozygous *HOXD13* mutation. **a, b** Dorsal and palmar views, respectively, showing very small hands; fusion of digits III–V with nail fusion; broad, very short thumb; and small, rudimentary digit II. **c** Corresponding radiograph. Enlarged carpal bones, hypoplastic/dysplastic metacarpals with carpal-like configurations (including thumbs), delta phalanx of the 4th proximal phalanx, duplication of digit V, and partial fusion with digit IV (left with bony synostosis). Soft tissue syndactyly III–V, right with distal bony fusion. **d** Foot of same individual. **e** Corresponding radiograph showing similar digital hypoplasia with some sparing of the great toe, shortening as well as absence of some metatarsals and phalanges, and tarsal-metatarsal fusion

Laurin–Sandrow Syndrome

MIM 135750

10

Synonyms
Sandrow syndrome
Mirror hands and feet with nasal defects
Tetramelic mirror-image polydactyly
Fibula and ulna, duplication of, with absence of tibia and radius

Includes
Mirror-Image Polydactyly

Major Clinical Findings
Mirror-image polydactyly refers to a duplication of all or most digits along a central axis (mirrored). In these cases, the thumb/hallux is in the center of the hand/foot, and the digits V are at the lateral sides. This may occur either as a complete duplication with 10 or more digits or as a partial duplication with several additional digits. Mirror-image polydactyly can occur as an isolated trait (in this case usually unilateral) or as part of a syndrome. Laurin–Sandrow syndrome has been described as the combination of mirror polysyndactyly of hands and feet together with facial anomalies involving the nasal alae and columella. Preaxial and postaxial polydactyly and mirror-image polydactyly are present to variable degrees, with up to 12 digits on one extremity. Malformation and synostosis of tarsal bones are seen. The fibula and tibia as well as the ulna and radius may appear alike, suggesting a duplication of one of the stylopod bones. Mental retardation may be present.

Differential Diagnosis
Laurin–Sandrow syndrome shows overlap with Haas-type syndactyly. Both conditions have similar cup-shaped syndactyly with polydactyly of the hands. In Haas-type syndactyly, however, the feet are relatively normal.

Genetic Transmission
Autosomal dominant.

Molecular Pathology
Laurin–Sandrow can be caused by small duplications encompassing the SHH regulating region, the zone of polarizing activity regulatory sequence (ZRS). The condition is thus allelic with triphalangeal thumb polydactyly syndrome, mesomelic dysplasia Werner type, and Haas syndactyly. Mirror-image duplications have been described in several mouse models such as the Doublefoot mouse and the Gli3 knockout mouse. The Doublefoot phenotype is caused by a misexpression of Indian hedgehog (Ihh) at the anterior margin of the limb bud in addition to the regular posterior expression of Shh in the zone of polarizing activity. Gli3 is the downstream effector of Shh, creating a gradient of repressor and activator activity across the limb bud.

References

Babbs C, Furniss D, Morriss-Kay GM, Wilkie AO (2008) Polydactyly in the mouse mutant Doublefoot involves altered Gli3 processing and is caused by a large deletion in cis to Indian hedgehog. Mech Dev 125(5–6):517–526

Kjaer KW, Hansen L, Eiberg H, Christensen KS, Opitz JM, Tommerup N (2005) Male-to-male transmission in Laurin–Sandrow syndrome and exclusion of RARB and RARG. Am J Med Genet A 137(2):148–152

Lohan S, Spielmann M, Doelken SC, Muhammad F, Baig SM, Wajid M et al (2014) Microduplications encompassing the Sonic Hedgehog limb enhancer ZRS are associated with Haas type polysyndactyly and Laurin–Sandrow syndrome. Clin Genet 2014 Oct;86(4):318–25

Mariño-Enríquez A, Lapunzina P, Omeñaca F, Morales C, Rodríguez JI (2008) Laurin–Sandrow syndrome: review and redefinition. Am J Med Genet A 146A(19):2557–2565

S. Mundlos, D. Horn, *Limb Malformations*,
DOI 10.1007/978-3-540-95928-1_10, © Springer-Verlag Berlin Heidelberg 2014

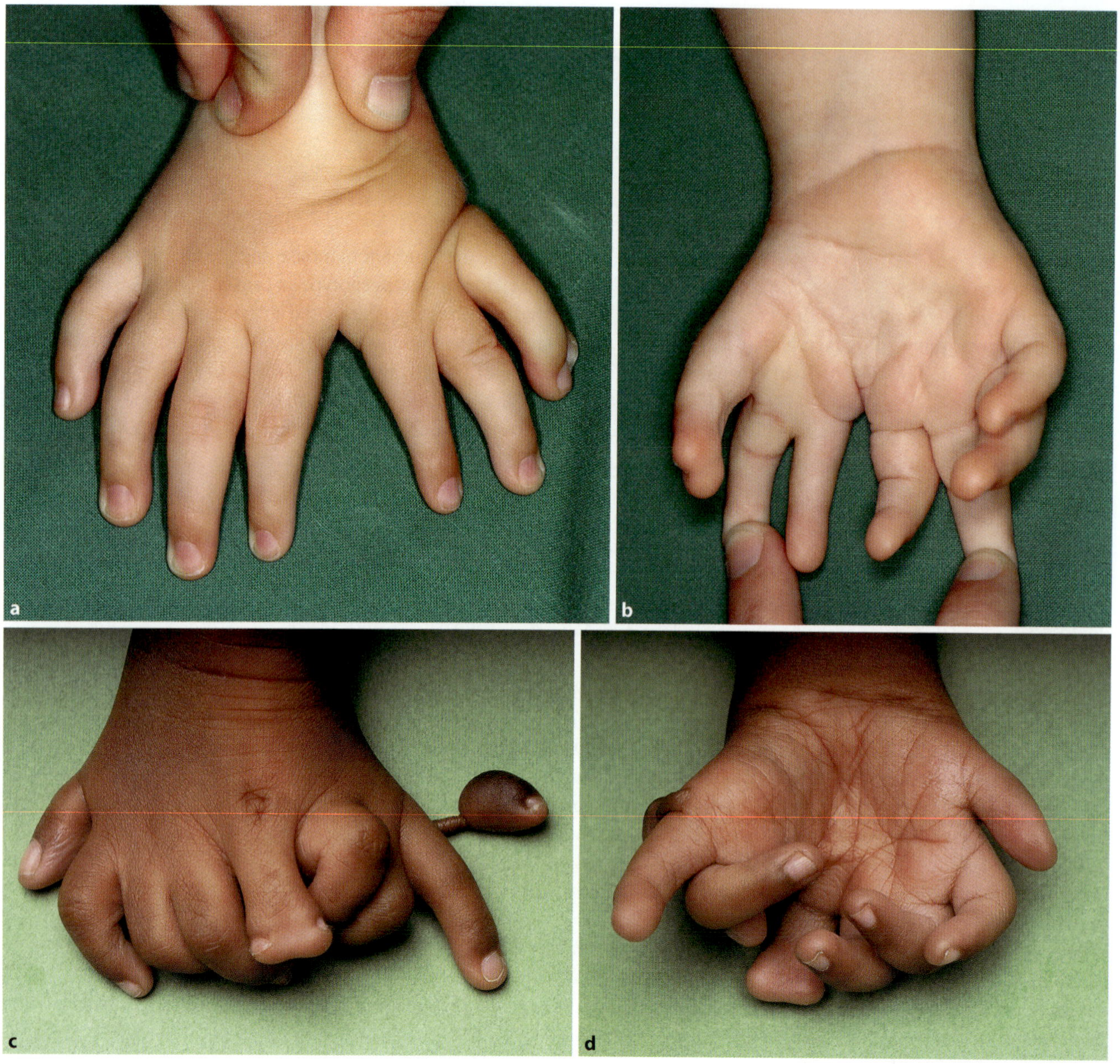

Fig. 10.1 Isolated mirror-image polydactyly. **a** Eight-fingered polydactyly with central cleft. The middle cleft is likely to correspond to the missing thumb(s). **b** Palmar view of same hand. (Courtesy of Rolf Habenicht, Kinderkrankenhaus Wilhelmstift, Hamburg, Germany.) **c, d** Complex 10-fingered mirror-image polydactyly in dorsal (**c**) and palmar (**d**) views. The duplicated digit in the middle represents two fused thumbs

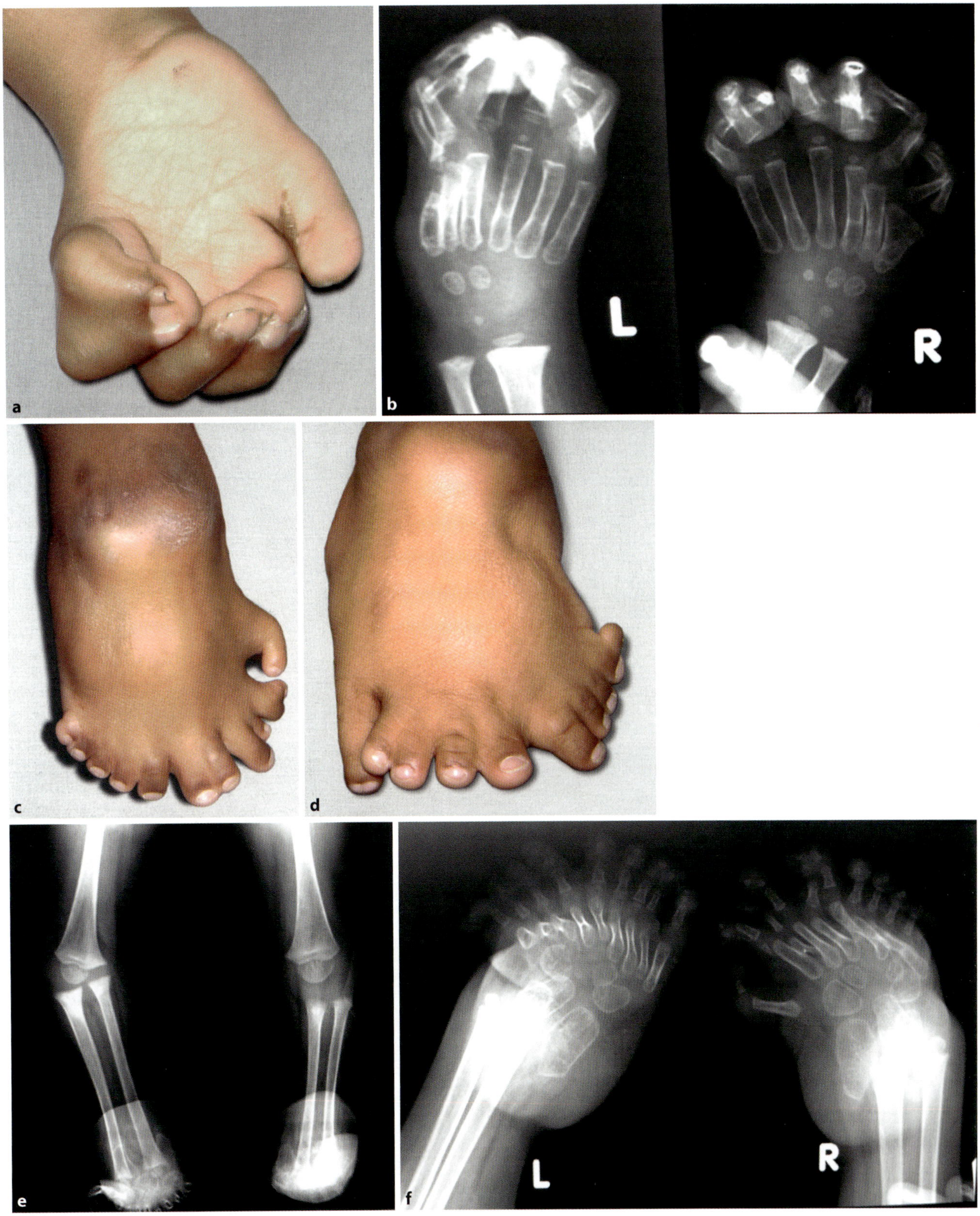

Fig. 10.2 Laurin–Sandrow syndrome. **a** Hand with complete synpolydactyly. **b** Corresponding radiograph of both hands showing six metacarpals and fusion of fingers (mirror image-like). **c, d** Feet of same individual with 12 and 11 toes. The most central toes appear as the largest, resulting in a mirror-image appearance. **e** Radiograph of the lower limb shows two bones of similar size (fibula-like) representing the tibia/fibula and mimicking the radius/ulna. **f** Radiograph of feet showing massive polydactyly and crowded/twisted metatarsals. (Courtesy of Siddram Patil, Narayana Hrudayalaya Hospitals, Bangalore, India)

Part III

Disorders: Polydactyly Associated

11 Ellis–Van Creveld Syndrome

MIM 225500

Synonyms
Chondroectodermal dysplasia

Major Clinical Findings
Ellis–van Creveld syndrome (EVC) comprises the combination of short stature, postaxial polydactyly, abnormal dentition, and cardiac defects. The short stature is of prenatal onset and is disproportionate, with progressive acromesomelic shortening of the limbs. The nails are hypoplastic. Radiologically there is postaxial polydactyly with or without fusion of the metacarpals/phalanges. The tubular bones are short and show distalward shortening with short and broad middle phalanges as well as hypoplastic distal phalanges. Also seen are cone-shaped epiphyses of the middle and distal phalanges; fusion of the capitate and hamate bones and extra carpal bones; a narrow thorax with short, poorly developed ribs; hypoplasia of the upper lateral tibia with knock-knee; and dysplasia of the pelvis with low iliac wings and spurlike downward projections at the medial and lateral aspects of the acetabulae.

Several abnormalities of the teeth and mouth may be present, including a short upper lip connected by multiple frenulae to the alveolar ridge, neonatal teeth, partial anodontia, enamel hypoplasia, and malocclusion. Cardiac defects are found in up to 50 % of patients, predominantly atrial septal defects and single atrium.

Occasional Findings
Intellectual disability, renal anomalies, fine hair, cryptorchidism, epispadias.

Genetic Transmission
Autosomal recessive.

Differential Diagnosis
Polydactyly, narrow thorax, and pelvic dysplasia are also observed in asphyxiating thoracic dysplasia (Jeune syndrome). Polydactyly is rare in Jeune syndrome but is a constant finding in EVC. In addition, the presence of frenulae, dysplastic nails, and congenital heart disease differentiate the two conditions. EVC and McKusick–Kaufman syndromes are clinically similar; both are recessively inherited disorders with postaxial polydactyly and a distinct congenital heart defect. Distinguishing characteristics are the osteochondrodysplasia and ectodermal anomalies in EVC and the hydrometrocolpos due to imperforate hymen or vaginal atresia in McKusick–Kaufman syndrome. McKusick–Kaufman syndrome is allelic to Bardet–Biedl syndrome type 6.

Molecular Pathology
Ellis–van Creveld syndrome can be caused by mutations in the *EVC* gene or by mutations in a nonhomologous gene, *EVC2* (LBN). Both genes are located in a head-to-head configuration. The clinical features appear to be identical regardless of whether the disorder is caused by mutation in *EVC* or in *EVC2*.

References

Ellis RWB, van Creveld S (1940) A syndrome characterized by ectodermal dysplasia, polydactyly, chondro-dysplasia and congenital morbus cordis: report of three cases. Arch Dis Child 15:65–84

McKusick VA (2000) Ellis–van Creveld syndrome and the Amish. Nature Genet 24:203–204

Ruiz-Perez VL, Ide SE, Strom TM, Lorenz B, Wilson D, Woods K et al (2000) Mutations in a new gene in Ellis–van Creveld syndrome and Weyers acrodental dysostosis. Nature Genet 24:283–286

Ruiz-Perez VL, Tompson SWJ, Blair HJ, Espinoza-Valdez C, Lapunzina P, Silva EO et al (2003) Mutations in two nonhomologous genes in a head-to-head configuration cause Ellis–van Creveld syndrome. Am J Hum Genet 72:728–732

S. Mundlos, D. Horn, *Limb Malformations*,
DOI 10.1007/978-3-540-95928-1_11, © Springer-Verlag Berlin Heidelberg 2014

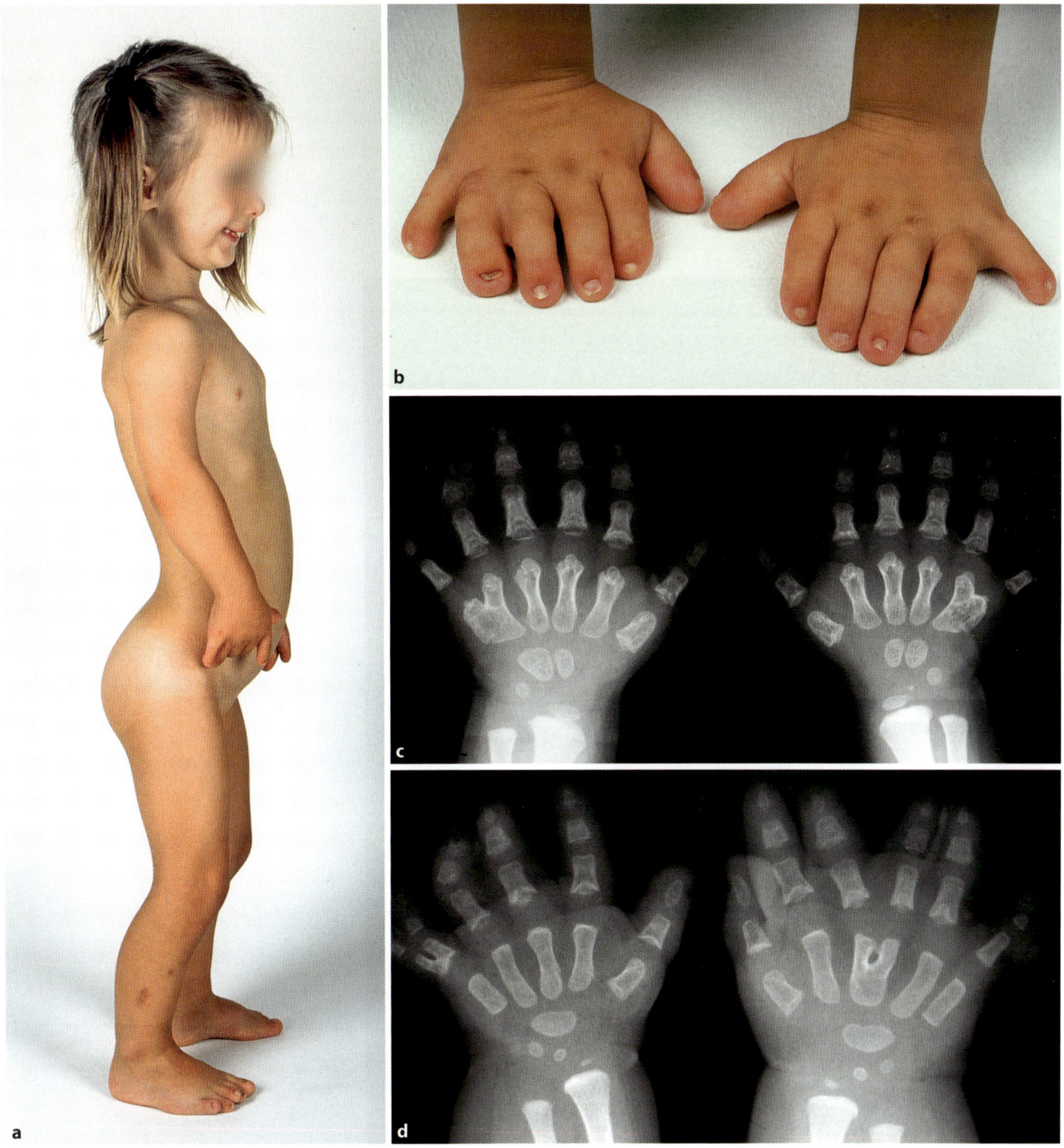

Fig. 11.1 **a** An 8-year-old girl with Ellis–van Creveld syndrome. Note short stature with a relatively long trunk, hyperlordosis, and inability to completely straighten her knees. **b** Hands of the same individual. Note postaxial polydactyly, short digits with distal hypoplasia, and dysplastic nails. **c** Corresponding radiograph. Note postaxial polydactyly with fusion of an additional metacarpal with metacarpal V, hypoplasia of the distal phalanges, cone-shaped epiphyses, duplication of the middle and distal phalanges of digit V on the left, and too close approximation of the carpal bones, suggesting the beginning of carpal fusion. **d** Variability in hand phenotypes. Radiographs show postaxial polydactyly with fusion of the proximal phalanges, hypoplasia of the distal phalanges, cone-shaped epiphyses, and os centralis on the left. The right hand shows fusion of metacarpals III and IV, postaxial polydactyly with additional postminimus, and fusion of carpal bones.

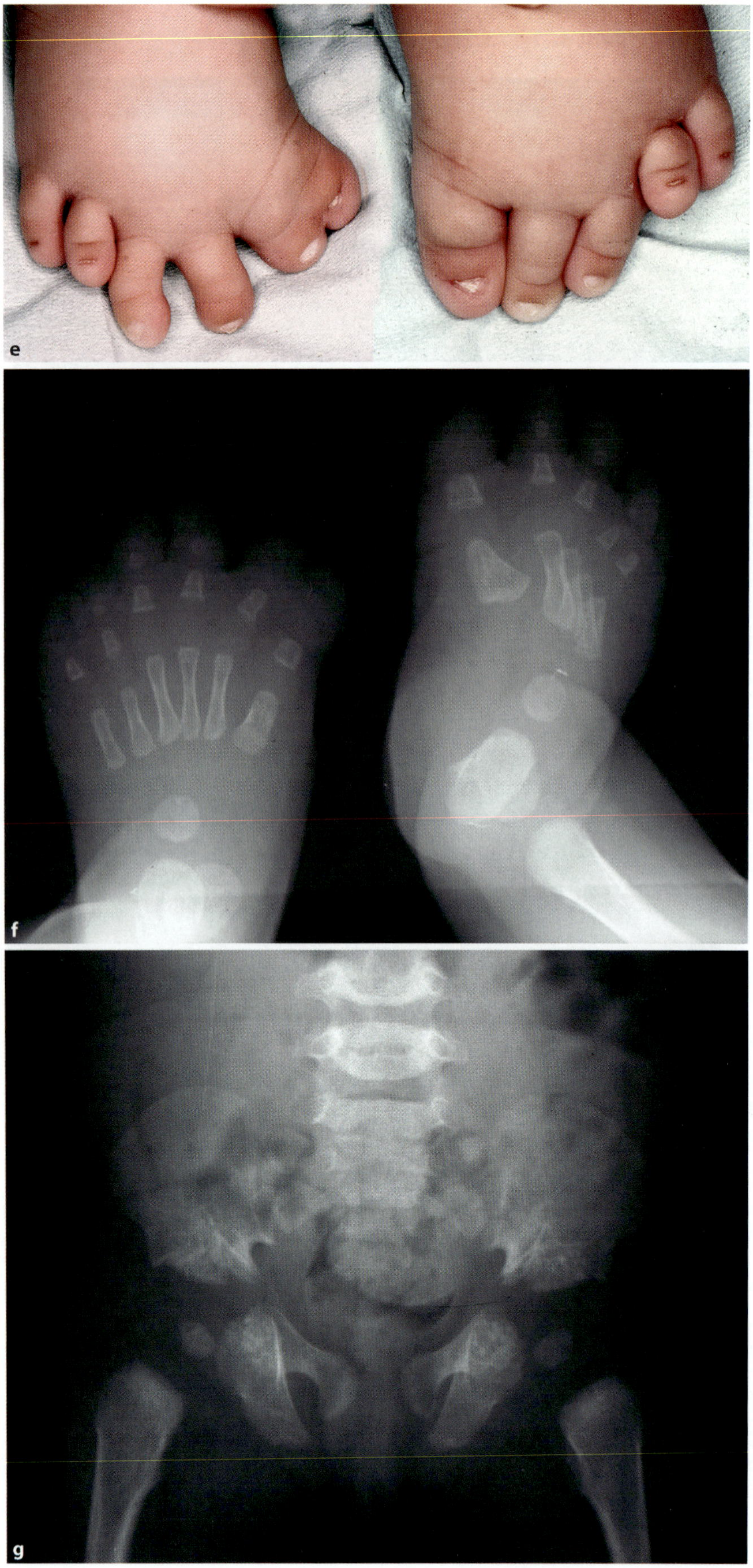

Fig. 11.1 (*continued*) **e** Feet showing preaxial polydactyly on the right and dysplasia of nails. **f** Corresponding radiograph showing preaxial polydactyly on the left; a broad, triangular metatarsal I on the right; small phalanges; and distal unossified phalanges. **g** Radiograph of pelvis showing narrow sacrosciatic notches, trident acetabulae, wide growth plates, and small epiphyses

Short Rib-Polydactyly Syndromes

12

Includes
Short Rib-Polydactyly Syndrome Type I, Saldino–Noonan Type
MIM 263530
Short Rib-Polydactyly Syndrome Type II, Majewski Type
MIM 263520
Short Rib-Polydactyly Syndrome Type III, Verma–Naumoff Type
MIM 263510
Short Rib-Polydactyly Syndrome Type IV, Beemer–Langer Type
MIM 269860

Major Clinical Findings
Short rib-polydactyly syndrome (SRPS) describes a group of skeletal dysplasias characterized by a hypoplastic thorax, short ribs, short limbs, polydactyly, and visceral abnormalities. They present at birth with severe short-limbed dwarfism, narrow thorax, protuberant abdomen, and variable degrees of hydrops. Malformations of the limbs include postaxial (rarely, preaxial and postaxial) polydactyly and brachydactyly. Multiple internal malformations are usually present, including abnormalities of the anus, renal hypoplasia, renal cysts, genital anomalies, Dandy–Walker malformation, bifid tongue, cleft upper lip, and esophageal atresia. Most patients die of respiratory insufficiency. Major radiological findings include very short, horizontally oriented ribs; very short tubular bones of the extremities with a pointed or ragged appearance (types I and III) or rounded ends (types II and IV); incomplete ossification of tubular bones; and small iliac bones with flattened acetabular roofs.

Genetic Transmission
Autosomal recessive.

Differential Diagnosis
Five types have been distinguished: SRPS I (Saldino–Noonan type), SRPS II (Majewski type), SRPS III (Verma–Naumoff type), SRPS IV (Beemer–Langer type), and SRPS V. Because of the phenotypic overlap among the subtypes (for instance, it is difficult, both clinically and radiologically, to separate types I and III), it is unclear whether the variants are due to variable expression or to genetic heterogeneity. In asphyxiating thoracic dysplasia (Jeune syndrome), the long bones are less severely affected, polydactyly is rare, and there are usually no internal malformations. Ellis–van Creveld syndrome also features polydactyly, but the involvement of the thorax is less severe.

Molecular Pathology
The short rib-polydactyly syndromes are heterogeneous in cause. Nevertheless, they all appear to be caused by mutations in genes that affect cilia function by reducing the number of cilia, altering cilia morphology, or both.

References

Elcioglu NH, Hall CM (2002) Diagnostic dilemmas in the short rib-polydactyly syndrome group. Am J Med Genet 111:392–400

Huber C, Cormier-Daire V (2012) Ciliary disorder of the skeleton. Am J Med Genet C Semin Med Genet 160C:165–174

Mill P, Lockhart PJ, Fitzpatrick E, Mountford HS, Hall EA, Reijns MAM et al (2011) Human and mouse mutations in WDR35 cause short-rib polydactyly syndromes due to abnormal ciliogenesis. Am J Hum Genet 88:508–515

Spranger J, Maroteaux P (1990) The lethal osteochondrodysplasias. Adv Hum Genet 19:331–332

S. Mundlos, D. Horn, *Limb Malformations*,
DOI 10.1007/978-3-540-95928-1_12, © Springer-Verlag Berlin Heidelberg 2014

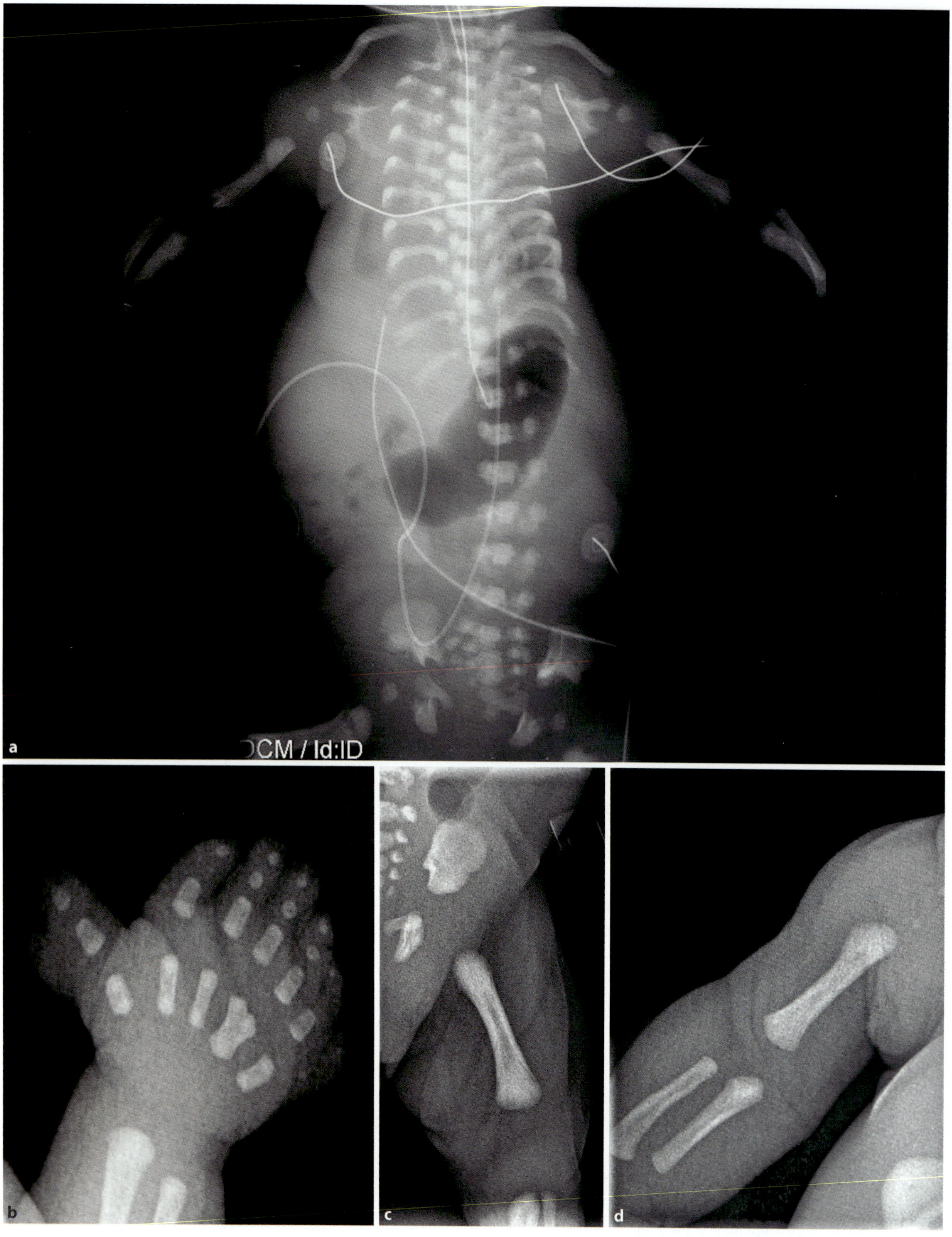

Fig. 12.1 **a,b** Short rib-polydactyly syndromes (SRPS) type I/III. **a** Anteroposterior (AP) body radiograph showing a very narrow thorax, precocious epiphyseal ossification of the proximal humeri and proximal femurs, trident acetabular roofs, and proximal femoral metaphyseal spurs. **b** AP radiograph of hand showing seven digits, postaxial polydactyly, round middle phalanges, and fused metacarpals IV/V. **c,d** SRPS type II. **c** AP radiograph of hips and femur showing proximal and distal femoral rounding. **d** AP radiograph of upper extremity showing round proximal humerus and precocious proximal humeral epiphyseal ossification

Bardet–Biedl Syndrome

MIM 209900

13

Major Clinical Findings

Bardet–Biedl syndrome (BBS) is characterized by polysyndactyly, mild to moderate psychomotor delay, mild to moderate intellectual disability, retinopathy developing during childhood, abnormalities of the renal system, hypogonadism, and obesity. Polysyndactyly is an almost consistent finding, with a frequency of 93–98 %. The polydactyly is usually of postaxial type and asymmetric, but it can also be preaxial. One to four limbs can be affected. Syndactyly occurs between the 2nd and 3rd toes as well as between the polydactylous fingers or toes. The hands and feet are broad.

Typical abnormalities of the renal system are symmetrical parenchymal reduction, fetal lobulation, noncommunicating cysts, and diverticula. Further renal anomalies include hypoplasia and hydronephrosis as well as focal scarring. Primary hypogenitalism is an almost consistent finding in males. Females show a broader spectrum of genital abnormalities, such as vaginal atresia and hydrometrocolpos. Obesity usually develops in infancy. Visual impairment starts to develop in the first and especially in the second decade and progresses to total blindness. Renal failure and myocardial infarction have been described as the major causes of death in BBS.

Occasional Findings

Ocular anomalies such as astigmatism, nystagmus, glaucoma, and cataracts; diabetes mellitus; hypertension; hip dysplasia; genua valga; cardiac defects; macrocephaly.

Genetic Transmission

Inheritance is autosomal recessive in most cases; however, triallelic inheritance has been described. In the latter, the clinical manifestation of some forms of BBS requires recessive mutations in one of several loci plus an additional mutation in another locus. This type of inheritance has also been described as recessive with a modifier of penetrance. Heterozygote carriers may have polydactyly or retinopathy.

Differential Diagnosis

Other syndromes that feature polydactyly, including Meckel–Gruber syndrome, Smith–Lemli–Opitz syndrome, and Pallister–Hall syndrome, have to be considered. Other conditions that show retinopathy, such as Cohen syndrome, need to be distinguished. Sonographic renal findings in an affected fetus or neonate are similar to those of autosomal recessive polycystic kidney disease.

Molecular Pathology

BBS is a genetically heterogeneous disorder. All BBS-associated genes (*BBS1*, *BBS2*, *ARL6*, *BBS4*, *BBS5*, *MKKS*, *BBS7*, *TTC8*, *PTHB1*, *BBS10*, *TRIM32*, *BBS12*, *MKS1*, *CEP290*) are involved in the function of the primary cilia. Accordingly, mutations in these genes compromise cilia structure and function or result in the loss of flagella.

References

Abu-Safieh L, Al-Anazi S, Al-Abdi L, Hashem M, Alkuraya H, Alamr M et al (2012) In search of triallelism in Bardet–Biedl syndrome. J Hum Genet 20:420–427

Beales PL, Elcioglu N, Woolf AS, Parker D, Flinter FA (1999) New criteria for improved diagnosis of Bardet–Biedl syndrome: results of a population survey. J Med Genet 36:437–446

Kim SK, Shindo A, Park TJ, Oh EC, Ghosh S, Gray RS et al (2010) Planar cell polarity acts through septins to control collective cell movement and ciliogenesis. Science 329:1337–1340

Stoetzel, C., Muller, J., Laurier, V., Davis, E. E., Zaghloul, N. A., et al. Identification of a novel BBS gene (*BBS12*) highlights the major role of a vertebrate-specific branch of chaperonin-related proteins in Bardet–Biedl syndrome. Am. J. Hum. Genet. 80:1–11, 2007.

S. Mundlos, D. Horn, *Limb Malformations*,
DOI 10.1007/978-3-540-95928-1_13, © Springer-Verlag Berlin Heidelberg 2014

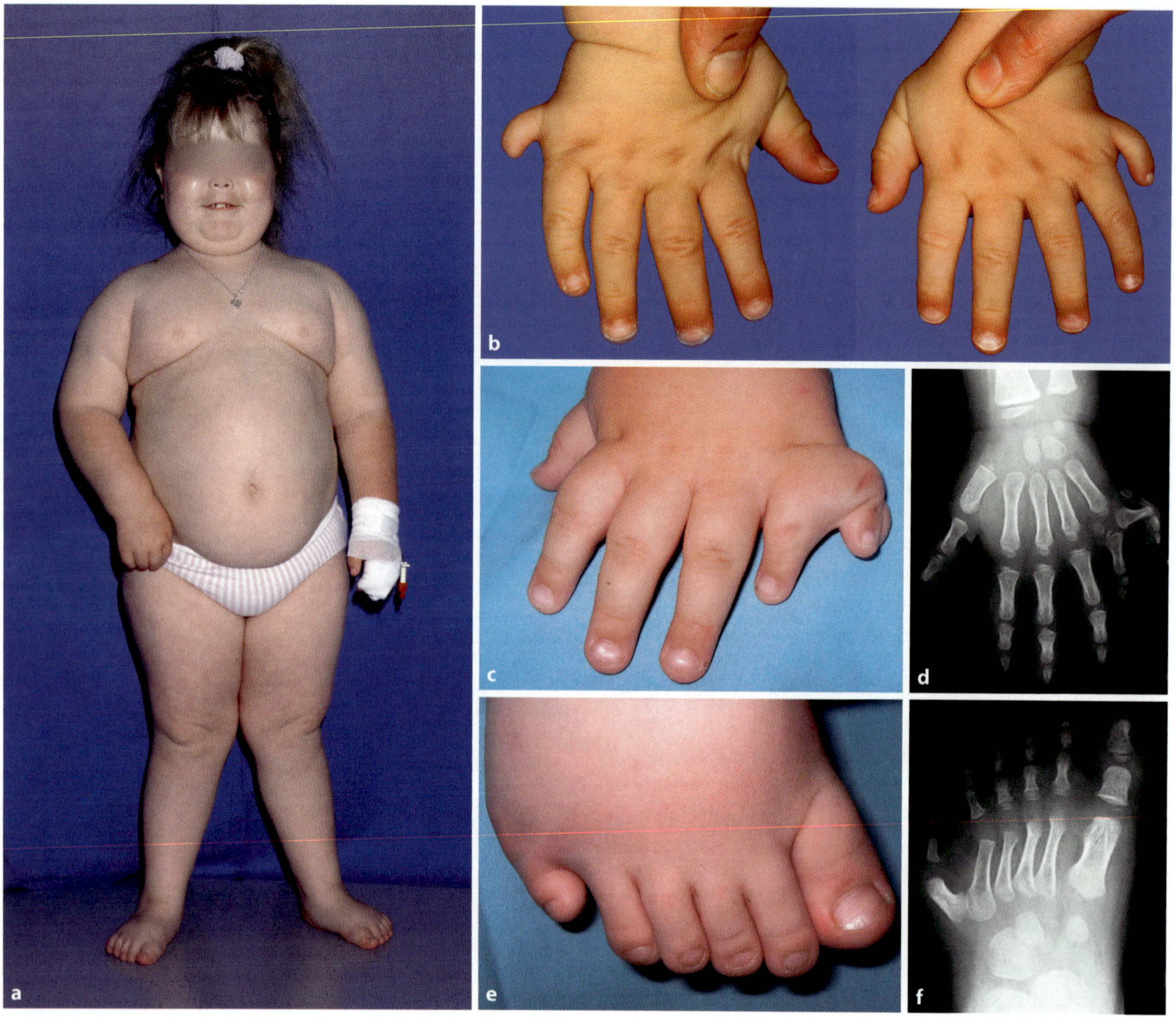

Fig. 13.1 **a** A 6-year-old girl with Bardet–Biedl syndrome. **b** Postaxial polydactyly with rudimentary 6th finger arising from the 5th metacarpal. **c** More complex postaxial synpolydactyly. **d** Corresponding radiograph shows postaxial polydactyly, additional rudimentary ossification (phalanx), and horizontal proximal phalanx that connects to the rest of the finger. **e** Postaxial polydactyly of the feet in the same individual. **f** Corresponding radiograph shows postaxial polydactyly with articulation/fusion of an additional metatarsal with a proximally broad 5th metatarsal

Meckel Syndrome

MIM 249000

14

Synonyms
Meckel–Gruber syndrome
Dysencephalia splanchnocystica

Major Clinical Findings
Meckel syndrome is a developmental disorder with extensive clinical variability. The classic triad includes occipital encephalocele, cystic kidneys, and fibrotic changes of the liver.

Minimum diagnostic criteria stated by different authors are cystic renal disease; a central nervous system malformation, most commonly occipital encephalocele; and polydactyly, which is most often postaxial. However, only about half of the affected individuals have polydactyly. Bowing of the limbs occurs.

Occasional Findings
Prenatal growth deficiency, Dandy–Walker malformation, microcephaly with sloping forehead, cerebellar hypoplasia, liver fibrosis, liver cysts.

Genetic Transmission
Autosomal recessive.

Differential Diagnosis
If the classic triad is not completely present, Joubert syndrome may be a differential diagnosis. Differential diagnoses for Meckel syndrome can also be etiologically unrelated to ciliopathies and include trisomy 13 and Smith–Lemli–Opitz syndrome, both characterized by brain anomalies and polydactyly.

Molecular Pathology
Extensive genetic heterogeneity has been documented. Homozygous and compound heterozygous mutations in different genes (*MSK1*, *TMEM216*, *TMEM67*, *CEP290*, *RPGRIP1L*, *CC2D2A*, *NPHP3*, *TCTN2*, *B9D1*, *B9D2*) have been reported. All of these mutations result in a dysfunction of primary cilia during embryogenesis. Primary cilia are an essential component of the hedgehog pathway.

References

Consugar, M.B., Kubly, V.J., Lager, D.J., Hommerding, C.J., Wong, W.C., Bakker, E., et al. Molecular diagnostics of Meckel–Gruber syndrome highlights phenotypic differences between MKS1 and MKS3. Hum. Genet. 121:591–599, 2007.

Kyttala, M., Tallila, J., Salonen, R., Kopra, O., Kohlschmidt, N., Paavola-Sakki, P., et al. *MKS1*, encoding a component of the flagellar apparatus basal body proteome, is mutated in Meckel syndrome. Nature Genet. 38:155–157, 2006.

Logan, C.V., Abdel-Hamed, Z., Johnson, C.A. Molecular genetics and pathogenic mechanisms for the severe ciliopathies: insights into neurodevelopment and pathogenesis of neural tube defects. Molec. Neurobiol. 43:12–26, 2011.

Seller, M.J. Phenotypic variation in Meckel syndrome. Clin. Genet. 20:74–77, 1981.

Wright, C., Healicon, R., English, C., Burn, J. Meckel syndrome: what are the minimum diagnostic criteria? J. Med. Genet. 31:482–485, 1994.

S. Mundlos, D. Horn, *Limb Malformations*,
DOI 10.1007/978-3-540-95928-1_14, © Springer-Verlag Berlin Heidelberg 2014

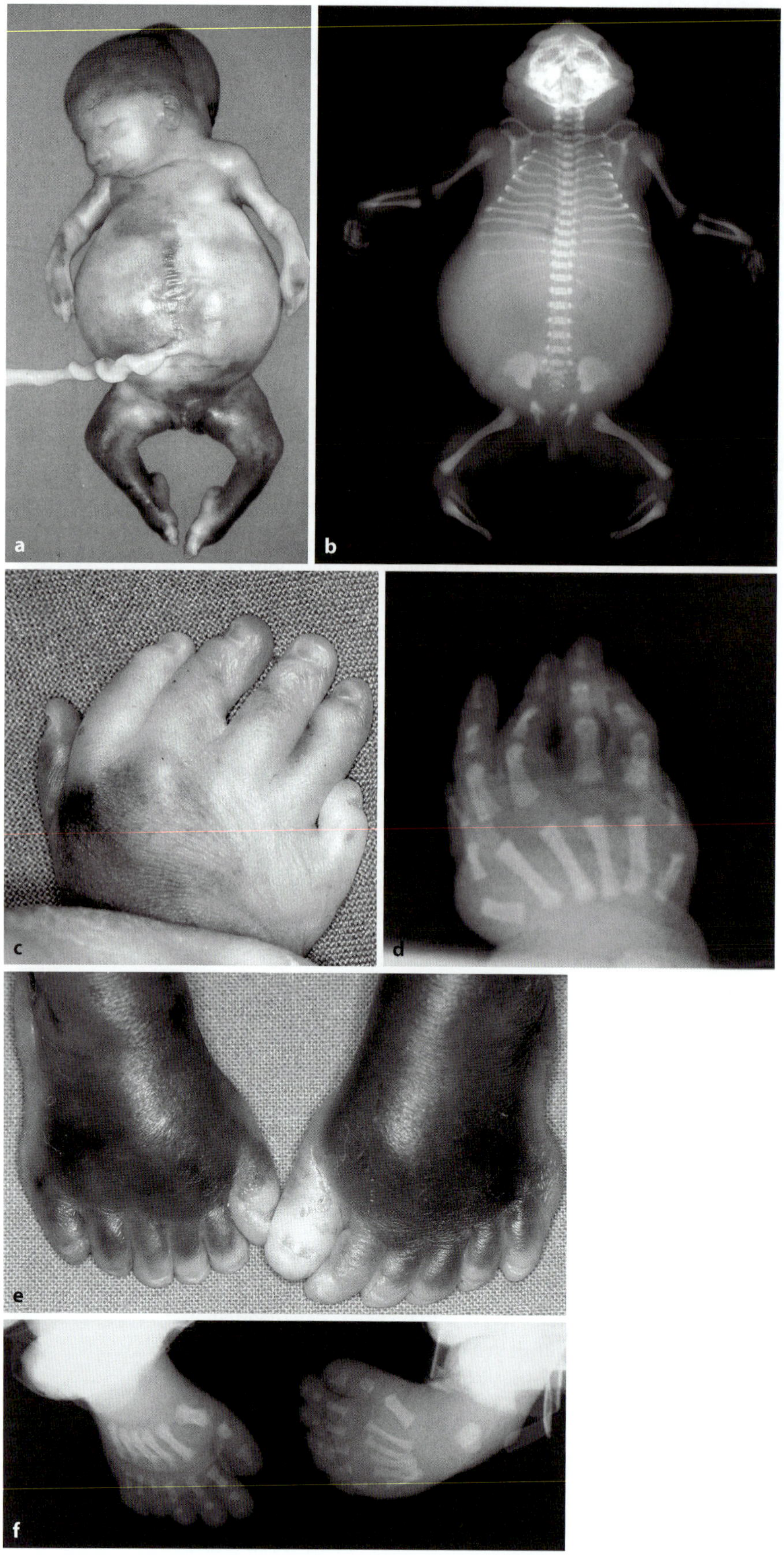

Fig. 14.1 **a** Stillborn infant with posterior encephalocele and enlarged abdominal masses caused by cystic and enlarged kidneys. **b** Corresponding radiograph reveals extreme microcephaly, thin clavicles, triangular thorax with wavy ribs, and relatively normal other bones. **c** Postaxial polydactyly, partial cutaneous syndactyly, and short digits. **d** Corresponding radiograph showing postaxial polydactyly with additional finger containing hypoplastic metacarpal and phalangeal bones. **e** Postaxial polydactyly of the feet. **f** Radiograph of the feet demonstrating postaxial polydactyly. (Courtesy of Peter Meinecke, Hamburg, Germany)

Carpenter Syndrome

MIM 201000

15

Synonyms
Acrocephalopolysyndactyly type 2

Major Clinical Findings
The combination of craniosynostosis with brachydactyly, polydactyly, and syndactyly is characteristic for Carpenter syndrome. Most commonly, the metopic, sagittal, and lambdoid sutures are affected, resulting in brachycephaly, a flat nasal bridge, and shallow supraorbital bridges. Severe cases may present with cloverleaf skull. Also seen are short and/or missing middle phalanges of fingers and toes II–V; flexion contractures of the interphalangeal joints; broad, partially duplicated thumbs; occasional postaxial polydactyly; preaxial polydactyly; and partial or complete syndactyly of the feet. Other features include obesity, postnatal growth retardation (< 25th percentile), variable delay in intellectual performance, low-set malformed ears, corneal opacity, microcornea, hypoplastic mandible and/or maxilla, hypogenitalism, and cryptorchidism. Cardiovascular defects occur in 50%.

Genetic Transmission
Autosomal recessive.

Differential Diagnosis
Unlike the other known craniosynostosis syndromes that most commonly affect the coronal sutures, Carpenter syndrome affects the midline sutures: metopic, sagittal, and lambdoid. The combination of craniosynostosis and limb anomalies occurs in Saethre–Chotzen, Pfeiffer, and Apert syndromes, but none of these conditions presents with polydactyly.

Molecular Pathology
Carpenter syndrome is caused by mutations in *RAB23*, which encodes a member of the RAB guanosine triphosphate (GTPase) family of vesicle transport proteins. RAB23 has been shown to act as a negative regulator of hedgehog signaling. A Carpenter subtype associated with defective left–right patterning has been reported to be caused by mutations in *MEGF8*.

References

Jenkins D, Seelow D, Jehee FS, Perlyn CA, Alonso LG, Bueno DF et al (2007) RAB23 mutations in Carpenter syndrome imply an unexpected role for hedgehog signaling in cranial-suture development and obesity. Am J Hum Genet 80(6):1162–70

Temtamy SA (1966) Carpenter's syndrome: acrocephalopolysyndactyly. An autosomal recessive syndrome. J Pediatr 69(1):111–120

S. Mundlos, D. Horn, *Limb Malformations*,
DOI 10.1007/978-3-540-95928-1_15, © Springer-Verlag Berlin Heidelberg 2014

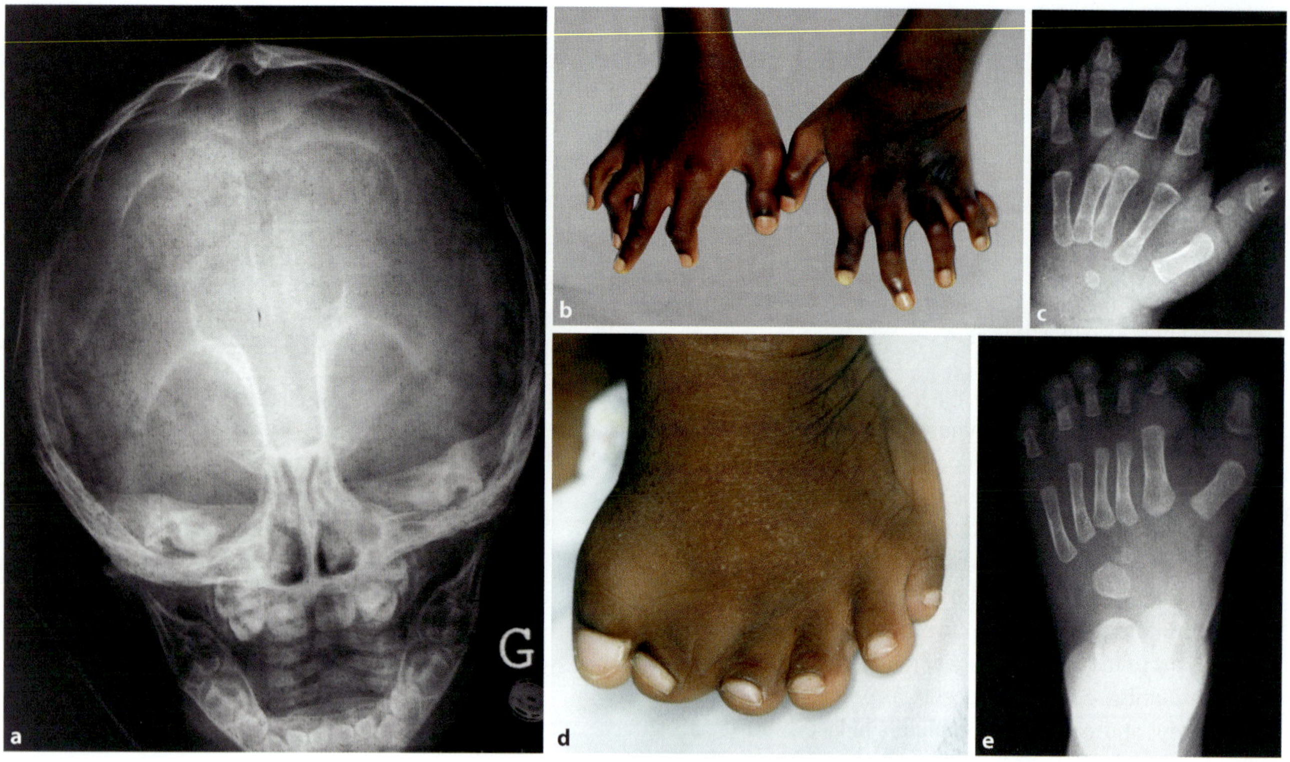

Fig. 15.1 **a** Radiograph of head showing fusion of sutures and orbital roof elevation. **b** Hands showing postaxial polydactyly, brachydactyly, and camptodactyly. **c** Radiograph of hand showing duplication of distal phalanx of the thumb, missing middle phalanges II–V, and medially misplaced middle phalanx of the thumb. **d** Foot showing preaxial polydactyly. **e** Radiograph of foot showing six digits with possible duplication of hallux, missing phalanges II–V, delta phalanx of the 2nd middle phalanx, and hypoplastic tufts. (Courtesy of Valerie Comier-Daire, Paris Descartes-Sorbonne Paris Cité, France)

16 Acrocallosal Syndrome

MIM 200990

Synonyms
Hallux duplication, postaxial polydactyly, and absence of corpus callosum
Schinzel–acrocallosal syndrome

Major Clinical Findings
Acrocallosal syndrome is characterized by polydactyly of the hands and feet in combination with brain abnormalities such as corpus callosum agenesis and Dandy–Walker malformation. Polydactyly of the hands is usually postaxial with an extra digit or pedunculated postminimus only. Cutaneous syndactyly of the 4th and 5th fingers and preaxial polydactyly of the feet are further characteristic features. Facial dysmorphic features include macrocephaly; large anterior fontanel; prominent forehead; hypertelorism; small, low-set, and malformed ears; short nose with a broad nasal bridge and anteverted nostrils; high arched palate; and open mouth with thick lips. Brain malformations are often cystic and may include cerebral atrophy, hypothalamic dysfunction, hypoplasia of the pons, abnormalities of the cerebellum, partial micropolygyria, partial pachygyria, and heterotopia.

Occasional Findings
Congenital heart defects, imperforate anus, hypospadias, cryptorchidism, rectovaginal fistula.

Genetic Transmission
Autosomal recessive.

Differential Diagnosis
The digital changes are similar to those in Greig cephalopolysyndactyly syndrome.

Molecular Pathology
Acrocallosal syndrome is caused by mutations in *KIF7*, which encodes a cilia-associated protein belonging to the kinesin family. As with many other cilia-associated proteins, it plays a role in the hedgehog signaling pathway through the regulation of GLI transcription factors. Acrocallosal syndrome is allelic with Joubert-12 syndrome and hydrolethalus syndrome.

References

Koenig R, Bach A, Woelki U, Grzeschik KH, Fuchs S (2002) Spectrum of the acrocallosal syndrome. Am J Med Genet 108:7–11

Putoux A, Thomas S, Coene KL, Davis EE, Alanay Y, Ogur G et al (2011) KIF7 mutations cause fetal hydrolethalus and acrocallosal syndromes. Nat Genet 43:601–606

Schinzel A (1979) Postaxial polydactyly, hallux duplication, absence of the corpus callosum, macrencephaly and severe mental retardation: a new syndrome? Helv Paediatr Acta 34:141–146

Schinzel A, Kaufmann U (1986) The acrocallosal syndrome in sisters. Clin Genet 30:399–405

S. Mundlos, D. Horn, *Limb Malformations*,
DOI 10.1007/978-3-540-95928-1_16, © Springer-Verlag Berlin Heidelberg 2014

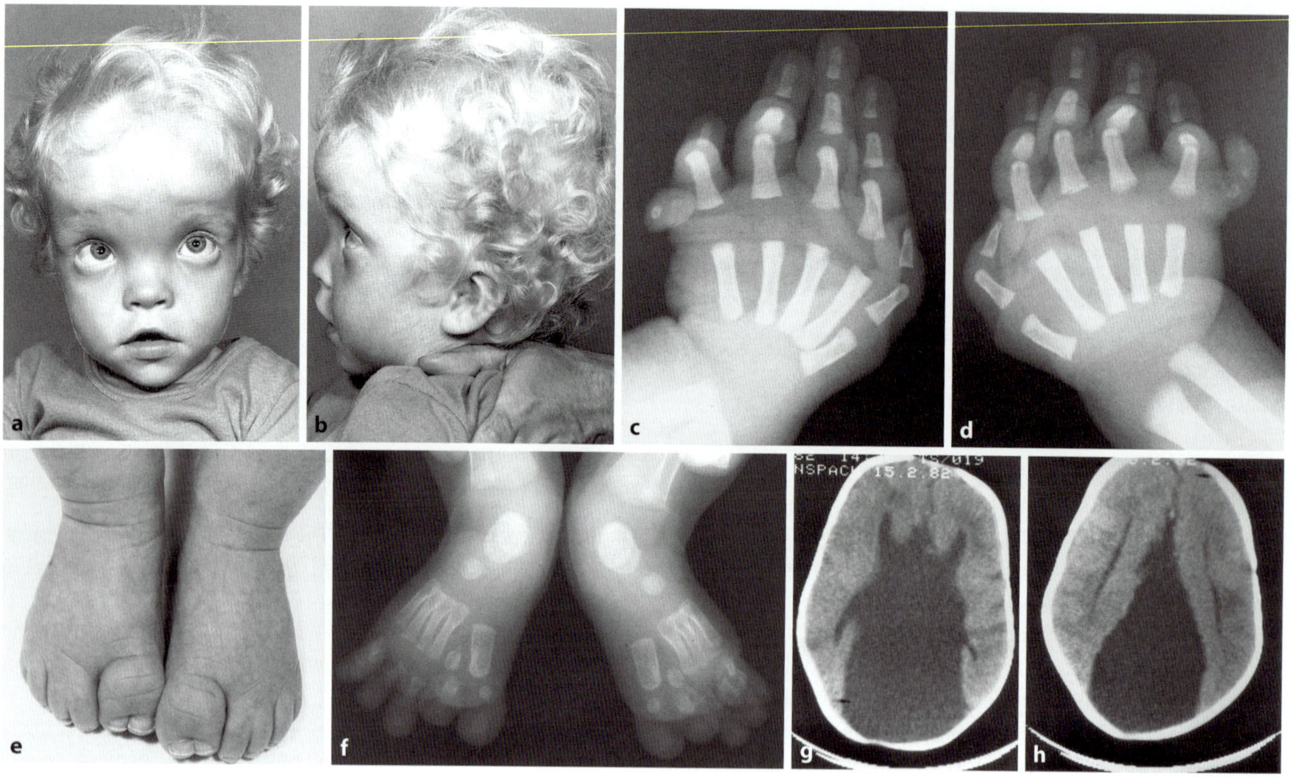

Fig. 16.1 **a** Facial features in acrocallosal syndrome. Note the large head with frontal bossing, frontal upsweep of hair, hypertelorism, and upturned nose with broad bridge. **b** Lateral view. **c, d** Radiographs of right and left hands. Postaxial polydactyly. **e** Feet at age 3 months. Duplication of halluces, syndactyly, fusion of nails, and partial cutaneous syndactyly of toes II and III. **f** Radiograph of feet shows symmetrical interaxial polydactyly, suggesting duplication of both halluces. **g, h** Computed tomography scan showing large supratentorial cyst and lateralization of anterior horns of lateral ventricles, indicating agenesis of corpus callosum. (From Schinzel 1979 and Schinzel and Kaufmann 1986)

17 Townes–Brocks Syndrome

MIM 107480

Synonyms
Renal-ear-anal-radial syndrome
REAR syndrome

Major Clinical Findings
Townes–Brocks syndrome is characterized by a combination of thumb, auricular, renal, and anal anomalies. The thumbs may be broad, bifid, triphalangeal, or (rarely) hypoplastic. The radius is not affected. Preaxial polydactyly is common. Also seen are pseudoepiphyses of the 2nd metacarpals; abnormalities of the carpal bones, including fusion of the triquetrum and hamate, and absent triquetrum and navicular bones; and syndactyly of fingers II–III and III–IV. The feet show fusion of metatarsals, short metatarsals, absent/hypoplastic 3rd toe, 5th toe clinodactyly, overlapping toes (2nd and 4th overlapping the 3rd), and syndactyly of toes III–IV. Auricular anomalies include preauricular tags, overfolding of the helix, and large ears. Hearing loss may be sensorineural, conductive, or mixed. Anal defects include imperforate anus, anterior placement, and stenosis. Renal anomalies are common, including renal hypoplasia, multicystic kidneys, ureterovesical reflux, urethral valves, and other types of malformations. Genital anomalies consist of cryptorchidism, bifid scrotum, and hypospadias in males, and rectovaginal fistula, vaginal aplasia, and bifid uterus in females. Heart defects may occur.

Genetic Transmission
Autosomal dominant.

Differential Diagnosis
The full clinical presentation leaves few differential diagnoses. However, Townes–Brocks syndrome is extremely variable, and any of the typical features may be missing. In these cases, the list of differential diagnoses is long. The preauricular tags are reminiscent of Goldenhar syndrome or hemifacial microsomia. The combination of polydactyly with renal defects raises the possibility of Meckel–Gruber syndrome. In cases with triphalangeal/duplicated thumb but without other apparent malformations, isolated polydactyly with triphalangeal thumb has to be considered.

Molecular Pathology
Townes–Brocks syndrome is caused by mutations in *SALL1*, a zinc finger transcription factor. The mutations are predominantly premature stop codons predicted to result in truncated proteins or a loss of function due to protein or mRNA degradation. *SALL1* is one of four functional *SALL* genes related to the *Drosophila spalt* (*sal*) gene. In the fly, *sal* is activated in the wing discs in response to hedgehog signaling. In vertebrates, Sall1 plays an important role in development and is expressed in the limb buds, the spinal cord, the genital tubercle, and the telencephalon during development. Inactivation of Sall1 in the mouse results in abnormal kidneys but no other defects. The introduction of a Townes–Brocks mutation, however, results in the typical phenotype involving anomalies of the limbs, kidneys, anus, and ears.

References

Kohlhase J (2000) SALL1 mutations in Townes–Brocks syndrome and related disorders. Hum Mutat 16(6):460–466

Kohlhase J, Wischermann A, Reichenbach H, Froster U, Engel W (1998) Mutations in the SALL1 putative transcription factor gene cause Townes–Brocks syndrome. Nat Genet 18(1):81–83

Powell CM, Michaelis RC (1999) Townes–Brocks syndrome. J Med Genet 36(2):89–93

Townes PL, Brocks ER (1972) Hereditary syndrome of imperforate anus with hand, foot, and ear anomalies. J Pediatr 81(2):321–326

S. Mundlos, D. Horn, *Limb Malformations*,
DOI 10.1007/978-3-540-95928-1_17, © Springer-Verlag Berlin Heidelberg 2014

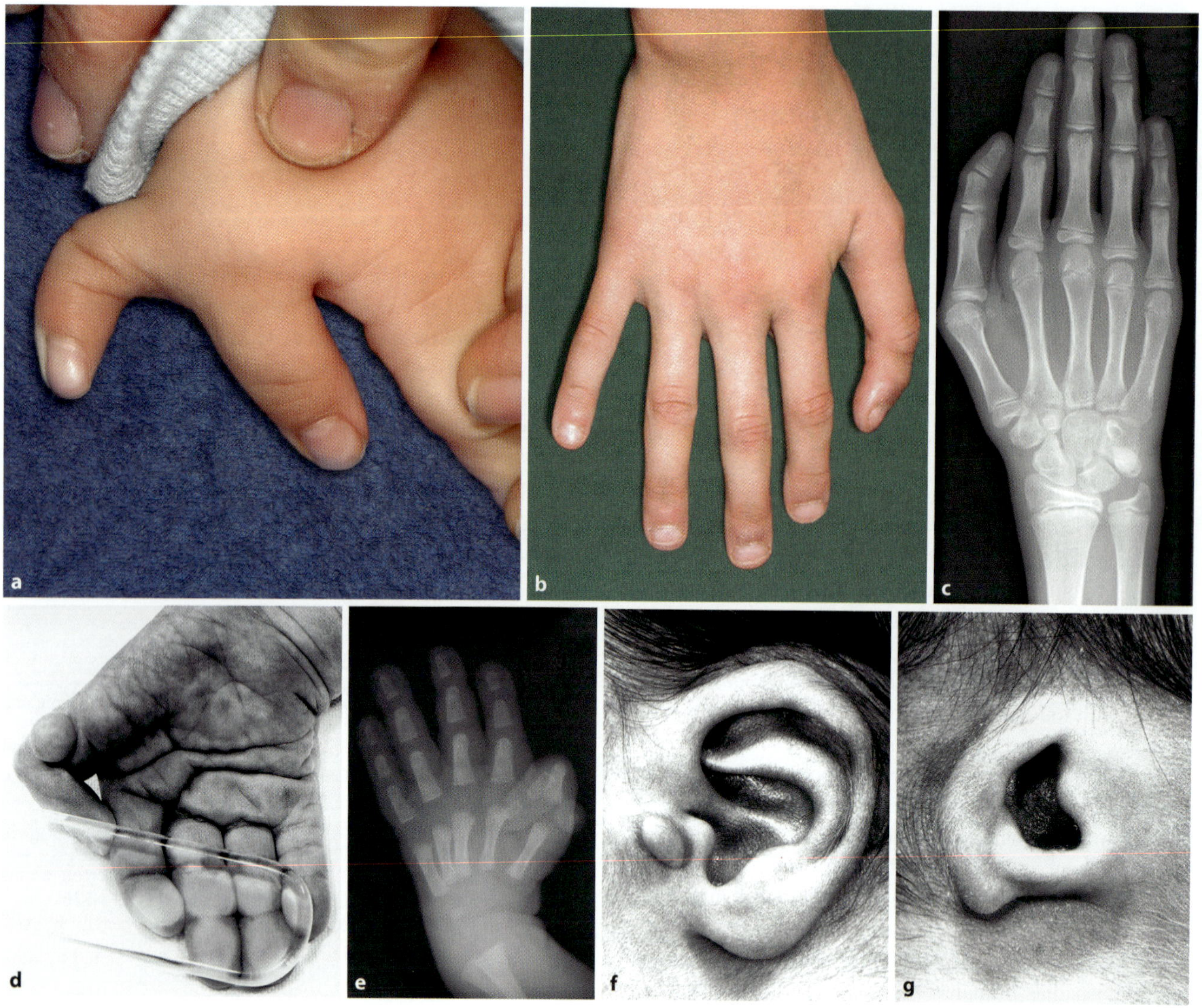

Fig. 17.1 **a–e** Variability in preaxial polydactyly phenotypes in Townes–Brocks syndrome. **a** Preaxial polydactyly. **b, c** Triphalangeal thumb without polydactyly. **d, e** Triphalangeal thumb (bent) with rudimentary polydactyly. **f, g** Ear abnormalities in Townes–Brocks syndrome. (**d–g** Courtesy of Rainer König, University of Frankfurt, Germany)

18 Pallister–Hall Syndrome

MIM 146510

Major Clinical Findings

Pallister–Hall syndrome (PHS) is characterized by the combination of polydactyly, hypothalamic hamartoma, hypopituitarism, and imperforate anus. In the limbs, various degrees of syndactyly, postaxial polydactyly, and central polydactyly may be present. Hypoplasia of the distal phalanges, together with nail hypoplasia, is common. The 4th metacarpal may be short, with one or two additional fingers associated with it. Shortening of the proximal upper limbs is also seen. Hypothalamic hamartoma is a benign tumor of the hypothalamus and does not need treatment from a tumor perspective. However, other problems are associated with these lesions, including treatment-resistant epilepsy (beginning with gelastic seizures but later including other seizure types), developmental and cognitive deficits, behavioral problems, and endocrine disturbances, most commonly central precocious (early) puberty. Pituitary abnormalities ranging from asymptomatic pituitary displacement to pituitary hypoplasia and panhypopituitarism are seen. Secondary to pituitary hypoplasia, adrenal gland hypoplasia may be present, resulting in a potentially life-threatening condition. The face shows a flat nasal bridge and midface; short nose; and abnormal ears, including posterior rotation, microtia, and absent external auditory canals. Abnormalities of the upper airways include bifid, hypoplastic, or absent epiglottis and dysplastic tracheal cartilage. Rectal atresia occurs in variable degrees. Other malformations such as renal disease (ectopia, dysplasia) and heart defects (ventricular septal defect, proximal aortic coarctation) may be present.

Other, less frequent features include abnormalities of the vertebrae; fused ribs; congenital luxation of the hip, knee, or radius; camptodactyly; holoprosencephaly with midline defect; Dandy–Walker malformation; polymicrogyria; encephalocele; frenulae between the alveolar ridge and the buccal mucosa; natal teeth; testicular underdevelopment with micropenis; hypoplasia of the pancreas; and small thyroid gland.

Genetic Transmission

Autosomal dominant.

Differential Diagnosis

There is substantial overlap with Greig syndrome, which is also caused by mutations in *GLI3*. However, Greig syndrome is generally confined to the limbs together with craniofacial anomalies. The characteristic broad, duplicated toe is not part of PHS. Acrocallosal syndrome also shows similar features, and distinguishing between the two conditions may be difficult. Agenesis of the corpus callosum and large intracranial cysts may serve in differentiating acrocallosal syndrome from PHS. Clinical overlap exists with the oral-facial-digital syndromes.

Molecular Pathology

PHS is caused by mutations in *GLI3*. The GLI family of zinc finger transcription factors is downstream of the hedgehog pathway and executes the signal. Upon exposure to hedgehog signal, Gli is transferred into the nucleus, where it activates target genes. In the absence of hedgehog signal, Gli is cleaved just after the DNA binding domain and is translocated into the nucleus. This time, however, it serves as a suppressor. Based on the asymmetry of hedgehog signal from the zone of polarizing activity, different concentrations of activating versus repressing forms of Gli exist, which form a gradient across the anterior–posterior axis of the limb. This gradient is essential to regulate digit number and identity. Nearly all patients with PHS have a truncating mutation (frameshift/nonsense or splicing) in *GLI3* in the middle third of the gene. In contrast, Greig syndrome is caused by many types of alterations, including translocations; large deletions; exonic deletions and duplications; small in-frame deletions; and missense, frameshift/nonsense, and splicing mutations that are predicted to result in loss of function. The PHS mutations predict a truncated functional repressor protein that is still active. However, overlapping phenotypes exist, and *GLI3* mutations should be considered in individuals who show one or more feature of either Greig syndrome or PHS.

References

Johnston JJ, Olivos-Glander I, Killoran C, Elson E, Turner JT, Peters KF et al (2005) Molecular and clinical analyses of Greig cephalopolysyndactyly and Pallister–Hall syndromes: robust phenotype prediction from the type and position of GLI3 mutations. Am J Hum Genet 76(4):609–622

Johnston JJ, Sapp JC, Turner JT, Amor D, Aftimos S, Aleck KA et al (2010) Molecular analysis expands the spectrum of phenotypes associated with GLI3 mutations. Hum Mutat 31(10):1142–1154

S. Mundlos, D. Horn, *Limb Malformations*,
DOI 10.1007/978-3-540-95928-1_18, © Springer-Verlag Berlin Heidelberg 2014

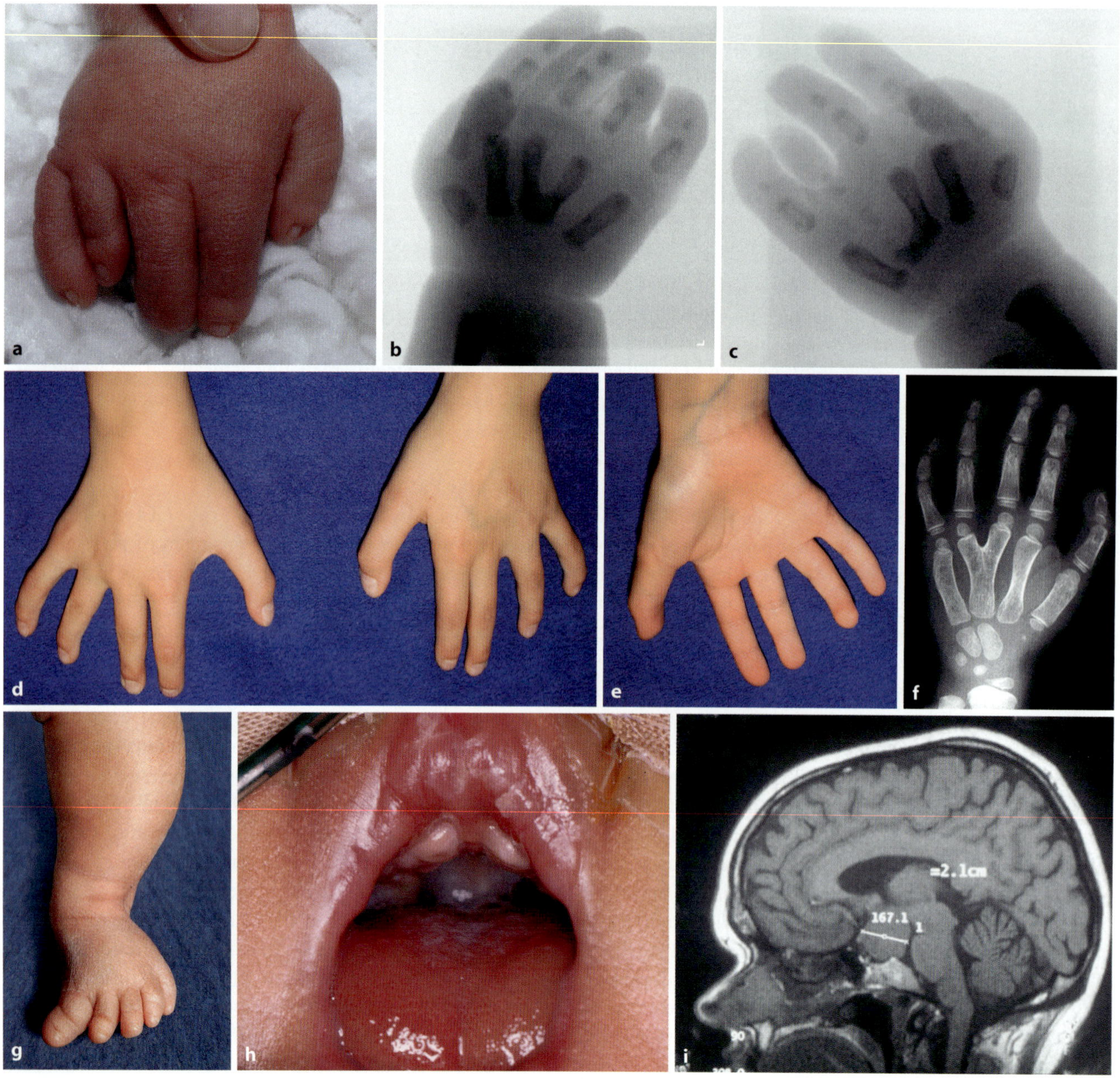

Fig. 18.1 **a** Newborn with Pallister–Hall syndrome. Note small digit IV and broad digit III. Hypoplastic nails. **b, c** Corresponding radiographs of hands showing Y-shaped branching of metacarpals III and IV, lack of ossification of distal phalanges on the right and L-shaped metacarpal III with minimal ossification of distal metacarpal IV, and minimal ossification in distal phalanges on the left. **d** Hands of 12-year-old girl after surgical release of metacarpal III/IV fusion. **e** Palmar view. Note similar length of digits II–V. **f** Corresponding radiograph before surgery showing Y-shaped branching of metacarpals III and IV, abnormally shaped and bent metacarpal V, and hypoplastic distal phalanges. **g** Foot of same individual as in **a** showing normal number of digits but medial deviation of toes. **h** Oral frenulae. **i** Magnetic resonance image showing hypothalamic hamartoblastoma

Part IV

Disorders: Syndactyly Isolated

19 Syndactyly Type Lueken

MIM 185900

Synonyms
Zygodactyly
Syndactyly type 1

Major Clinical Findings
Syndactyly type Lueken is characterized by variable syndactyly of the digits of the hands and feet. The least severely affected show syndactyly type I, also called zygodactyly, a term referring to complete or partial webbing between digits III and IV and/or complete or partial webbing between toes II and III. In the most severe cases, there is complete syndactyly of fingers II–V, the thumb is spared, and there is syndactyly of all toes, including the hallux. In severe cases, bony fusion of the distal phalanges can be observed. Penetrance is incomplete.

Genetic Transmission
Autosomal dominant.

Differential Diagnosis
The condition shows overlap with craniosynostosis Philadelphia type, which features craniosynostosis together with syndactyly type 1 and may reflect a phenotypic spectrum of this condition. The term syndactyly type I/zygodactyly is descriptive and does not describe a genetic entity. Syndactyly type I also occurs in mild forms of *HOXD13*-associated synpolydactyly.

Molecular Pathology
Syndactyly Lueken type has been shown to be caused by duplications involving the *Indian hedgehog* (*IHH*) gene and adjacent regulatory regions on chromosome 2q.

References

Bosse K, Betz RC, Lee Y-A, Wienker TF, Reis A, Kleen H et al (2000) Localization of a gene for syndactyly type 1 to chromosome 2q34-q36. Am J Hum Genet 67:492–497

Klopocki E, Lohan S, Brancati F, Koll R, Brehm A, Seemann P et al (2011) Copy-number variations involving the IHH locus are associated with syndactyly and craniosynostosis. Am J Hum Genet 88:70–75

S. Mundlos, D. Horn, *Limb Malformations*,
DOI 10.1007/978-3-540-95928-1_19, © Springer-Verlag Berlin Heidelberg 2014

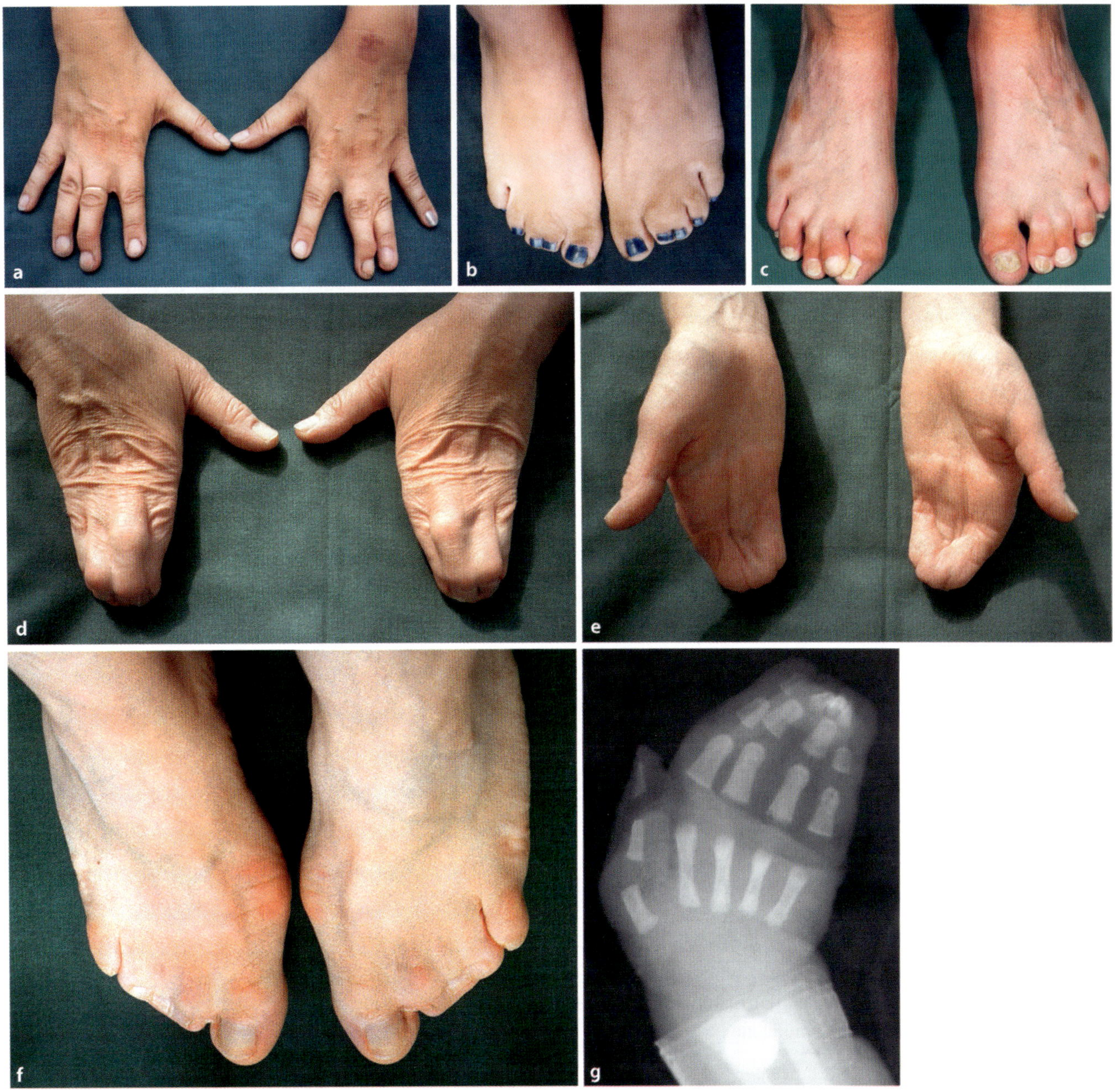

Fig. 19.1 **a** Syndactyly type Lueken III/IV on the left side, proximal syndactyly of digits II/III bilaterally. Contracture deformity of distal interphalangeal joints of digits III. **b** Feet of same individual. Note partial to complete syndactyly, sparing toe V. **c** Feet of an individual with normal hands. Moderate involvement of feet; note lateral deviation of hallux and partial syndactyly of toes II/III on right and III/IV/V on left. **d** Severely affected individual from same family with complete syndactyly sparing the thumbs. **e** Palmar view. **f** Feet of same individual. **g** Hand radiograph of child with syndactyly type Lueken. Note complete soft tissue syndactyly II–V and bony fusion of distal phalanges III, IV, and V. (Courtesy of K. Bosse, University of Cologne, Germany)

20 Metacarpal 4–5 Fusion Syndrome

MIM 309630

Includes

Syndactyly Type V

MIM 186300

Synonyms

Metacarpal fusion postaxial

Major Clinical Findings

Metacarpal 4–5 fusion (MF4) syndrome is characterized by fusion of the metacarpals IV and V. Metacarpal V is often hypoplastic, and finger V is flexed in a 45° ulnar deviation. Movement of finger V is restricted, but flexion is possible. Radiographs show variable degrees of metacarpal IV/V fusion. In the severe cases, the proximal phalanx of finger V rests on a lateral and distal part of a single Y-shaped metacarpal. In other cases, there is fusion of the proximal half of the 4th and 5th metacarpals with separated distal epiphyses. Unilaterality may occur. No other abnormalities have been reported.

Genetic Transmission

X-linked recessive.

Differential Diagnosis

MF4 has been described in association with a specific mutation (p.Q317R) in *HOXD13*. Complete syndactyly of digits IV and V, usually without metacarpal fusion, is a characteristic sign of oculodentodigital syndrome.

Molecular Pathology

MF4 is caused by mutations in the *FGF16* gene on chromosome Xq21.

References

Anneren G, Amilon A (1994) X-linked recessive fusion of metacarpals IV and V and hypoplastic metacarpal V. (Letter). Am J Med Genet 52:248–250

Jamsheer A, Zemojtel T, Kolanczyk M, Stricker S, Hecht J, Krawitz P et al (2013) Whole exome sequencing identifies FGF16 nonsense mutations as the cause of X-linked recessive metacarpal 4/5 fusion. J Med Genet 50:579–584

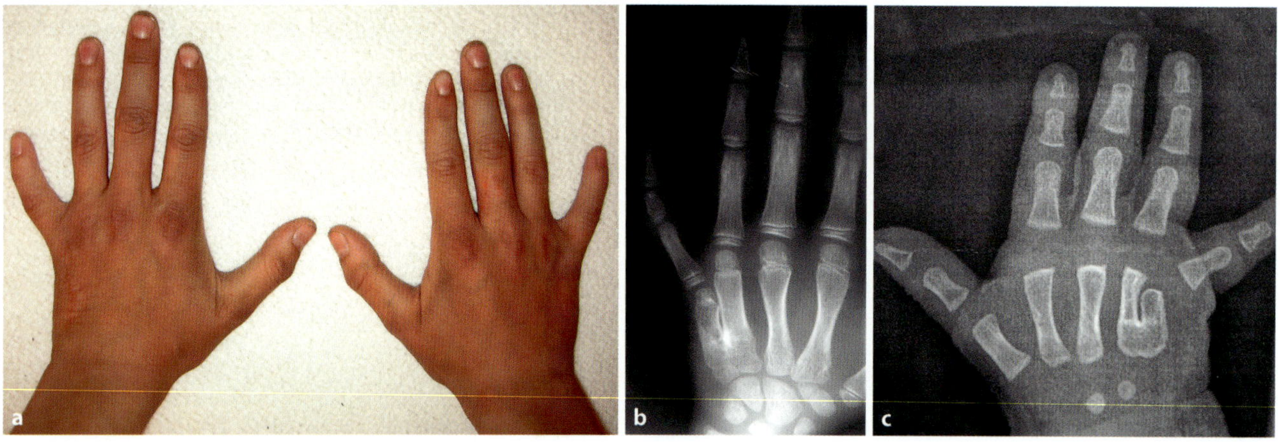

Fig. 20.1 **a** Short, distally placed digits V. **b** Anteroposterior hand radiograph showing proximal fusion of metacarpals IV and V with short metacarpal V. **c** Radiograph in younger individual showing golf-club-shaped metacarpals IV and V with proximal fusion. (From Jamsheer et al. 2013)

S. Mundlos, D. Horn, *Limb Malformations*,
DOI 10.1007/978-3-540-95928-1_20, © Springer-Verlag Berlin Heidelberg 2014

Syndactyly Type Haas

MIM 186200

21

Synonyms
Syndactyly type IV
Polysyndactyly, Haas type

Major Clinical Findings
Syndactyly type Haas is characterized by complete syndactyly affecting all digits of the hand together with polydactyly that includes metacarpals and phalanges. Flexion of the fingers gives the hands a cup-shaped form. The feet may show variable but much milder involvement, with partial cutaneous syndactyly of toes.

Genetic Transmission
Autosomal dominant.

Differential Diagnosis
There is phenotypic overlap with Laurin–Sandrow syndrome. Both conditions show severe, cup-shaped polysyndactyly of the hands. The feet show severe mirror-image polydactyly in Laurin–Sandrow syndrome, which is not a feature of Haas syndactyly. Both conditions result from similar mutations and are likely to represent a phenotypic spectrum. There is similarity to Apert syndrome.

Molecular Pathology
Haas-type syndactyly can be caused by mutations in a *Sonic hedgehog* (*SHH*) regulatory element (the zone of polarizing activity regulatory sequence, or ZRS) that resides in intron 5 of the *LMBR1* gene. Duplications encompassing the ZRS result in the same phenotype. The ZRS is a highly conserved genomic region located in an intron of the *LMBR1* gene, some 1 Mb away from *SHH*. The sequence serves as an enhancer regulating the limb expression of Shh. Deletions of the ZRS result in a loss of Shh expression and thus truncated limbs, whereas mutations and duplications result in a series of conditions, including polydactyly-triphalangeal thumb syndrome, Werner mesomelic dysplasia, Laurin–Sandrow syndrome, and Haas-type syndactyly.

References

Gillessen-Kaesbach G, Majewski F (1991) Bilateral complete polysyndactyly (type IV Haas). Am J Med Genet 38(1):29–31

Lohan S, Spielmann M, Doelken SC, Muhammad F, Baig SM, Wajid M et al (2014) Microduplications encompassing the Sonic Hedgehog limb enhancer ZRS are associated with Haas type polysyndactyly and Laurin–Sandrow syndrome. Clin Genet 2014 Oct;86(4):318–25

Wieczorek D, Pawlik B, Li Y, Akarsu NA, Caliebe A, May KJ et al (2010) A specific mutation in the distant sonic hedgehog (SHH) cis-regulator (ZRS) causes Werner mesomelic syndrome (WMS) while complete ZRS duplications underlie Haas type polysyndactyly and preaxial polydactyly (PPD) with or without triphalangeal thumb. Hum Mutat 31(1):81–89

S. Mundlos, D. Horn, *Limb Malformations*,
DOI 10.1007/978-3-540-95928-1_21, © Springer-Verlag Berlin Heidelberg 2014

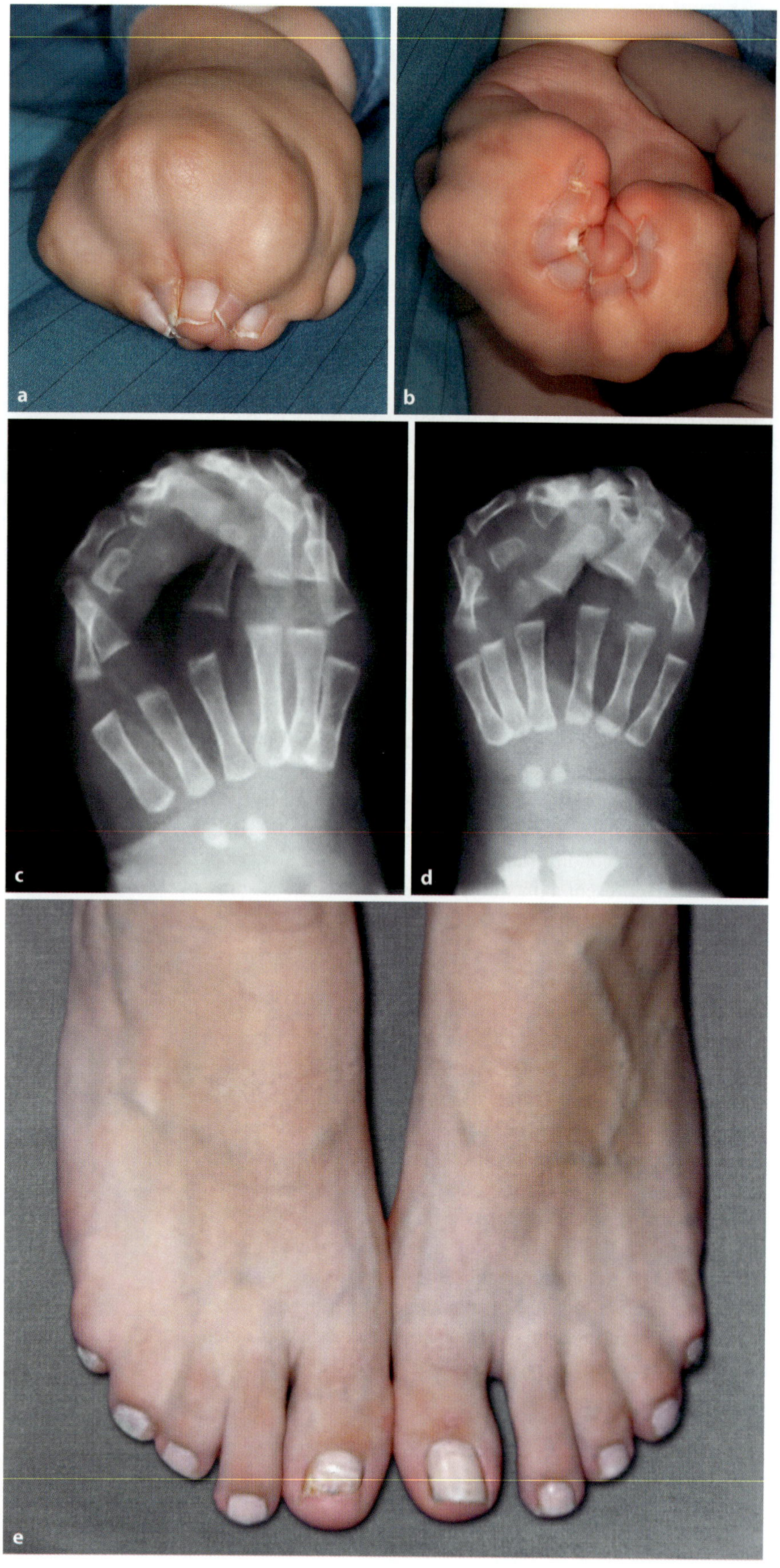

Fig. 21.1 **a, b** Cup-shaped hands with syndactyly of all fingers and nail fusion (due to a duplication of the *SHH*-regulating ZRS). **a** Dorsal view of right hand. **b** Palmar view of left hand. **c, d** Corresponding radiographs showing six metacarpals. Note disorganization of phalanges with distal fusions bilaterally. **e** Feet of individual with similar hand phenotype as in **a** (due to point mutation in the ZRS). Note syndactyly of toes, which is more severe toward the lateral side, but no polydactyly. (**e** Courtesy of Dagmar Wieczorek, University of Essen, Germany)

22 Acropectorovertebral Dysplasia

MIM 102510

Synonyms
F-syndrome

Major Clinical Findings
Acropectorovertebral dysplasia features complex malformations of the hands and feet. A characteristic feature in the hands is an abnormal segmentation of the 1st ray with broad, short thumbs that are partially fused with the index finger. In some individuals the thumb is very short, and finger II is radially deviated due to the soft tissue webbing; in others, the tips of digits I and II show bony fusion with soft tissue webbing between the digits. Fingers II–V are less severely affected and may be normal except for finger V clinodactyly. Fusion of the capitate and hamate, and sometimes other carpals, is seen. The feet show a complex malformation pattern with fusion of metatarsals IV and V, duplications of distal phalanges, and lack of metatarsal II that arises from the metatarsophalangeal joint I. Sternal deformity and spina bifida occulta at L5 or S1 have been observed.

Genetic Transmission
Autosomal dominant.

Differential Diagnosis
Other forms of syndactyly. However, the fusion of fingers I and II is very rare.

Molecular Pathology
The condition has been mapped to chromosome 2q36.

References

Camera G, Camera A, Pozzolo S, Costa M, Mantero R (1995) F-syndrome (F-form of acro-pectoro-vertebral dysplasia): report on a second family. Am J Med Genet 57(3):472–475

Grosse FR, Herrmann J, Opitz JM (1969) The F-form of acropectorovertebral dysplasia: the F-syndrome. Birth Defects Orig Art Ser V(3):48–63

Thiele H, McCann C, van't Padje S, Schwabe GC, Hennies HC, Camera G et al (2004) Acropectorovertebral dysgenesis (F syndrome) maps to chromosome 2q36. J Med Genet 41(3):213–218

S. Mundlos, D. Horn, *Limb Malformations*,
DOI 10.1007/978-3-540-95928-1_22, © Springer-Verlag Berlin Heidelberg 2014

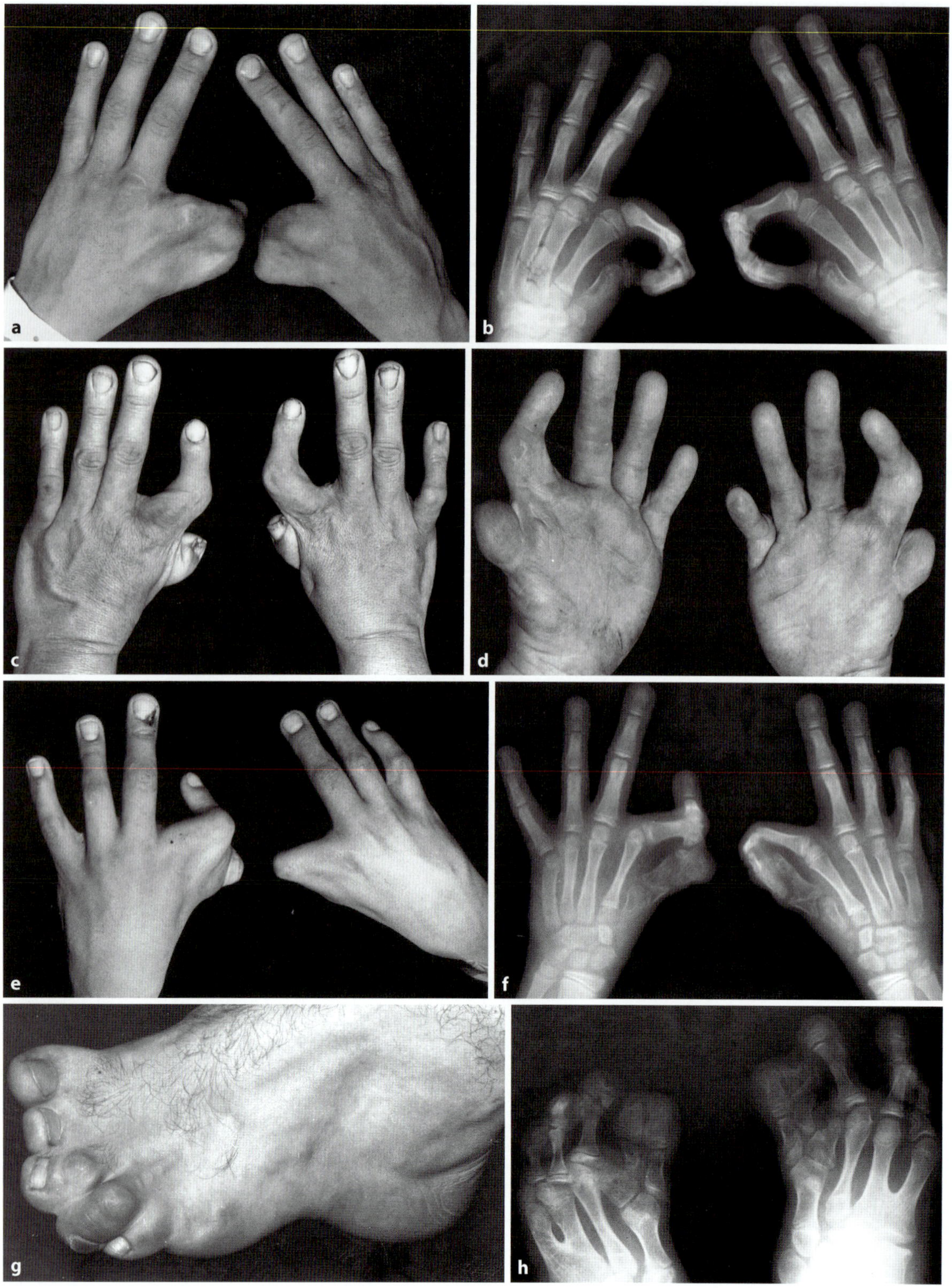

Fig. 22.1 **a** Fingers I and II are fused and form one broad finger. **b** Corresponding radiograph shows that both digits are distally fused, leaving the more proximal structures intact. Short and abnormally shaped 1st metacarpal; unusually large pseudoepiphyses of metacarpal II. **c, d** Dorsal and palmar views, respectively, of additional member of same family. Note very short digit I and radially deviated digit II. **e** Digits I and II are completely fused in the right hand. The left hand also shows fusion but with a distally located terminal phalanx. **f** Corresponding radiograph shows very abnormal digit I with multiple ossification sites and longitudinally oriented growth plates (delta phalanges). There is distal fusion with the middle/proximal phalanges of digits II. The middle and terminal phalanx appear to escape this fusion on the left side and form a separate rudimentary finger. Carpal fusions are also present. **g** Feet with complete syndactyly. **h** Corresponding anteroposterior radiograph of both feet: enlarged 1st metatarsal dividing into paired double digits containing several delta phalangeal epiphyses, as well as medially dislocated and fused hallux phalanges and proximal fusion of metatarsals IV and V. (Courtesy of John Opitz, University of Utah, USA)

Part V

Disorders: Syndactyly Associated

23 Apert Syndrome

MIM 101200

Synonyms
Acrocephalosyndactyly, type 1

Major Clinical Findings
Apert syndrome comprises craniosynostosis, midface hypoplasia, and symmetrical severe syndactyly of the hands and feet, minimally involving digits II, III, and IV. The 1st and 5th fingers may be joined to the mid-digital hand mass. Associated synonychia often occurs. Some patients have preaxial or postaxial polydactyly. Osseous symphalangism of the proximal interphalangeal joints and synostosis of adjacent distal phalanges develop with age. In the feet, syndactyly involves the 2nd, 3rd, and 4th toes in most cases. The big toes are broad and enlarged. Acrobrachycephaly, midface underdevelopment, proptosis, shallow orbits, hypertelorism, and downward slanting palpebral fissures are commonly observed. About half of the affected individuals have intellectual disability. A craniectomy performed early in life is likely to improve psychomotor development.

Occasional Findings
Postaxial and preaxial polydactyly, fusion of cervical vertebrae, malformations of the corpus callosum, ventriculomegaly, strabismus, ametropia, high arched palate, cleft palate, crowded teeth, hyperhidrosis, acne vulgaris at adolescence.

Genetic Transmission
Autosomal dominant. Most cases are sporadic, representing new mutations, but transmission with complete penetrance has been reported.

Differential Diagnosis
The Apert syndrome phenotype is quite specific in most cases; differential diagnoses play no major role. In some cases Apert syndrome should be distinguished from other syndromes with craniosynostosis and syndactyly, such as Crouzon and Carpenter syndromes.

Molecular Pathology
Two mutations in the *FGFR2* gene (Ser252Trp, Pro253Arg) encoding for fibroblast growth factor receptor 2 are responsible for almost all cases of Apert syndrome. Other *FGFR2* mutations are rarely found. These mutations are exclusively paternal in origin. Apert syndrome is allelic to Crouzon syndrome.

FGFR2 belongs to a family of growth factor receptors that belong to the family of tyrosine kinase receptors. They have a similar protein structure consisting of an extracellular domain with three immunoglobulin-like domains, a transmembrane domain, and an intracellular domain that harbors the tyrosine kinase domain. Upon binding of the ligand, these receptors form dimers, resulting in activation of the tyrosine kinase and the corresponding signaling cascades. The Apert mutations are located in the linker between the second and third extracellular immunoglobulin domains of FGFR2. Mutant receptors were shown to have an increased affinity for specific FGF ligands, leading to activation of signaling. Thus, as in most other *FGFR*-related conditions, the mutations appear to result in activation of the receptor. Investigations of the Apert *FGFR2* mutations in calvarial osteoblasts were shown to alter the balance between precursor cells and mature osteoblasts, leading to increased bone matrix formation that ultimately results in premature calvaria ossification and closure of sutures.

References

Lajeunie E, Cameron R, El Ghouzzi V, de Parseval N, Journeau P, Gonzales M et al (1999) Clinical variability in patients with Apert's syndrome. J Neurosurg 90:443–447

Oldridge M, Lunt PW, Zackai EH, McDonald-McGinn DM, Muenke M, Moloney DM et al (1997) Genotype-phenotype correlation for nucleotide substitutions in the IgII-IgIII linker of FGFR2. Hum Molec Genet 6:137–143

Wilkie AOM, Slaney SF, Oldridge M, Poole MD, Ashworth GJ, Hockley AD et al (1995) Apert syndrome results from localized mutations of FGFR2 and is allelic with Crouzon syndrome. Nature Genet 9:165–172

S. Mundlos, D. Horn, *Limb Malformations*,
DOI 10.1007/978-3-540-95928-1_23, © Springer-Verlag Berlin Heidelberg 2014

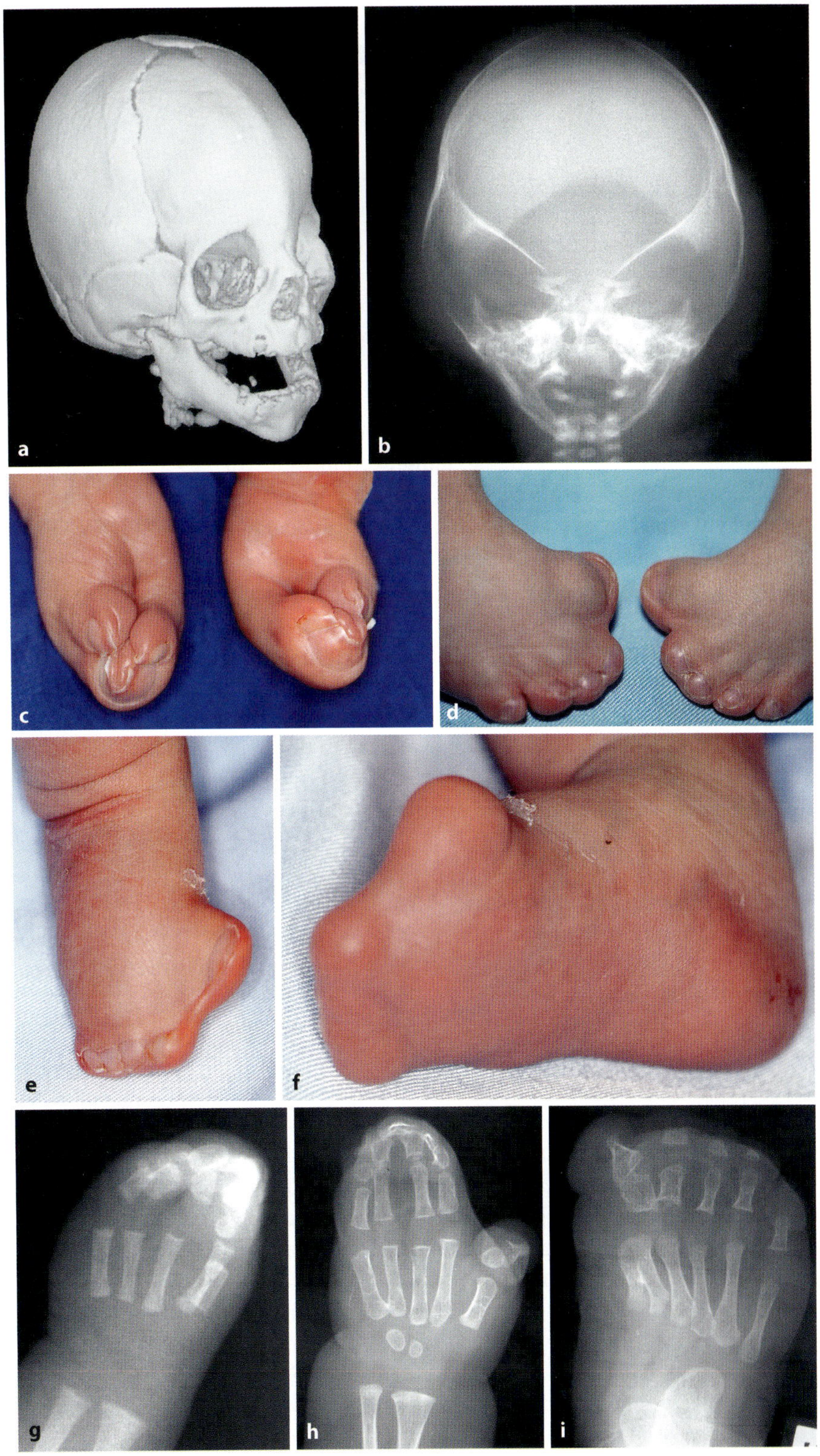

Fig. 23.1 **a** Three-dimensional computed tomography scan of skull showing turricephaly due to early fusion of at least the metopic suture and partial fusion of the coronal suture. **b** Radiograph of newborn skull showing typical deformity and fusion of sutures. **c** Cup-shaped hands with complete fusion of nails. **d** Feet showing fusion of toes and very broad hallux but separate nails. **e, f** Plantar and anteroposterior view of feet showing more severe involvement with complete fusion of toes and medially deviated, broad hallux. **g** Hand radiograph of a fetus showing cup-shaped syndactyly with distal bony fusion and normal number of metacarpals but round and oval bony structures in fusion. **h** Radiograph of "mitten hand" showing distal bony syndactyly of digits II–V replacing the middle and distal phalanges. Note separate thumb with round hypoplastic middle phalanx. **i** Radiograph of foot showing diffuse soft tissue and distal bony fusion, including an enlarged hallux and duplication of the 1st metatarsal

24 Craniosynostosis, Philadelphia Type

MIM 185900

Synonyms
Chromosome 2q35 duplication syndrome
Syndactyly type 1 with or without craniosynostosis

Major Clinical Findings
In this condition, syndactyly occurs together with craniosynostosis. Syndactyly is variable, ranging from mild III/IV syndactyly in the hands and II/III syndactyly in the feet (syndactyly type I or zygodactyly) to complete syndactyly of fingers II–V and toes I–V. The thumbs are always spared, but the halluces may be involved. The syndactyly is usually cutaneous, but in cases with complete syndactyly, bony fusions of the distal phalanges may occur. Preaxial polydactyly of the feet with fusion and shape abnormalities of the 1st metatarsal are seen. Cranial synostosis is variable, ranging from mild fusion of the sagittal suture to premature fusion of all sutures and Kleeblattschädel (cloverleaf skull). Overall, the limb phenotype appears to be more penetrant than the cranial phenotype.

Genetic Transmission
Autosomal dominant.

Differential Diagnosis
Other types of syndactyly and craniosynostosis. Syndactyly type Lueken shows a similar limb phenotype.

Molecular Pathology
Philadelphia-type craniosynostosis is caused by structural variations involving the *Indian hedgehog* (*IHH*) locus. Ihh belongs to the family of hedgehog proteins, developmentally important secreted signaling molecules that play major roles in cell differentiation and morphogenesis. Whereas Sonic hedgehog (Shh) has widespread roles in many developmental processes, Ihh's function is restricted to the skeleton and gut. In the skeleton, Ihh plays an essential role in regulating chondrocyte differentiation via the Pthlh/Ihh loop, thereby regulating growth plate morphology and function. Furthermore, Ihh is important for joint formation and the development of cortical bone. Both are absent in Ihh-deficient mice. Ihh also plays a role in osteoblast differentiation of the cranial sutures.

Philadelphia-type craniosynostosis has been shown to be caused by duplications upstream of the *IHH* gene involving regulatory sites that are located within an intron of the next flanking gene, *NHEJ1*. This region contains enhancers that show activity at the Ihh-specific sites: the growth plates, the digit tips, and the cranial sutures. The size and location of the duplications are likely to determine whether the phenotype consists of syndactyly with craniosynostosis or only syndactyly.

References

Klopocki E, Lohan S, Brancati F, Koll R, Brehm A, Seemann P et al (2011) Copy-number variations involving the IHH locus are associated with syndactyly and craniosynostosis. Am J Hum Genet 88(1):70–75

Robin NH, Segel B, Carpenter G, Muenke M (1996) Craniosynostosis, Philadelphia type: a new autosomal dominant syndrome with sagittal craniosynostosis and syndactyly of the fingers and toes. Am J Med Genet 62(2):184–191

S. Mundlos, D. Horn, *Limb Malformations*,
DOI 10.1007/978-3-540-95928-1_24, © Springer-Verlag Berlin Heidelberg 2014

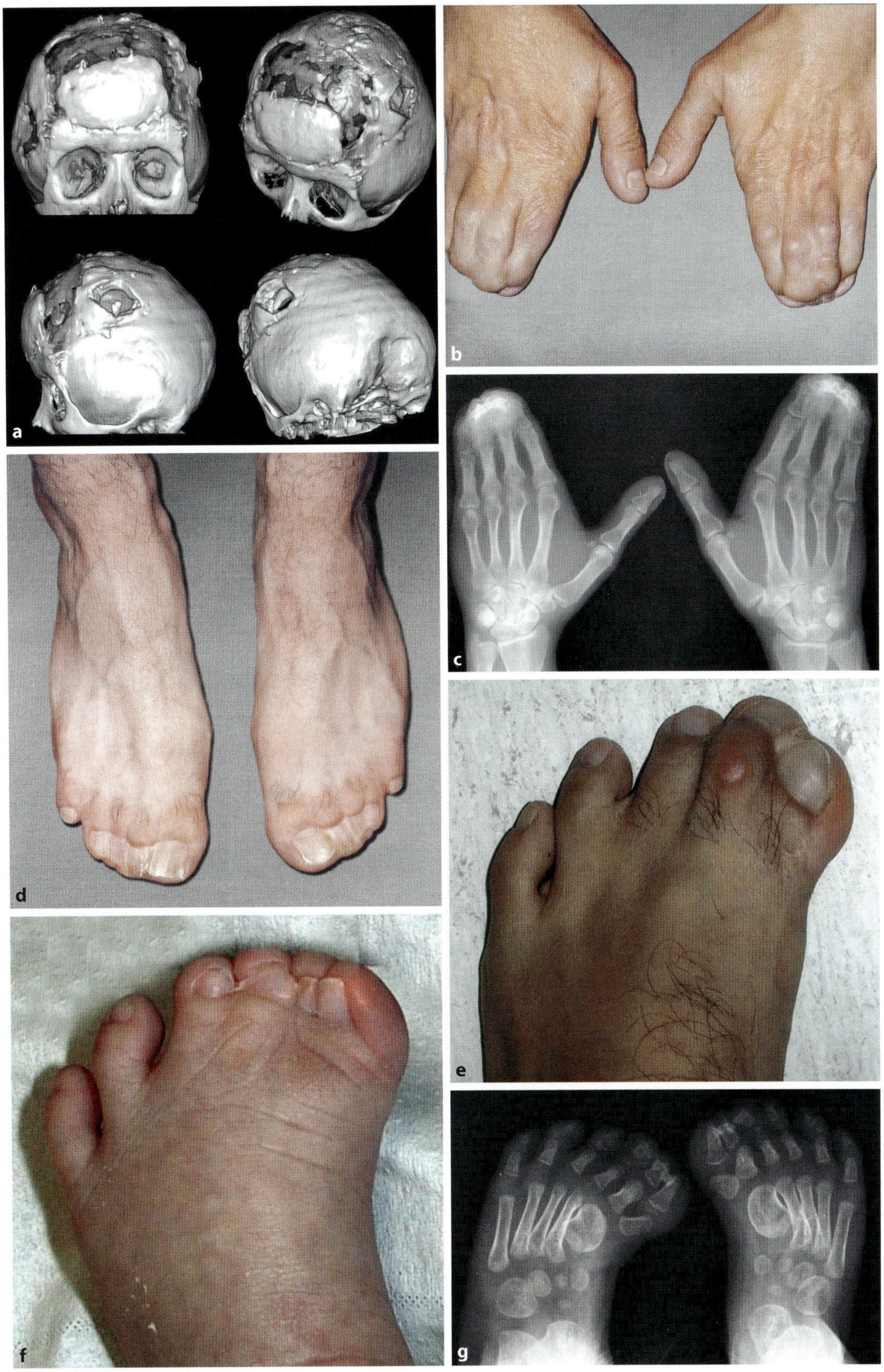

Fig. 24.1 **a** Three-dimensional computed tomography scan of skull after partial correction of multiple suture synostosis. **b** Complete syndactyly II–V bilaterally. **c** Corresponding radiographs showing distal bony fusion of phalanges II–V. **d–f** Foot phenotypes. **d** Complete syndactyly of all toes with fusion of nails (same individual as in **b**). **e** Syndactyly of toes I–III, malformation of great toe. **f** Newborn with preaxial polydactyly of feet. **g** Corresponding radiograph showing preaxial polydactyly; broad, round metatarsal I; and distal bony fusion of phalanges. (**a**, **f** from Klopocki et al. 2011, **b–d** from Robin et al. 1996)

25 Fraser Syndrome

MIM 219000

Synonyms
Cryptophthalmos–syndactyly syndrome

Major Clinical Findings
Fraser syndrome is characterized by cryptophthalmos, syndactyly, ear malformations, and abnormal genitalia. Cryptophthalmos is found in the majority of cases and may be unilateral. Eyelashes, Meibomian glands, and lacrimal glands are absent. Soft tissue syndactyly is seen in two-thirds of affected individuals. In most cases, fingers and toes are affected. Intellectual disability is observed in approximately 50%.

Occasional Findings
Cleft lip/palate, abnormal eyebrows and nose, laryngeal and tracheal abnormalities, encephalocele, umbilical hernia, urogenital anomalies.

Genetic Transmission
Autosomal recessive.

Differential Diagnosis
Fraser syndrome should be distinguished from isolated cryptophthalmos as well as from ablepharon–macrostomia syndrome.

Molecular Pathology
Fraser syndrome is genetically heterogeneous and can be caused by homozygous or compound heterozygous mutation in the *FRAS1* gene, the *FREM2* gene, or the *GRIP1* gene.

References

McGregor L, Makela V, Darling SM, Vrontou S, Chalepakis G, Roberts C et al (2003) Fraser syndrome and mouse blebbed phenotype caused by mutations in FRAS1/Fras1 encoding a putative extracellular matrix protein. Nature Genet 34:203–208

Shafeghati Y, Kniepert A, Vakili G, Zenker M (2008) Fraser syndrome due to homozygosity for a splice site mutation of FREM2. Am J Med Genet 146A:529–531

Thomas IT, Frias JL, Felix V, Sanchez de Leon L, Hernandez RA, Jones MC (1986) Isolated and syndromic cryptophthalmos. Am J Med Genet 25:85–98

van Haelst MM, Maiburg M, Baujat G, Jadeja S, Monti E, Bland E et al (2008) Molecular study of 33 families with Fraser syndrome: new data and mutation review. Am J Med Genet 146A:2252–2257

Vogel MJ, van Zon P, Brueton L, Gijzen M, van Tuil MC, Cox P et al (2012) Mutations in GRIP1 cause Fraser syndrome. J Med Genet 49:303–306

S. Mundlos, D. Horn, *Limb Malformations*,
DOI 10.1007/978-3-540-95928-1_25, © Springer-Verlag Berlin Heidelberg 2014

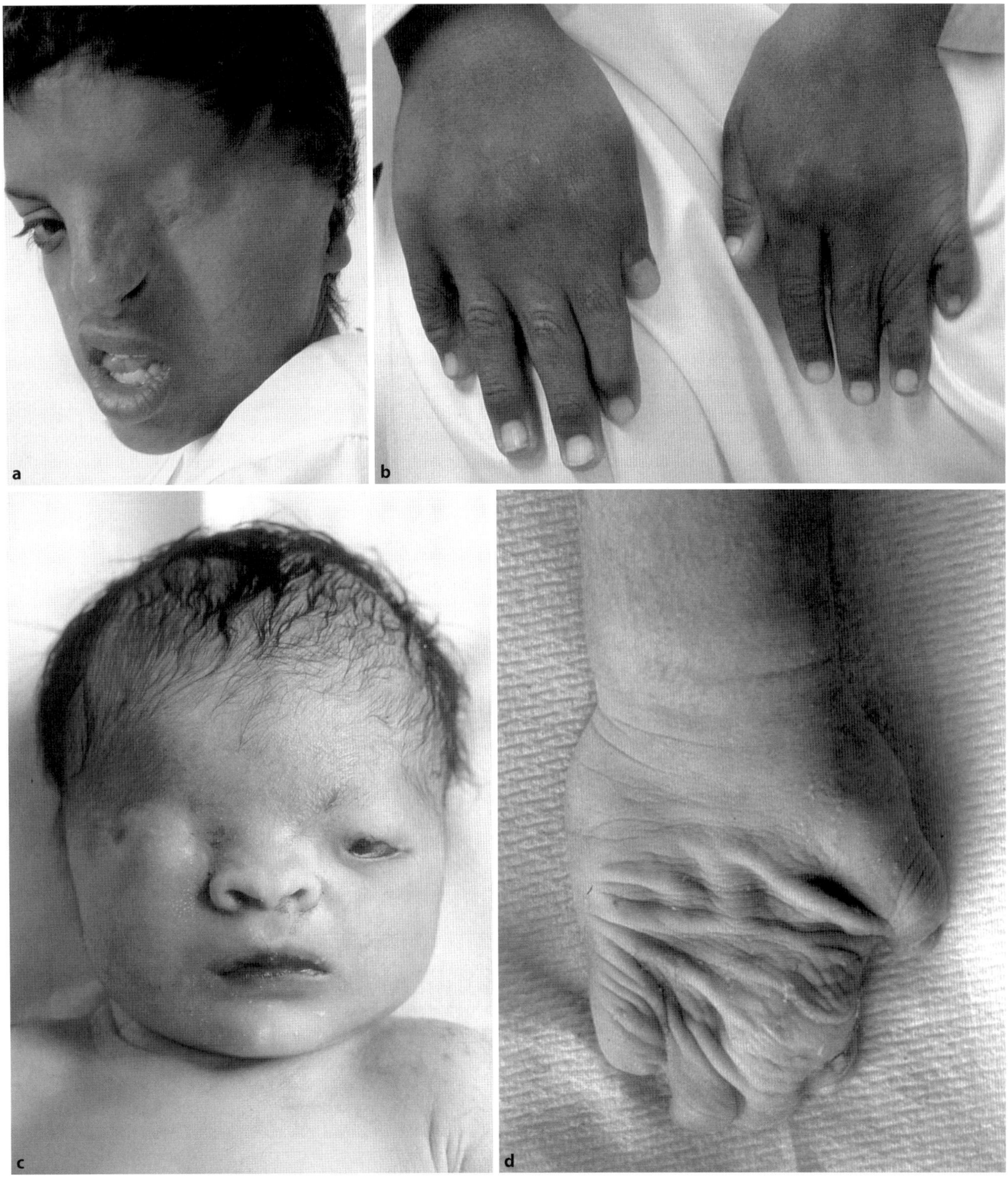

Fig. 25.1 **a** Unilateral cryptophthalmos and ear malformation. **b** Hands of same individual showing partial syndactyly II/III on the right and cutaneous syndactyly III/IV on the left. **c** Newborn showing cryptophthalmos on the right, microphthalmus, and malformation of eyelids on the left. **d** Syndactyly of digits II–V

26 Cenani–Lenz Syndrome

MIM 212780

Synonyms

Cenani syndactylism
Cenani–Lenz syndactyly
Syndactyly, type VII

Major Clinical Findings

Cenani–Lenz syndrome is a complex limb malformation featuring synostoses of the metacarpals and phalanges with oligodactyly. Radiography shows complete disorganization of the metacarpals and phalanges and partial absence of the carpals. Variable findings include shortening of the ulna and radius with fusion. In the most severe cases, this results in a single cuboid-shaped bone replacing the radius and ulna. The feet are less severely affected but also show syndactyly. Abnormalities of the spine with hemivertebrae and rib fusions occur. A specific facial appearance has been reported, consisting of a high, prominent forehead; hypertelorism; downward slanting palpebral fissures; a short nose; a short, prominent philtrum; deep-set eyes; low-set ears; retrognathia; and malar hypoplasia. Renal aplasia/hypoplasia has been reported in approximately 50 % of patients.

Genetic Transmission

Autosomal recessive.

Differential Diagnosis

The clinical findings are rather specific. Considerable clinical variability may cause diagnostic problems.

Molecular Pathology

Cenani–Lenz syndrome is caused by loss of function mutations in LRP4. LRP4 is a multifunctional receptor implicated in the regulation of several molecular pathways, including Wnt and Bmp signaling. It is expressed in the apical ectodermal ridge in the developing limb bud, and its inactivation in mice results in polysyndactyly. Structural variations at the *GREM1–FMN1* locus may cause a similar phenotype.

References

Cenani A, Lenz W (1967) Totale Syndaktylie und totale radioulnare Synostose bie zwei Bruedern. Ein Beitrag zur Genetik der Syndaktylien. Ztschr Kinderheilk 101:181–190

Dimitrov BI, Voet T, De Smet L, Vermeesch JR, Devriendt K, Fryns JP et al (2010) Genomic rearrangements of the GREM1-FMN1 locus cause oligosyndactyly, radio-ulnar synostosis, hearing loss, renal defects syndrome and Cenani–Lenz-like non-syndromic oligosyndactyly. J Med Genet 47:569–74

Li Y, Pawlik B, Elcioglu N, Aglan M, Kayserili H, Yigit G et al (2010) LRP4 mutations alter Wnt/beta-catenin signaling and cause limb and kidney malformations in Cenani–Lenz syndrome. Am J Hum Genet 86:696–706

Fig. 26.1 Phenotypic variability in Cenani–Lenz syndrome. **a** Short, small hands; broad digit on radial side; three very short digits on the right and two on the left. **b** Corresponding radiograph of right hand showing complete disorganization of phalanges and four metacarpals, of which the ulnar one is broad and probably represents a fusion of metacarpals IV/V. The rudimentary thumb is fused with residual phalanges of digit II. There is bony fusion of proximal phalanges III and IV, and a rudimentary digit V is visible. Multiple delta phalangeal development. **c** Hands with only three digits: a broad thumb and two rudimentary digits. **d** Corresponding radiograph showing a loss of organization of phalanges. There is fusion of the proximal phalanges to a single bone with laterally placed (delta phalangeal) epiphyses. The phalanges of the 1st digit are abnormally shaped, with laterally placed epiphyses. Only three metacarpals are present. The most ulnar one is broad and probably represents the fusion of two. **e** Radiograph of severely affected individual showing fusions of metacarpals II–V to a single bone; digit I remains as the only single digit. There are fusions of phalanges to round structures with lateral or circular epiphyses (fused delta phalangeal epiphyses). **f** Foot phenotype of individual in **a**. Short toes, with syndactyly of toes I–III on the right and II/III on the left. **g** Corresponding radiograph. Note fusion of metatarsals IV/V bilaterally. **h** Radiograph of severely affected fetus. Note complete fusion of radius and ulna to a single bone on the left and a single cuboid-shaped forearm bone on the right. Few bony structures of the hands are visible (note that fibula is also present on the right). (Courtesy of Bernd Wollnik, University of Cologne, Germany, and Hülya Kayserili, Istanbul University, Turkey)

S. Mundlos, D. Horn, *Limb Malformations*,
DOI 10.1007/978-3-540-95928-1_26, © Springer-Verlag Berlin Heidelberg 2014

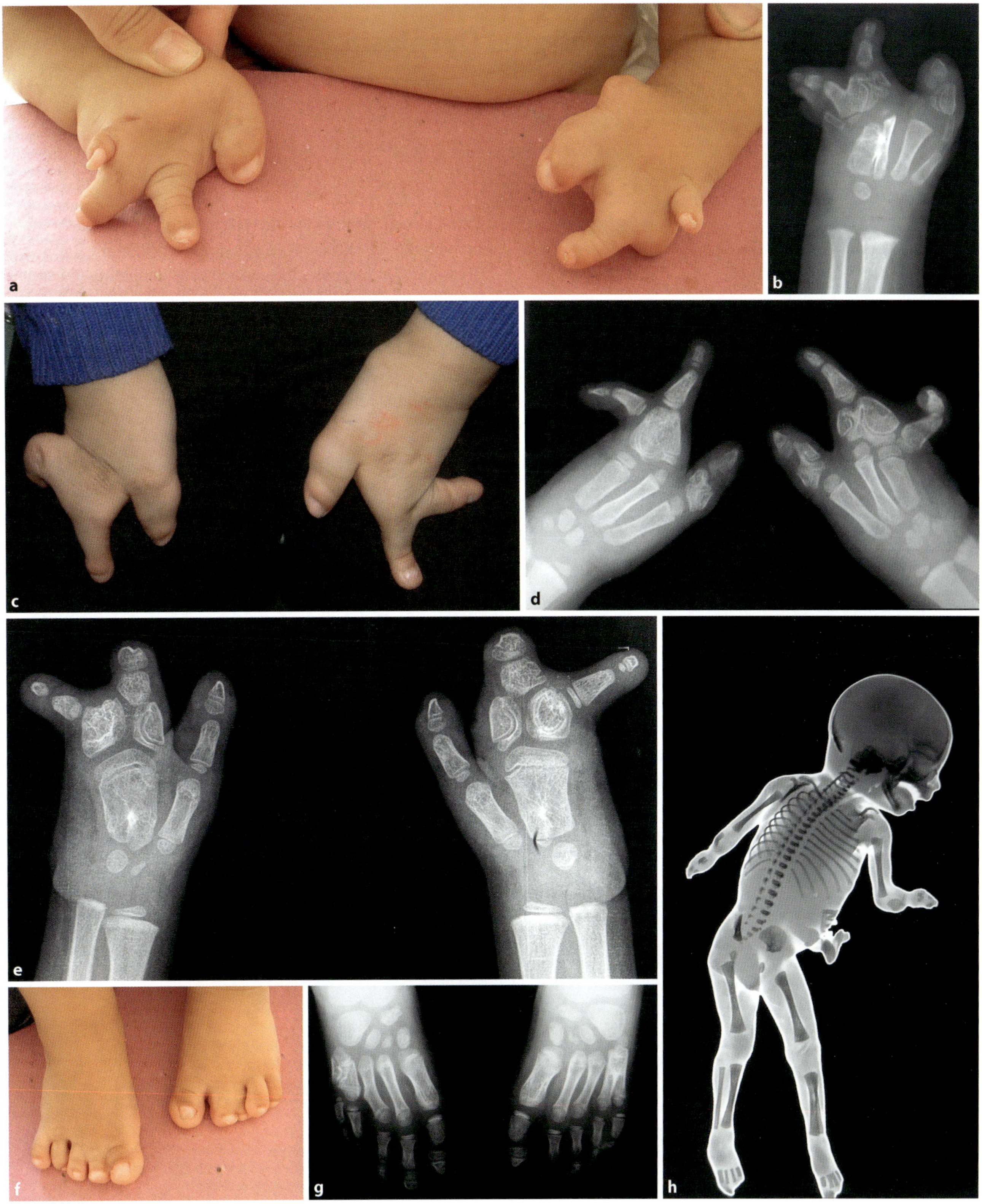
a
b
c
d
e
f
g
h

27 Oculodentodigital Dysplasia

MIM 164200

Included
Isolated Syndactyly Type III
MIM 186100

Synonyms
Oculodentoosseous dysplasia

Major Clinical Findings
Oculodentodigital dysplasia (ODDD) is a complex malformation syndrome exhibiting distinct craniofacial and limb anomalies. Syndactyly involving digits IV and V, which has also been termed syndactyly III, is the most common feature in this condition. However, additional digits may be involved. Affected individuals have a characteristic facial appearance with a pinched, narrow nose and/or hypoplastic alae nasi. The teeth are often small and carious due to enamel hypoplasia. Selective tooth agenesis and microdontia may be present. Typical eye findings include microphthalmia, microcornea, cataracts, and anomalies of the iris. Neurological defects include dysarthria, neurogenic bladder disturbances, spastic paraparesis, ataxia, anterior tibial muscle weakness, and seizures. Other features include conductive hearing loss, diffuse yellow-orange nonepidermolytic hyperkeratosis on the palms and soles, and fine, dry, sparse, slow-growing hair. An autosomal recessive variant of ODDD exists with a similar but more severe phenotype.

Occasional Findings
Cleft palate, hyperkeratosis of the palms and soles, cardiac abnormalities including atrioseptal defect and cardiac conduction abnormalities, hyperostosis of the skull and vertebrae.

Genetic Transmission
Autosomal dominant, autosomal recessive (rare).

Differential Diagnosis
ODDD and "isolated" syndactyly type III (MIM 186100) are likely to represent a disease spectrum rather than separate genetic conditions. The recessive form of ODDD has been reported to show overlap with Hallermann–Streiff syndrome.

Molecular Pathology
ODDD is caused by mutations in the connexin 43 gene (*GJA1*). Connexins are the pore-forming subunits of gap junction channels. Cx43 allows cell networks to respond to extracellular stimuli via the propagation of specific signals converging on connexin-sensitive transcriptional units. These are important for many tissues and cells, including myocytes, neurons, and osteoblasts. GJA1 is strongly expressed in the distal part of early limb buds and in the developing digits and regions of precartilage condensation, corresponding to the phenotype. The recessive form of ODDD is also caused by mutations in *GJA1*.

References

Paznekas WA, Boyadjiev SA, Shapiro RE, Daniels O, Wollnik B, Keegan CE et al (2003) Connexin 43 (*GJA1*) mutations cause the pleiotropic phenotype of oculodentodigital dysplasia. Am J Hum Genet 72:408–418

Richardson RJ, Joss S, Tomkin S, Ahmed M, Sheridan E, Dixon MJ (2006) A nonsense mutation in the first transmembrane domain of connexin 43 underlies autosomal recessive oculodentodigital syndrome. J Med Genet 43:e37

Schrander-Stumpel CTRM, De Groot-Wijnands JBG, De Diesmulders CEM, Fryns JP (1993) Type III syndactyly and oculodentodigital dysplasia: a clinical spectrum. Genet Counsel 4:271–276

S. Mundlos, D. Horn, *Limb Malformations*,
DOI 10.1007/978-3-540-95928-1_27, © Springer-Verlag Berlin Heidelberg 2014

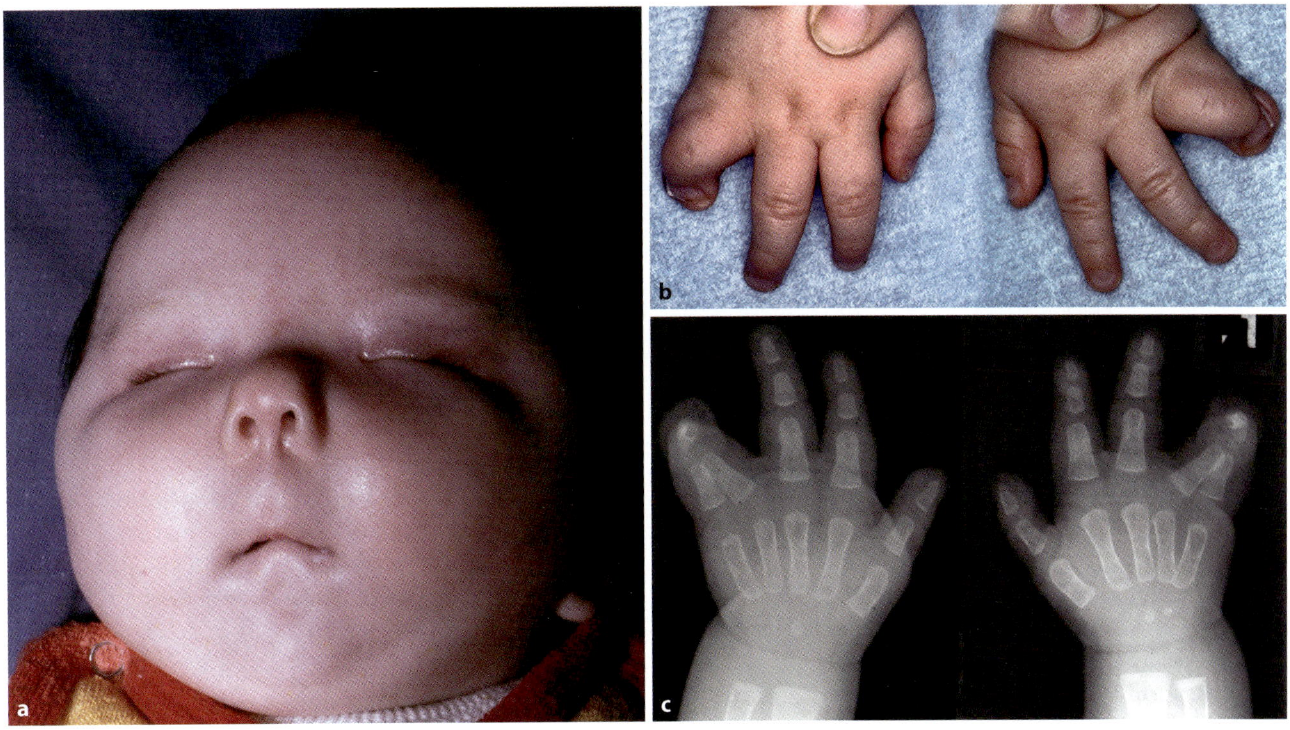

Fig. 27.1 **a** Typical facial appearance in oculodentodigital dysplasia. Narrow, upturned, laterally pinched nose with hypoplastic alae nasi, narrow nasal bridge, long and prominent columella, and small mouth. **b** Syndactyly IV/V bilaterally. **c** Corresponding radiograph of hands reveals soft tissue syndactyly and bony synostosis of fingers IV/V with a distal reduction defect

28 Oro-Facial-Digital Syndrome, Type 1

MIM 311200

Major Clinical Findings

Oro-facial-digital syndrome type I (OFD1) is characterized by oral, facial, and digital abnormalities. The facial aspect consists of a broad nasal root, hypertelorism, dystopia canthorum, abnormalities of the upper lip, hypoplasia of the alar cartilages, and sparse scalp hair. Evanescent milia of the face occur in the first years of life. Characteristic oral manifestations are hyperplastic frenulae; irregular margin of the lips with a median cleft lip (in approximately 50%); abnormalities of the tongue, including lobulated or bifid tongue, tongue nodules, and tongue hamartomas (in approximately 70%); and cleft palate. Irregular lobulation of the tongue and hamartoma formation on the ventral surface are seen in most affected females. Digital abnormalities include brachydactyly, clinodactyly, and syndactyly. Toe malformations are observed in 25% and include unilateral or bilateral preaxial polysyndactyly, brachydactyly, and syndactyly. In some instances, postaxial polydactyly of the hands and feet has been documented. Radiographs of the hands and feet show short and thick tubular bones, an irregular pattern of radiolucency and/or spicule-like formation in the metacarpal and phalangeal bones, and cone-shaped epiphyses of phalanges.

Adult-onset bilateral polycystic kidneys and medullary cystic renal disease are present in approximately 50%. Progressive renal insufficiency occurs in some instances, as does fibrocystic liver with dilatation of the intrahepatic bile ducts resulting in hepatic fibrosis. Mild developmental delay is observed in about 40%. Various malformations of the central nervous system are seen (hydrocephaly, porencephaly, agenesis of corpus callosum).

Occasional Findings

Malposition of teeth, small mandible, aplasia of mandibular lateral incisors.

Genetic Transmission

X-linked dominant with lethality in males.

Differential Diagnosis

Clinical features overlap with those reported in other forms of orofaciodigital syndromes. OFD1 can be distinguished from other forms of orofaciodigital syndrome by its X-linked dominant inheritance pattern and by polycystic kidney disease, which seems to be specific for this type. Most clinical overlap exists between type 1 and type 2, which is autosomal recessively inherited. Patients with OFD2 do not show hyperplastic frenulae. Hyperplastic frenulae, a mild cleft of the upper lip, and brachydactyly can be seen in Ellis–van Creveld syndrome.

Molecular Pathology

OFD1 is caused by mutations in the *OFD1* gene. Because the OFD1 protein localizes to the centrosome and basal body of primary cilia, OFD1 is considered to be a ciliopathy. Ofd1 is essential for primary cilia function in mice and zebrafish.

References

Ferrante MI, Giorgio G, Feather SA, Bulfone A, Wright V, Ghiani M et al (2001) Identification of the gene for oral-facial-digital type I syndrome. Am J Hum Genet 68:569–576

Ferrante MI, Romio L, Castro S, Collins JE, Goulding DA, Stemple et al (2009) Convergent extension movements and ciliary function are mediated by ofd1, a zebrafish orthologue of the human oral-facial-digital type 1 syndrome gene. Hum Molec Genet 18:289–303

Gurrieri F, Franco B, Toriello H, Neri G (2007) Oral-facial-digital syndromes: review and diagnostic guidelines. Am J Med Genet 143A:3314–3323

Thauvin-Robinet C, Cossee M, Cormier-Daire V, Van Maldergem L, Toutain A, Alembik Y et al (2006) Clinical, molecular, and genotype-phenotype correlation studies from 25 cases of oral-facial-digital syndrome type 1: a French and Belgian collaborative study. (Letter). J Med Genet 43:54–61

S. Mundlos, D. Horn, *Limb Malformations*,
DOI 10.1007/978-3-540-95928-1_28,

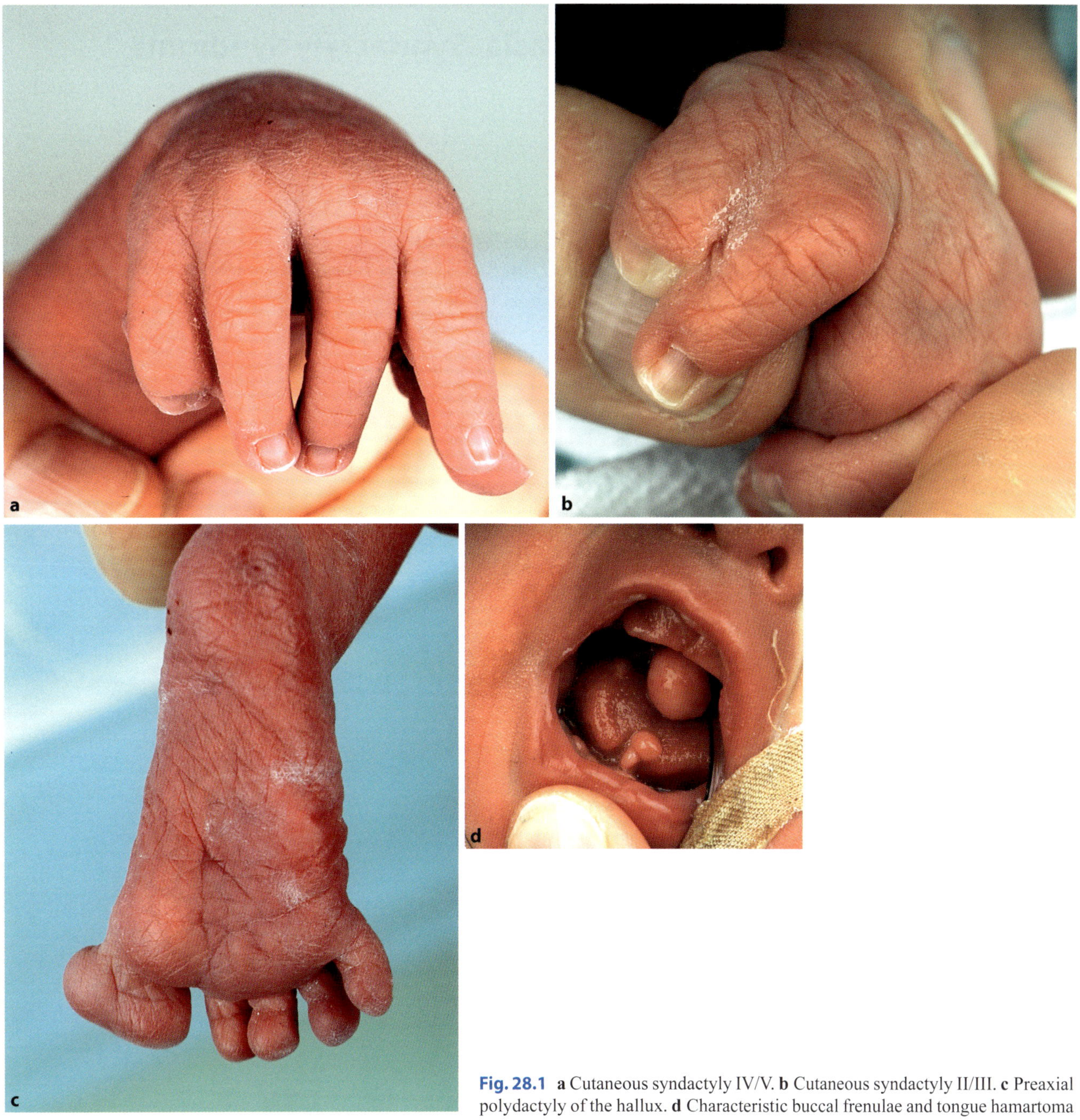

Fig. 28.1 **a** Cutaneous syndactyly IV/V. **b** Cutaneous syndactyly II/III. **c** Preaxial polydactyly of the hallux. **d** Characteristic buccal frenulae and tongue hamartoma

29 Ectodermal Dysplasia–Syndactyly Syndrome

MIM 613573

Major Clinical Findings
Ectodermal abnormalities in this condition consist of sparse scalp hair, sparse to absent eyebrows and eyelashes, and conical and cylindrical teeth with enamel hypoplasia. Hair loss progresses to nearly complete or even complete alopecia in the second decade of life. All affected individuals manifest cutaneous syndactyly of fingers II/III and/or III/IV and of toes II/III and/or III/IV. Most patients have hyperkeratosis of the palms.

Occasional Findings
Morphological hair abnormalities, hypoplastic and thickened nails with abnormal color.

Genetic Transmission
Autosomal recessive.

Differential Diagnosis
Normal sweating differentiates this syndrome from other types of syndromic ectodermal dysplasia with limb abnormalities, such as ectrodactyly–ectodermal dysplasia–cleft lip/palate (EEC) syndrome.

Molecular Pathology
Ectodermal dysplasia–syndactyly syndrome 1 is caused by homozygous or compound heterozygous mutations in the *PVRL4* gene. *PVRL4* encodes for nectin-4, a cell adhesion molecule mainly implicated in the formation of cadherin-based adherens junctions.

References

Brancati F, Fortugno P, Bottillo I, Lopez M, Josselin E, Boudghene-Stambouli O et al (2010) Mutations in PVRL4, encoding cell adhesion molecule nectin-4, cause ectodermal dysplasia-syndactyly syndrome. Am J Hum Genet 87:265–273

S. Mundlos, D. Horn, *Limb Malformations*,
DOI 10.1007/978-3-540-95928-1_29, © Springer-Verlag Berlin Heidelberg 2014

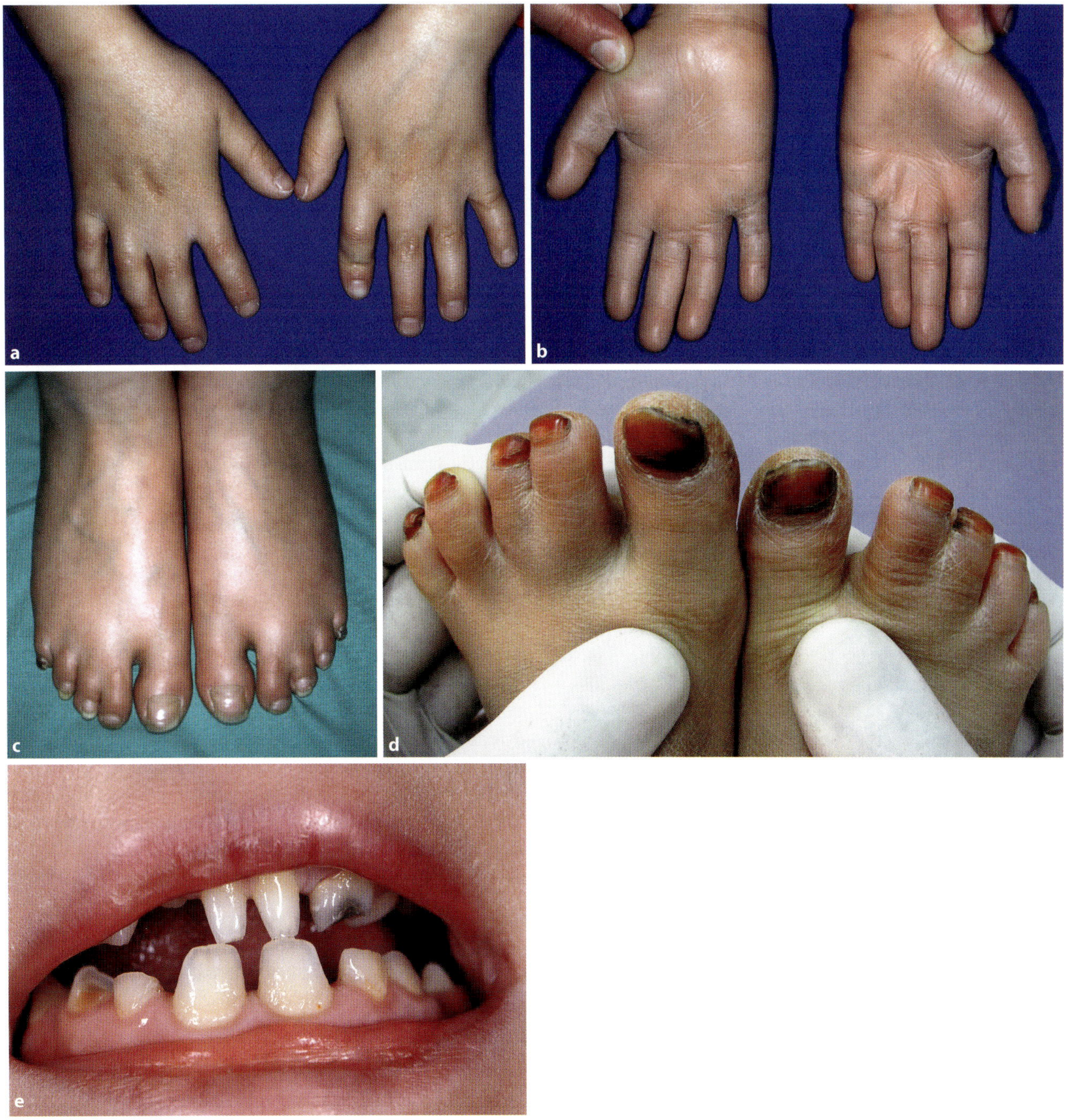

Fig 29.1 **a** Hands with mild syndactyly II–V. **b** Palmar view. Note dry skin with hyperkeratosis and a relatively long palm due to partial webbing. **c** Syndactyly of toes II/III and, to a lesser degree, IV/V. **d** Syndactyly of toes II/III and hyperkeratosis. **e** Hypodontia and abnormally shaped incisors

30 Smith–Lemli–Opitz Syndrome

MIM 270400

Major Clinical Findings

Smith–Lemli–Opitz syndrome (SLOS) is a multiple congenital malformation and intellectual disability syndrome with a broad clinical spectrum and phenotypes ranging from mild to severe. SLOS occurs in approximately 1 in 20,000–30,000 births in populations of northern and central European background. SLOS is mainly characterized by growth retardation, microcephaly, psychomotor delay, soft tissue syndactyly of the 2nd and 3rd toes, and genital abnormalities. In males, genital findings range from mild anomalies to sex reversal. Severely affected individuals exhibit multiple malformations in the central nervous system (including the eye), heart, kidney, and bowel. Individuals with a severe phenotype may die in the neonatal period because of failure to thrive and hepatic dysfunction. More mildly affected patients show a better prognosis. Characteristic facial features include ptosis, strabismus, a flat nasal bridge, anteverted nares, and micrognathia. Cleft palate has been observed in about 50%.

Postaxial polydactyly of the hands and feet is observed in 25% of mildly affected individuals and in 75% of those severely affected. Soft tissue syndactyly of the 2nd and 3rd toes has been documented in about 80%. Because of a short 1st metacarpal, the thumb appears to be short; a short 1st metatarsal is a frequent radiographic feature. Dislocated hips occur in about 50% of the affected individuals. Positional foot abnormalities are frequent.

Individuals with SLOS show a characteristic behavioral profile of psychomotor delay, language impairment, sleep disturbance, self-injurious behavior, and autism spectrum of behavior. Cholesterol supplementation may improve the clinical course.

Occasional Findings

Clinodactyly of fingers, holoprosencephaly, partial agenesis of the cerebellar vermis, agenesis of the corpus callosum, seizures, lung abnormalities, hypoplastic labia majora, upper urinary tract anomalies, renal cysts, hypoplasia of the kidneys, various congenital heart defects, broad maxillary alveolar ridges, and increased photosensitivity.

Genetic Transmission

Autosomal recessive.

Differential Diagnosis

Pallister–Hall syndrome can be distinguished by the presence of a hypothalamic hamartoblastoma.

Molecular Pathology

SLOS is caused by homozygous or compound heterozygous mutations in the *DHCR7* gene encoding sterol delta-7-reductase, the penultimate enzyme of mammalian sterol biosynthesis that converts 7-dehydrocholesterol (7-DHC) to cholesterol. Deficiency of 7-dehydrocholesterol reductase is the causative factor of SLOS. The mutation spectrum of *DHCR7* varies significantly among populations.

References

Opitz JM, Penchaszadeh VB, Holt MC, Spano LM (1987) Smith–Lemli–Opitz (RSH) syndrome bibliography. Am J Med Genet 28:745–750

Wassif CA, Maslen C, Kachilele-Linjewile S, Lin D, Linck LM, Connor WE et al (1998) Mutations in the human sterol delta-7-reductase gene at 11q12–13 cause Smith–Lemli–Opitz syndrome. Am J Hum Genet 63:55–62

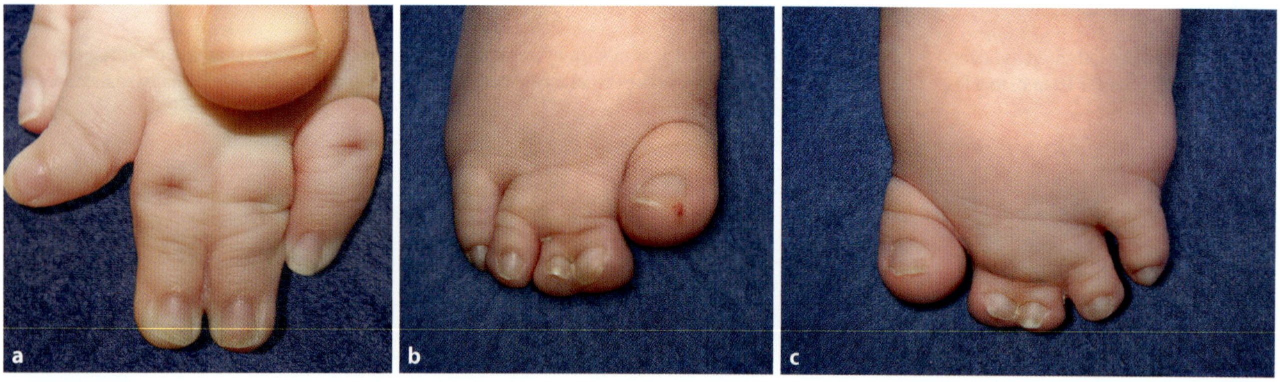

Fig. 30.1 **a** Syndactyly of digits III/IV, radial deviation of digit II. **b, c** Feet of the same individual showing typical syndactyly of toes II/III as well as partial syndactyly with toe IV

S. Mundlos, D. Horn, *Limb Malformations*,
DOI 10.1007/978-3-540-95928-1_30, © Springer-Verlag Berlin Heidelberg 2014

Part VI

Disorders: Brachydactyly Isolated

31 Brachydactyly Type A1

MIM 112500

Synonyms
BDA1
Farabee type brachydactyly

Major Clinical Findings
Brachydactyly type A1 (BDA1) is characterized by short broad hands with proportionate shortening of all digits (the thumb is less affected) due to small or missing middle phalanges. Interphalangeal creases are often missing, and bending in the interphalangeal joints is diminished. Radiographs show primarily short or absent middle phalanges, but commonly short distal phalanges, symphalangism, and small proximal phalanges with broad epiphyses. The 2nd and 5th digits are the most severely affected. The metacarpals are frequently short and show broad epiphyses. Also seen are additional carpals adjacent to the metacarpal bases; short, absent middle phalanges of the toes; and short proximal phalanges of the great toe. In severely affected individuals the entire skeleton is affected, and short stature is observed.

Occasional Findings
Some affected individuals may have involvement of the proximal phalanges with overlaps to brachydactyly type C.

Genetic Transmission
Autosomal dominant.

Differential Diagnosis
In some affected individuals, there is considerable overlap with brachydactyly type C. In fact, families have been described in which both conditions appear to coexist. Shortening of the middle phalanges may also occur in other brachydactylies, in particular types C and B, and in brachydactyly-associated conditions including the various acrocephalosyndactyly syndromes and in trichorhinophalangeal syndrome. In the latter, however, characteristic cone-shaped epiphyses are present.

Molecular Pathology
BDA1 is caused by mutations in *Indian hedgehog* (*IHH*), which belongs to the family of hedgehog signaling proteins. Its expression is restricted to the cartilaginous anlagen, the digit tips, and prehypertrophic chondrocytes in the growth plate. Ihh is a central signaling molecule for skeletal development that is essential for chondrocyte differentiation, development of joints, and bone formation. Like Shh, Ihh binds to its receptor Ptch, which, by binding to Smo, activates Gli transcription factors that regulate downstream target genes. The changes identified in BDA1 are missense mutations that cluster in certain areas of the Ihh molecule, suggesting a specific mutational mechanism. In a mouse model carrying a human BDA1 mutation, it was shown that the mutation results in a gain of function because of impaired binding to the hedgehog inhibitor Hip and the receptor Ptch. This results in a change in the potency and range of hedgehog signaling in the digits, which interferes with normal digit and joint development. At least one other locus for BDA1 is known.

Remarks
This trait was the first in humans to be interpreted in Mendelian dominant terms, by Farabee in 1903. BDA1 is allelic to acrocapitofemoral dysplasia, a recessive disorder with cone-shaped epiphyses in the hands and hips.

References

Gao B, Guo J, She C, Shu A, Yang M, Tan Z et al (2001) Mutations in IHH, encoding Indian hedgehog, cause brachydactyly type A-1. Nat Genet 28(4):3864–3868

Gao B, Hu J, Stricker S, Cheung M, Ma G, Law KF et al (2009) A mutation in Ihh that causes digit abnormalities alters its signalling capacity and range. Nature 458(7242):1196–1200

McCready ME, Sweeney E, Fryer AE, Donnai D, Baig A, Racacho L et al (2002) A novel mutation in the IHH gene causes brachydactyly type A1: a 95-year-old mystery resolved. Hum Genet 111:3684

S. Mundlos, D. Horn, *Limb Malformations*,
DOI 10.1007/978-3-540-95928-1_31, © Springer-Verlag Berlin Heidelberg 2014

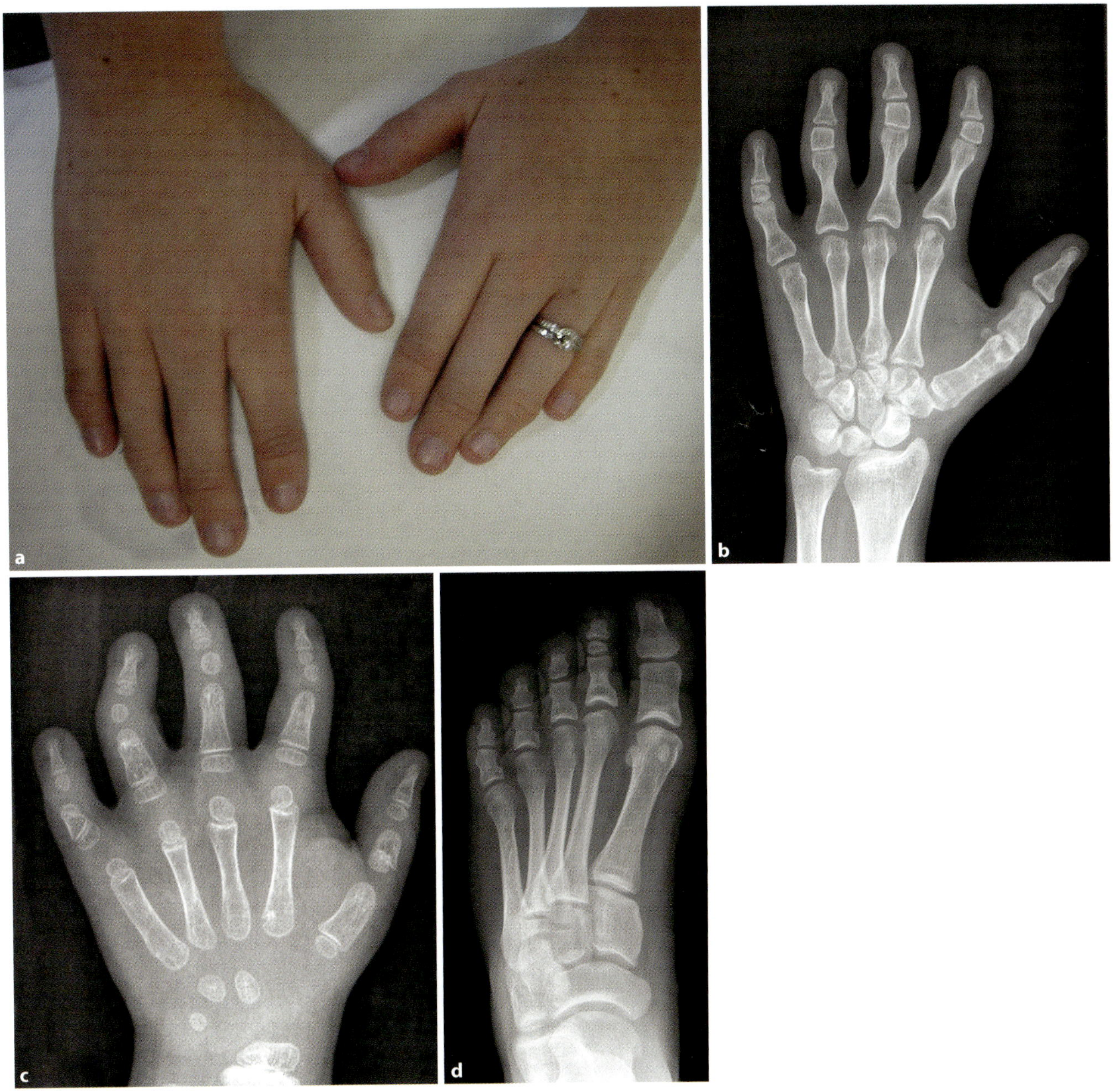

Fig. 31.1 **a** Very short or missing middle phalanges in brachydactyly type A1. **b** Radiograph shows classic short, cuboidal middle phalanges II–V in an adult. **c** Radiograph at age 39 months demonstrates short, bullet-shaped proximal phalanges with relatively large epiphyses; round, rudimentary ossification centers of the middle phalanges; and round, enlarged epiphyses of distal phalanges I and V. The thumb is the least affected digit. **d** Radiograph of foot shows small middle phalanx in toe II and missing middle phalanges in toes III–V

32 Brachydactyly Type A2

MIM 112600

Synonyms

BDA2
Brachymesophalangy II
Mohr–Wriedt type brachydactyly

Major Clinical Findings

Brachydactyly type A2 (BDA2) is characterized by short or absent middle phalanges of the 2nd finger and, to a lesser degree, the 5th finger. The index finger is short and frequently deviated medially due to the abnormal triangular shape of the middle 2nd phalanx. There is variable 5th-finger clinodactyly due to the abnormal shape of the middle phalanx, as well as short and broad laterally deviated halluces and medially deviated 2nd toes.

Occasional Findings

Syndactyly, delta-shaped epiphyses of the middle and proximal phalanges of fingers II and III, broad terminal phalanx of finger II.

Genetic Transmission

Autosomal dominant.

Differential Diagnoses

BDA2 shows overlap with brachydactyly type C (BDC). Mild forms of BDC may resemble BDA2, and vice versa. Brachydactyly with short 2nd and 5th fingers has also been called brachydactyly type A4 and is part of the phenotypic spectrum of BDA2. Brachydactyly type A3 is a normal variant affecting only digit V.

Molecular Pathology

BDA2 is genetically heterogenous. Specific mutations in *GDF5* that result in a selective inactivation of the binding to the BMP receptor 1B (BMPR1B) are a cause, as well as dominant negative mutations in the *GDF5* high-affinity receptor (BMPR1B) itself. A variant of BDA2 has also been shown to be caused by mutations in *GDF5* that interfere with cleavage of the GDF5 prodomain from the mature peptide. Furthermore, duplications of a regulatory region of BMP2 result in BDA2. Together, these findings suggest that BDA2 is caused by a deregulation of BMP signaling in the developing digits.

References

Dathe K, Kjaer KW, Brehm A, Meinecke P, Nurnberg P, Neto JC et al (2009) Duplications involving a conserved regulatory element downstream of BMP2 are associated with brachydactyly type A2. Am J Hum Genet 84:483–492

Lehmann K, Seemann P, Boergermann J, Morin G, Reif S, Knaus P et al (2006) A novel R486Q mutation in BMPR1B resulting in either a brachydactyly type C/symphalangism-like phenotype or brachydactyly type A2. Eur J Hum Genet 14(12):1248–1254

Lehmann K, Seemann P, Stricker S, Sammar M, Meyer B, Süring K et al (2003) Mutations in bone morphogenetic protein receptor 1B cause brachydactyly type A2. Proc Natl Acad Sci U S A 100(21):12277–12782

Plöger F, Seemann P, Schmidt-von Kegler M, Lehmann K, Seidel J, Kjaer KW et al (2008) Brachydactyly type A2 associated with a defect in proGDF5 processing. Hum Mol Genet 17(9):122–133

Seemann P, Schwappacher R, Kjaer KW, Krakow D, Lehmann K, Dawson K et al (2005) Activating and deactivating mutations in the receptor interaction site of GDF5 cause symphalangism or brachydactyly type A2. J Clin Invest 115(9):2373–2381

S. Mundlos, D. Horn, *Limb Malformations*,
DOI 10.1007/978-3-540-95928-1_32, © Springer-Verlag Berlin Heidelberg 2014

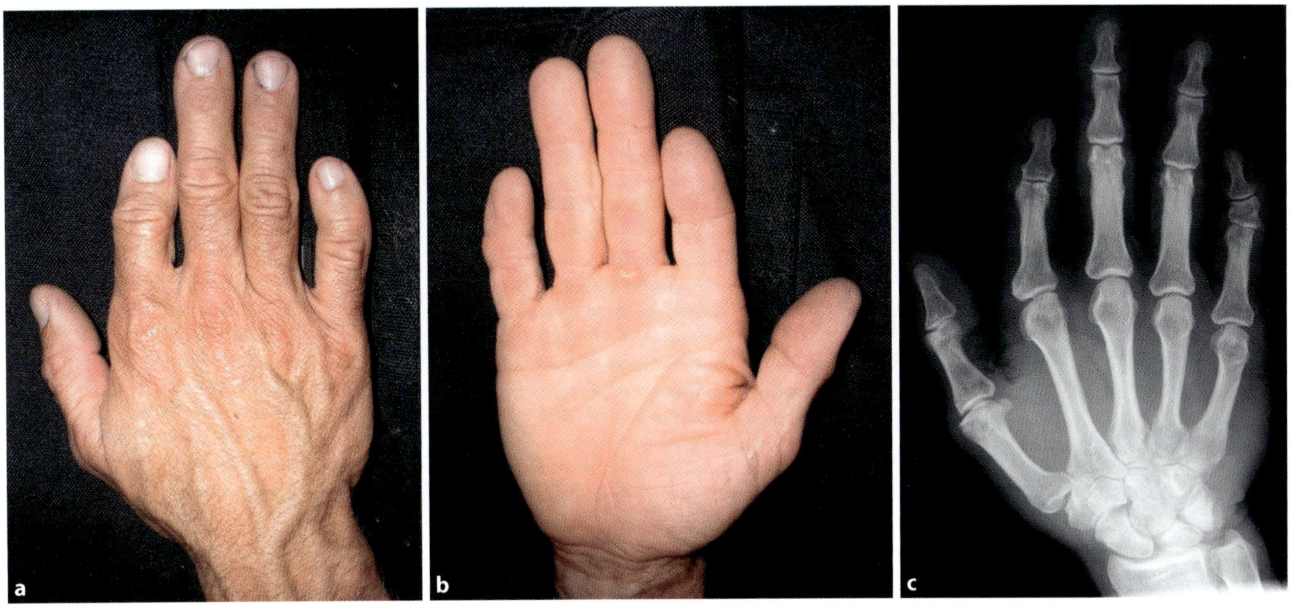

Fig. 32.1 Dorsal (**a**) and palmar (**b**) views of hand in an individual with brachydactyly type A2 and a mutation in *BMPR1B*. Note short digit II with missing interdigital crease and small middle phalanx of digit V. **c** Radiograph shows missing middle phalanx II and small middle phalanx V

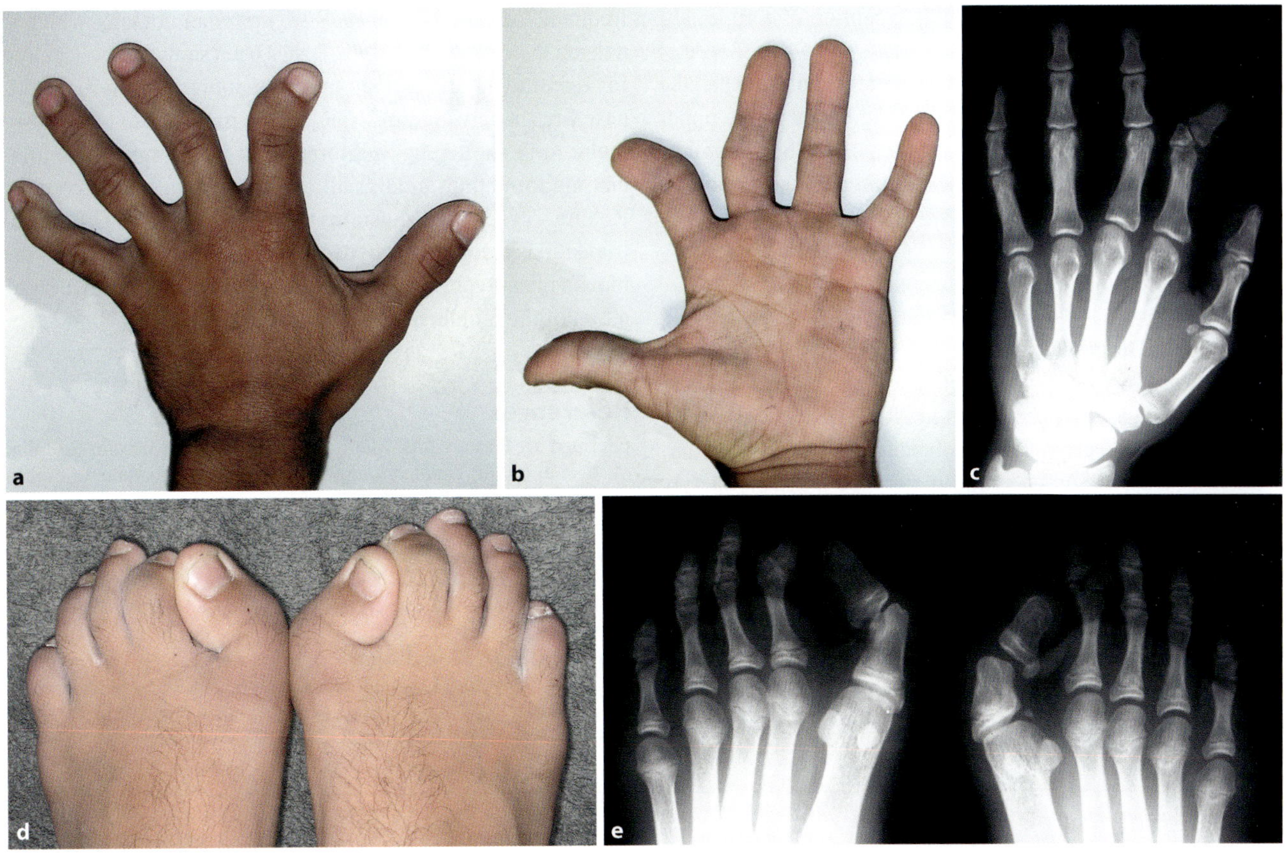

Fig. 32.2 Dorsal (**a**) and palmar (**b**) views of hand of an individual with brachydactyly type A2 and a duplication at the *BMP2* locus. Note absent middle phalanx II and radial deviation of distal phalanx. **c** Radiograph shows hypo/dysplastic, almost triangular middle phalanx II, resulting in the radial deviation of the distal phalanx. There is mild ulnar deviation of middle phalanx III at the proximal interphalangeal joint. **d,e** Feet showing lateral deviation of halluces due to (**e**) abnormally shaped proximal phalanx I. Note abnormally shaped middle phalanges of toes II and deviation of distal phalanx of left foot

33 Brachydactyly Type B1

MIM 113000

Major Clinical Findings

Brachydactyly type B1 (BDB1) is characterized by shortening/hypoplasia of the distal and, less frequently, middle phalanges of fingers II–V, resulting in an amputation-like phenotype. Additional findings include nail dysplasia, distal tapering of digits, syndactyly, camptodactyly, and variable degrees of distal and proximal symphalangism. Broad thumbs with or without distal duplication/clefts and syndactyly occur in severe cases. The feet show similar hypoplastic/aplastic distal phalanges. Fusion of carpal bones may occur. The motion of the hands is remarkably good, and patients adapt well to the deformity. A homozygous patient has been described who showed severe distal limb malformations with absence of all phalanges and nails with the exception of a rudimentary finger V. The metacarpals and metatarsals were of normal number but were hypoplastic and deformed, and some had the characteristics of carpal bones. The long bones of the upper limbs were normal in structure and shape but short. In addition, vertebral malformations and a small penis were noted.

Genetics Transmission

Autosomal dominant.

Differential Diagnosis

BDB1 shows overlap with brachydactyly type B2 (BDB2), a condition caused by mutations in NOGGIN. The presence of syndactyly and proximal symphalangism, however, is suggestive of BDB2. Sorsby syndrome is type B brachydactyly in association with symphalangism and macular colobomas. Cooks syndrome is somewhat similar to BDB1, featuring nail hypoplasia and distal symphalangism. However, in this condition the terminal phalanges are present.

Molecular Pathology

BDB1 is caused by mutations in the receptor tyrosine kinase ROR2 and is thus allelic to Robinow syndrome. The changes in BDB1 are frameshift and nonsense mutations predicted to result in truncation of the receptor, either the N-terminal or C-terminal of the tyrosine kinase (TK) domain. Mutations located in the C-terminal of the TK domain are associated with a more severe phenotype, that is, aplasia of the terminal and middle phalanges of digits II–V as well as duplications of the terminal phalanges of the thumb. The alterations located in the N-terminal of the TK are invariably frameshift mutations. In these individuals the thumbs are usually not affected, the terminal digits may be present to variable degrees, and terminal symphalangism is frequently observed. The ROR2 C-terminal domain, which is deleted in brachydactyly type B, has been shown to be required for recruitment and activation of the nonreceptor tyrosine kinase Src. Inactivation of ROR2 in the mouse results in mesomelic limb shortening, malformations of the spine, craniofacial malformations, and small external genitals, thus copying Robinow syndrome. Mutations that copy the human C-terminal truncations result in brachydactyly. However, in contrast to the human phenotype, the mutation is recessive, and the mice show a loss of the middle but not the distal phalanges.

References

Oldridge M, Fortuna AM, Maringa M, Propping P, Mansour S, Pollitt C et al (2000) Dominant mutations in ROR2, encoding an orphan receptor tyrosine kinase, cause brachydactyly type B. Nat Genet 24(3):275–278

Schwabe GC, Tinschert S, Buschow C, Meinecke P, Wolff G, Gillessen-Kaesbach G et al (2000) Distinct mutations in the receptor tyrosine kinase gene ROR2 cause brachydactyly type B. Am J Hum Genet 67(4):822–831

Schwabe GC, Trepczik B, Suring K, Brieske N, Tucker AS, Sharpe PT et al (2004) Ror2 knockout mouse as a model for the developmental pathology of autosomal recessive Robinow syndrome. Dev Dyn 229:400–410

Fig. 33.1 Phenotypes and variability in brachydactyly type B1. **a** Moderately affected individual showing absent distal phalanx of digit IV on the right and hypoplasia on the left. **b** Palmar view shows absent distal interphalangeal creases in digits IV and distal tapering and a rudimentary crease in the right digit III. **c** An individual from the same family showing missing distal phalanges of both digits IV, tapering of distal digits III, and broadening of distal digit II with nail hypoplasia. **d** The corresponding radiograph shows a normal thumb, abnormally shaped distal phalanx II with missing or fused middle phalanx, fusion of the middle phalanx with the distal phalanx in digit III, missing distal phalanx in digit IV, and fusion of the hypoplastic distal with the middle phalanx in digit V. **e** Close-up of distal phalanges II, III, and IV with fusion and abnormal shapes. **f** More severely affected individual with truncation in the middle phalanx of digits IV and distal hypoplasia and fusion in all digits. **g** The most severe form, with truncation at the level of the middle (digits II, III, and V) or even proximal phalanges (digit IV)

S. Mundlos, D. Horn, *Limb Malformations*,
DOI 10.1007/978-3-540-95928-1_33, © Springer-Verlag Berlin Heidelberg 2014

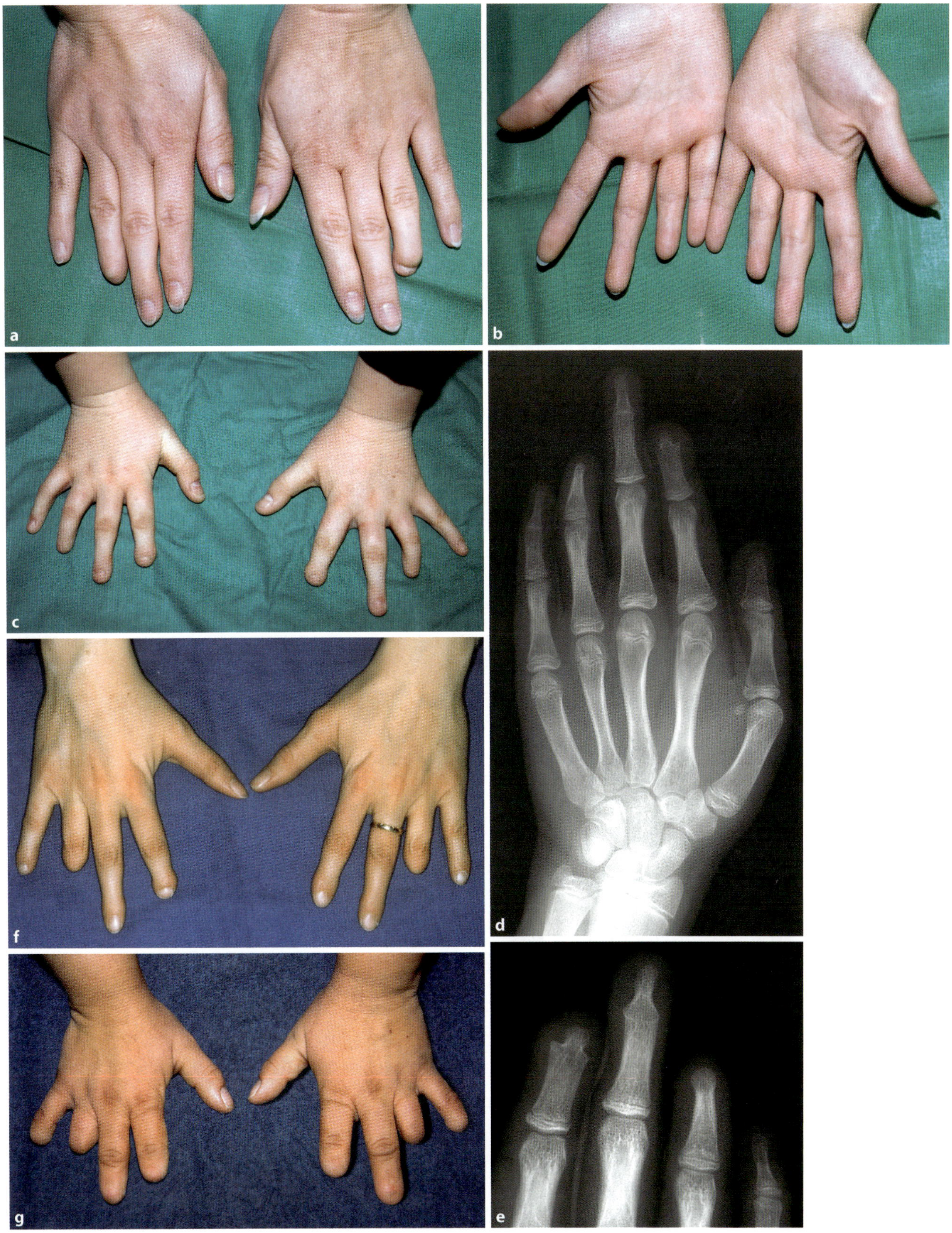
a
b
c
d
f
g
e

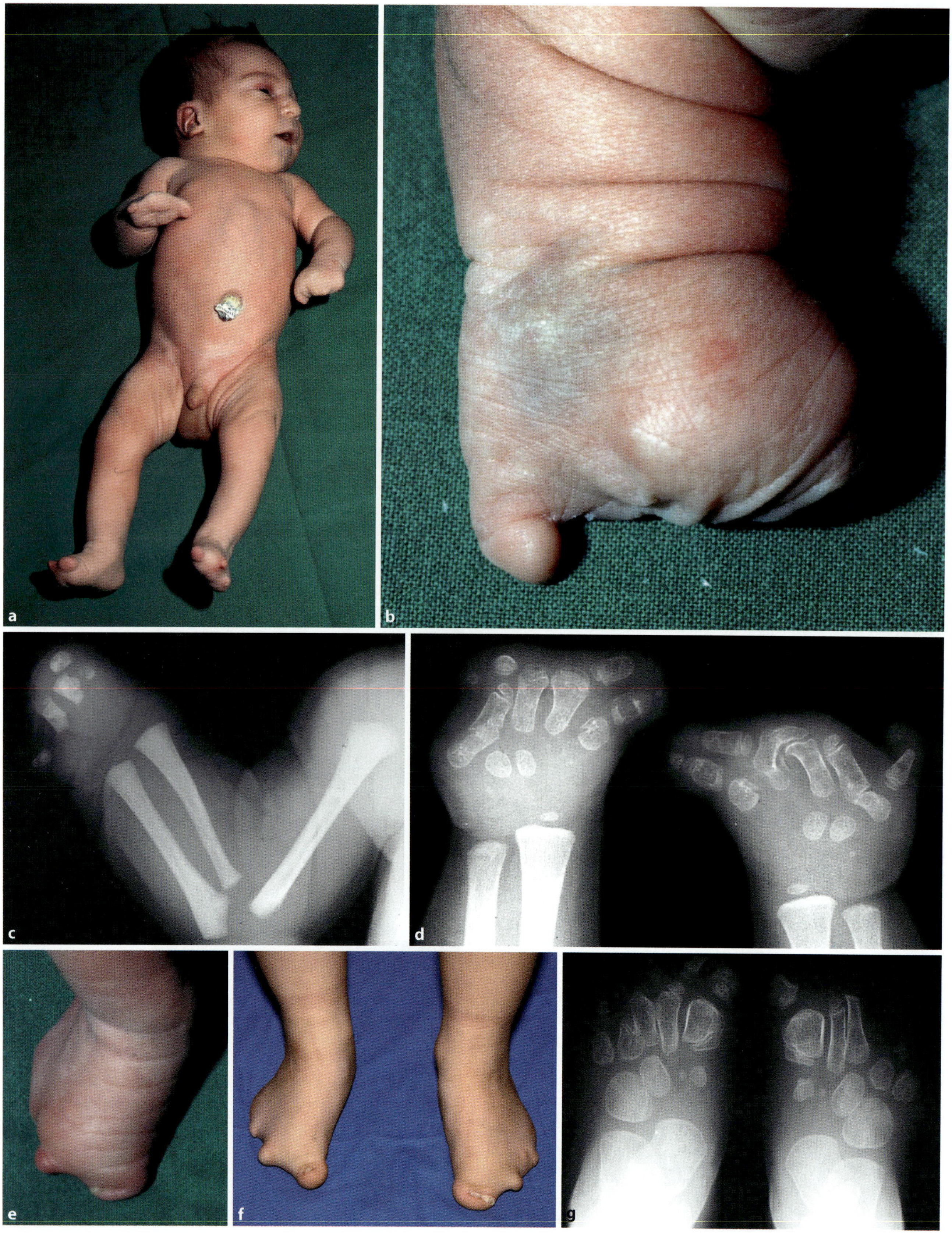

Fig. 33.2 Homozygous brachydactyly type B1 in newborn (**a–c, e**) and at age 6 (**d, f, g**). Note almost complete absence of digits with the exception of a fused broad thumb and a rudimentary digit V in the hands. **c, d** Radiographs of arm in newborn and hands at age 6, respectively. Note the absence of distal structures, disorganization of metacarpals, fusion of digits I and II, and normal carpal bones with delayed ossification. **e** Feet of newborn show absence of toes with rudimentary hallux. **f** Feet at age 6 years and corresponding radiograph (**g**) show loss of phalanges and highly abnormal round metatarsals with delta phalanx of the 1st metatarsal. (From Schwabe et al. 2000)

Brachydactyly Type B2

MIM 611377

34

Major Clinical Findings

Brachydactyly type B2 (BDB2) is characterized by hypoplasia/aplasia of the distal phalanges in combination with symphalangism, fusion of carpal/tarsal bones, and partial cutaneous syndactyly. Characteristically, fingers IV and V show a transverse distal reduction, whereas fingers II and III are less severely affected. In those fingers in which the distal phalanges are present, abnormal proximal interphalangeal joints are frequently observed, resulting in inability to bend the fingers and missing flexion creases. In more severely affected individuals, the distal and middle phalanges of digits II–V may be entirely absent. Fusion of the proximal and/or distal interphalangeal joints may be present, as well as a coalition of carpal and tarsal bones leading in the hands to a small metacarpus with abnormally configured bones. Acceleration of bone age may be present. The thumbs are proximally set in the majority of patients due to short 1st metacarpal bones. Cutaneous syndactyly, particularly between fingers II, III, and IV, can be observed as an associated feature. Symmetrical constrictions imitating amniotic bands have been observed. Sensorineural hearing loss and farsightedness have been observed in a few patients.

Genetic Transmission

Autosomal dominant.

Differential Diagnosis

The absence of terminal and/or middle phalanges, imitating an amputation-like phenotype, is similar to brachydactyly type B1. Proximal symphalangism is a typical feature of symphalangism (SYM1) . In these cases, however, the terminal phalanges are not affected. Amniotic bands may produce a similar phenotype, and bandlike constriction rings have been described in BDB2.

Molecular Pathology

Missense mutations in NOGGIN (NOG) are the cause for BDB2. It is predominantly expressed in neural tissues as well as during skeletal development. NOG is a glycosylated secreted protein that acts as a homodimer and hides both receptor binding interfaces when it is bound to bone morphogenetic proteins (BMPs), thus inhibiting binding of BMPs to their receptors. BDB2 is allelic to SYM1 and multiple synostoses syndrome (SYNS1). In contrast to the symphalangism-associated mutations, BDB2 mutations do not result in a major loss of function as indicated by calculation of free binding energy of the modeled NOG-GDF5 complex and functional testing in cell culture systems. Rather, they are expected to alter NOG's ability to bind to BMPs, thus disturbing the intricate balance of BMP signaling.

References

Lehmann K, Seemann P, Silan F, Goecke TO, Irgang S, Kjaer KW et al (2007) A new subtype of brachydactyly type B caused by point mutations in the bone morphogenetic protein antagonist NOGGIN. Am J Hum Genet 81(2):388–396

S. Mundlos, D. Horn, *Limb Malformations*,
DOI 10.1007/978-3-540-95928-1_34, © Springer-Verlag Berlin Heidelberg 2014

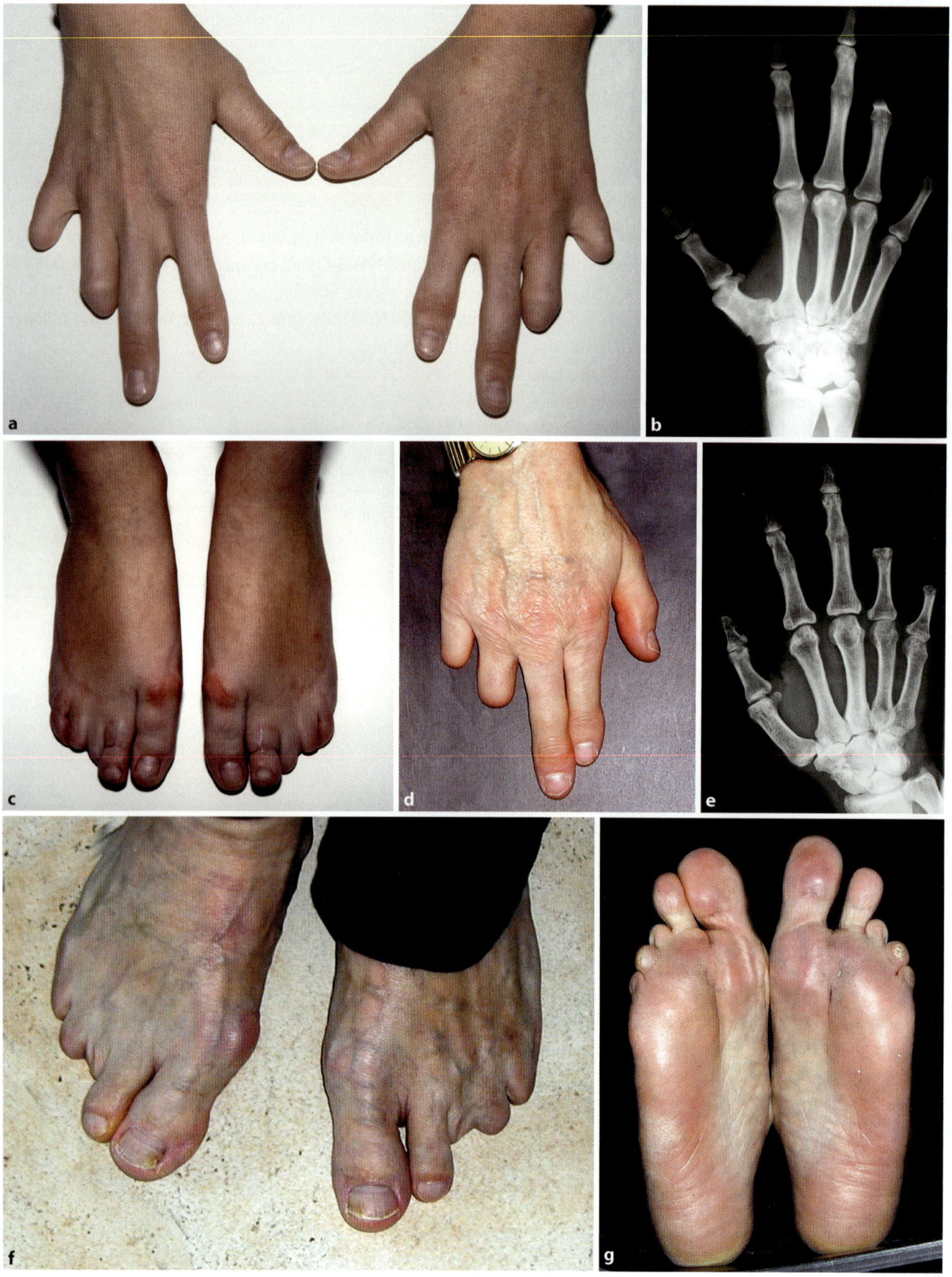

Fig. 34.1 **a** Individual with brachydactyly type B2 (BDB2) showing normal thumbs, partial syndactyly of digits II/III on the right, missing proximal interphalangeal creases, and truncation of digits at the level of the proximal phalanx in digits IV and V. **b** Corresponding radiograph. Note complete fusion of the proximal interphalangeal joints of digits II–IV, as well as distal truncation of digits IV and V. **c** Feet of the same individual showing normal halluces, bandlike constrictions at toes II, absence of distal phalanges, and syndactyly of toes III–V. **d** Variability in phenotype. BDB2 hand with truncation of digits IV and V at the level of the proximal phalanx and short digits II and III with missing proximal interphalangeal creases. **e** Corresponding radiograph. Note symphalangism of proximal interphalangeal joints II and III and amputation-like truncation of digits II and V at the level of the interphalangeal joint. **f** Feet of the same individual with truncation of toes III–V. **g** Plantar view

Brachydactyly Type C

MIM 113100

35

Synonyms

Brachydactyly, Haws type

Major Clinical Findings

Brachydactyly type C (BDC) is characterized by brachymesophalangy of the 2nd, 3rd, and 5th fingers; hyperphalangy (more than three phalanges per digit) of the 2nd and/or 3rd finger; and shortening of the 1st metacarpal. There is limited flexion in the distal interphalangeal joints, 5th-finger clinodactyly, and ulnar deviation of the 2nd and 3rd fingers. Generally, the 4th finger is the least affected and is therefore the longest digit in BDC. Typical radiographic signs are an extra wedge-shaped bone at the base of the proximal phalanx in the index fingers, corresponding to an abnormally shaped large epiphysis and extra ossification centers at, within, or between the phalanges, resulting in the appearance of an extra phalanx (hyperphalangism). With age, these ossification centers fuse with the remainder of the phalanx. The 1st metacarpals are often plump and short. Accompanying skeletal or nonskeletal features such as short stature, talipes equinovalgus/equinovarus, Perthes disease, hip dysplasia, and spine deformities have been described.

Genetic Transmission

Autosomal dominant.

Differential Diagnosis

Mild BDC shows overlapping features with brachydactyly type A2 (BDA2).

Molecular Pathology

Heterozygous frameshift or nonsense mutations affecting the cartilage-derived morphogenetic protein-1 (CDMP1), also called growth and differentiation factor 5 (GDF5), are responsible for dominant BDC. A recessive form of BDC has been described, caused by a homozygous missense mutation located within the CDMP1 prodomain. BDC-like phenotypes have been reported in association with mutations in BMPR1B, the high-affinity receptor for GDF5. Bone morphogenetic proteins (BMPs) act as homodimers or heterodimers that bind to two different types of membrane-spanning serine/threonine kinase receptors, the type I BMP receptors (ACVRL1, ACVR1, BMPR1A, BMPR1B), and the type II BMP receptors (BMPR2, ACVR2). Binding of BMPs to heterotetrameric receptor complexes activates the SMADs, as well as other intracellular signaling pathways such as the MAPK pathway. The high-affinity receptor for Gdf5 is BMPR1B, whereas BMP2 signals mainly through BMPR1A. BMP and GDF signaling are precisely regulated by a large number of antagonists, such as NOG, which act extracellularly on the membrane level as well as intracellularly. Gdf5 is expressed along early cartilage condensations, in the joint interzone, and in the perichondrium during limb development. Mice with an inactivating mutation in Gdf5 (brachypodism, bp) show severe shortening of all bones of the limb, aplasia of the fibula, and absence of interphalangeal joints, resembling acromesomelic dysplasia of the Hunter–Thompson/Grebe type.

References

Everman DB, Bartels CF, Yang Y, Yanamandra N, Goodman FR, Mendoza-Londono JR et al (2002) The mutational spectrum of brachydactyly type C. Am J Med Genet 112(3):291–296

Lehmann K, Seemann P, Boergermann J, Morin G, Reif S, Knaus P et al (2006) A novel R486Q mutation in BMPR1B resulting in either a brachydactyly type C/symphalangism-like phenotype or brachydactyly type A2. Eur J Hum Genet 14(12):1248–1254

Polinkovsky A, Robin NH, Thomas JT, Irons M, Lynn A, Goodman FR et al (1997) Mutations in CDMP1 cause autosomal dominant brachydactyly type C. Nat Genet 17(1):18–19

Schwabe GC, Turkmen S, Leschik G, Palanduz S, Stover B, Goecke TO et al (2004) Brachydactyly type C caused by a homozygous missense mutation in the prodomain of CDMP1. Am J Med Genet 124A:356–363

Storm EE, Huynh TV, Copeland NG, Jenkins NA, Kingsley DM, Lee SJ (1994) Limb alterations in brachypodism mice due to mutations in a new member of the TGF-beta superfamily. Nature 368:639–643

S. Mundlos, D. Horn, *Limb Malformations*,
DOI 10.1007/978-3-540-95928-1_35, © Springer-Verlag Berlin Heidelberg 2014

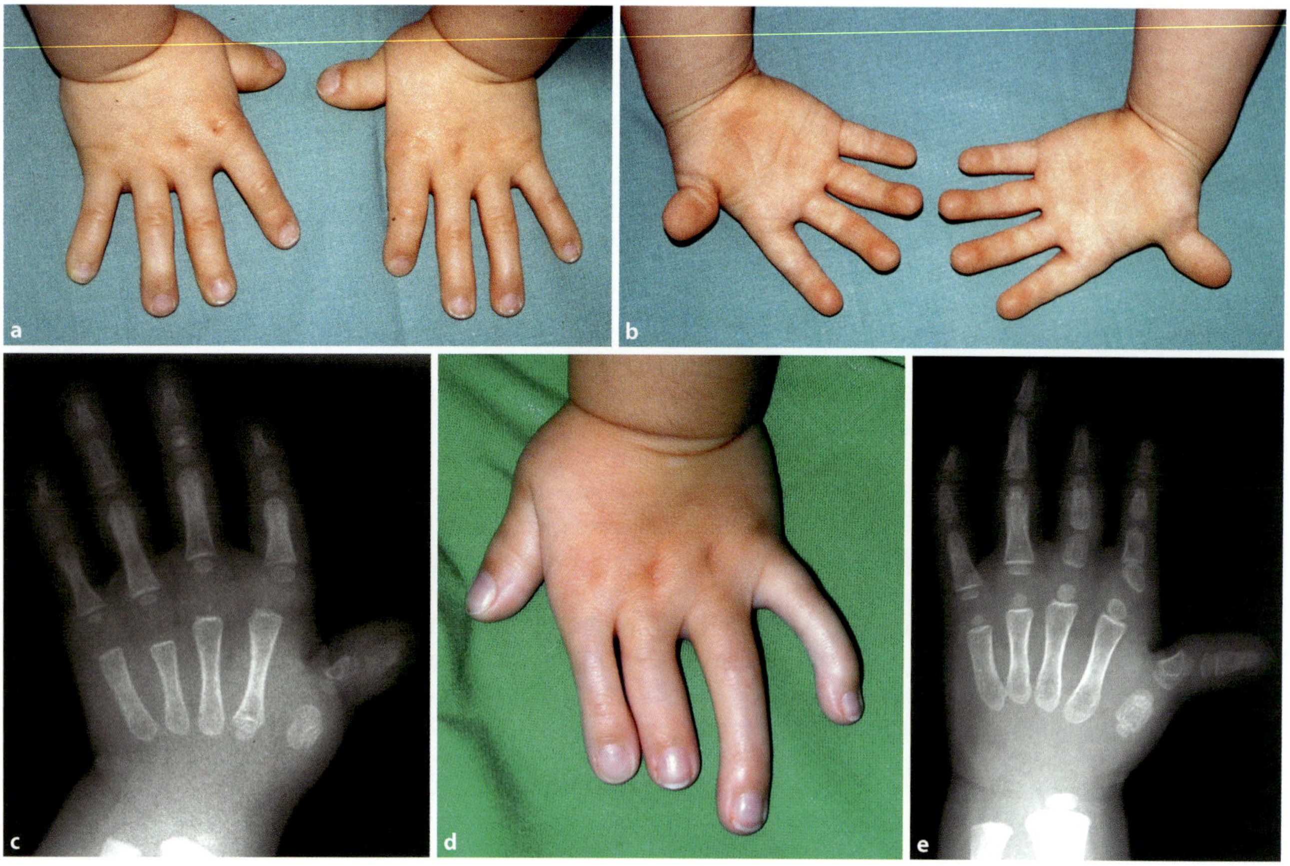

Fig. 35.1 Variability in brachydactyly type C (BDC). Dorsal (**a**) and palmar (**b**) views of hands showing short digit I with radial deviation. **c** Corresponding radiograph shows small, round metacarpal I with abnormal laterally placed epiphysis; small, modified delta-shaped epiphysis of proximal phalanx I; short 2nd proximal phalanx; and small, abnormally formed middle phalanges in digits II, III, and V. **d** Typical BDC hand. Digit IV is the least affected and the longest digit. Note short thumb and abnormally thin digit II. **e** Corresponding radiograph shows rounded and short metacarpal I and short proximal phalanx of the thumb with triangular and laterally placed epiphysis (delta phalanx). Digit II shows hyperphalangy with an accessory ossification center. Digit III shows abnormally shaped proximal and middle phalanges

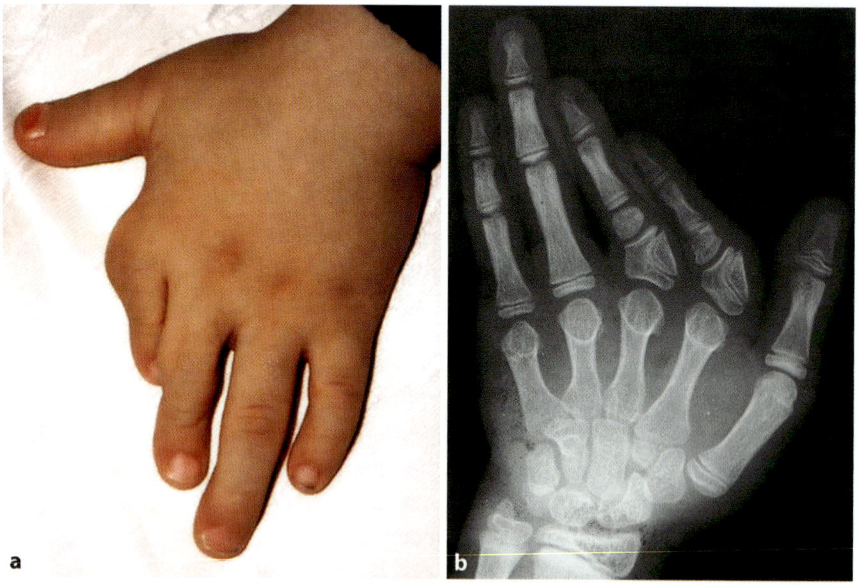

Fig. 35.2 Recessive brachydactyly type C with more severe manifestation. **a** Very short, almost rudimentary digit II with ulnar deviation. **b** Radiograph shows a normal thumb, short metacarpals III–V, and hyperphalangy of digits II and III with abnormally shaped proximal phalanges that show a triangular, laterally placed growth plate (delta phalanx)

36 Brachydactyly Type E; Brachydactyly Type D

MIM 113300; MIM 113200

Major Clinical Findings

In brachydactyly type E (BDE), the 3rd, 4th, and 5th metacarpals and/or metatarsals are short and the most frequently affected. The phalanges may also be involved. There is wide variability in the number of digits affected, even within the same family. The metacarpals make up the knuckles of the hand and normally form a line. A typical clinical sign of BDE can be seen if a fist is made that reveals the shortness of the affected metacarpals. In a subgroup of BDE with mutations in *PTHLH*, abnormalities of dentition may occur, including oligodontia and delayed eruption of the primary and secondary teeth. Short stature can be an associated feature.

In brachydactyly type D (BDD), the distal phalanx of the thumb is shortened to various degrees. The toes are broad. Penetrance is complete in females and incomplete in males. About three-fourths of affected persons, both males and females, express the trait bilaterally. BDD is often a component of BDE.

Genetic Transmission

Autosomal dominant.

Differential Diagnosis

Shortening of the 3rd, 4th, and 5th metacarpals is a feature of many conditions. BDE occurs as an isolated trait or as part of more complex syndromic conditions such as hypertension–brachydactyly syndrome (MIM 112410), Turner syndrome, and Albright hereditary osteodystrophy (AHO; MIM 103580). AHO is caused by haploinsufficiency of the signaling protein $G\alpha_s$ encoded by the *GNAS1* gene in nonimprinted tissues. Clinically AHO is characterized by short stature, BDE, BDD, and heterotopic ossifications. Pseudohypoparathyroidism (PHP) and pseudopseudohypoparathyroidism (PPHP) are conditions associated with AHO. The BDE phenotype in these conditions is very similar to that of isolated BDE, and differentiation on a clinical basis may be impossible. The appearance of the face may help to discriminate some cases, but round faces have also been described in BDE. Calcifications and mental retardation should not occur in BDE. Short stature and obesity suggest a diagnosis of PHP. Many individuals with BDE also show shortening of the distal phalanx of the thumb (BDD), but this can also be seen in PHP and PPHP.

BDE is part of the brachydactyly mental retardation syndrome (MIM 600430). This condition presents with a range of features including intellectual disability, behavioral abnormalities, developmental delay, and sleep disturbance, as well as a specific facial dysmorphism. BDE is a variable feature in this condition and may be missing. BDE may also occur in association with hypertension, as in BDE hypertension syndrome.

Molecular Pathology

BDE is a genetically heterogenous condition. Mutations in *HOXD13* can cause a BDE and BDD phenotype. However, this seems to be very rare. Many isolated cases are due to mutations or deletions in the parathyroid hormone-related peptide (PTHRH) gene *PTHLH*. PTHRP has PTH-like growth regulatory activity and is able to activate the same receptor as PTH (that is, the PTH/PTHRP receptor), leading to stimulation of both the Gs and Gq families of heteromeric G proteins. Thus, the PTH signaling pathway appears to be of particular importance for the growth of metacarpals and digits.

Brachydactyly mental retardation syndrome has been shown to be associated with deletions on chromosome 2q37.3. The responsible gene within this deletion is histone deacetylase 4 (*HDAC4*). *HDAC4* interacts with key players of skeletogenesis, including Runx2 and Mef2c.

References

Johnson D, Kan S, Oldridge M, Trembath RC, Roche P, Esnouf RM et al (2003) Missense mutations in the homeodomain of HOXD13 are associated with brachydactyly types D and E. Am J Hum Genet 72:984–997

Klopocki E, Hennig BP, Dathe K, Koll R, de Ravel T, Baten E et al (2010) Deletion and point mutations of PTHLH cause brachydactyly type E. Am J Hum Genet 86(3):434–439

Williams SR, Aldred MA, Der Kaloustian VM, Halal F, Gowans G, McLeod DR et al (2010) Haploinsufficiency of HDAC4 causes brachydactyly mental retardation syndrome, with brachydactyly type E, developmental delays, and behavioral problems. Am J Hum Genet 87(2):219–228

S. Mundlos, D. Horn, *Limb Malformations*,
DOI 10.1007/978-3-540-95928-1_36, © Springer-Verlag Berlin Heidelberg 2014

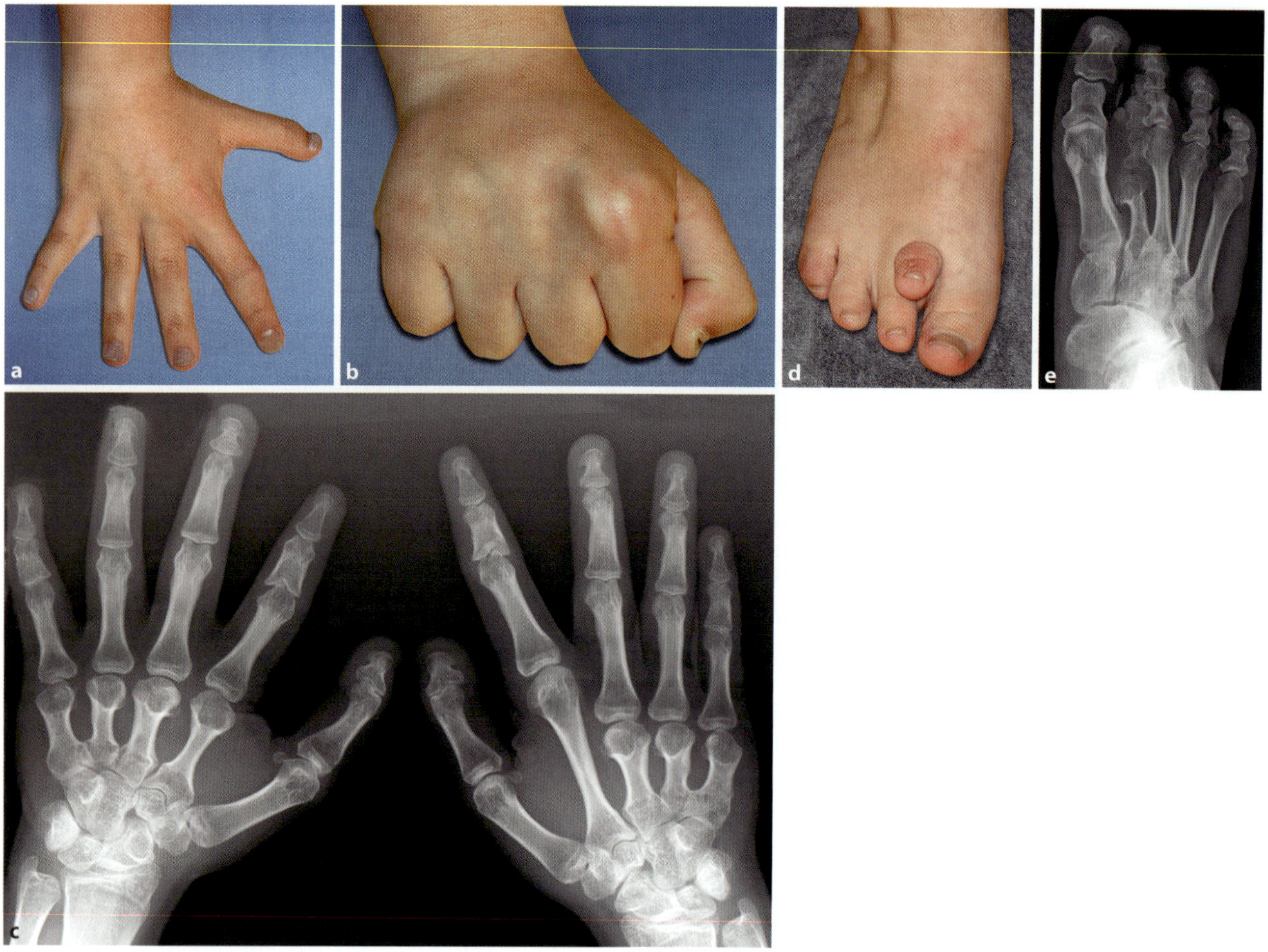

Fig. 36.1 Brachydactyly type E (BDE) with mutation in *PTHLH*. **a** Typical BDE with small hand and short metacarpals. **b** Knuckle sign showing differences in metacarpal length. **c** Corresponding radiograph shows very short metacarpals II–V on the left and III–V on the right. (Variable degrees of metacarpal shortening are common in BDE.) The thumbs show short and broad distal phalanges (brachydactyly type D component). The proximal interphalangeal joints of digits II are abnormal, reflecting remnants of cone-shaped epiphyses of the middle phalanges, with short distal phalanges of digits III. **d** BDE of feet with short and dorsally placed 2nd toe. **e** Corresponding radiograph shows a very short 2nd metatarsal

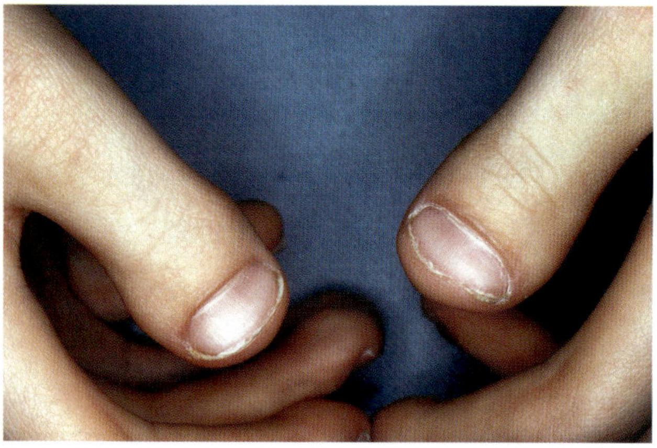

Fig. 36.2 Brachydactyly type D. Short and broad distal phalanx of the thumbs with short nails

Cooks Syndrome

MIM 106995

37

Synonyms
Anonychia/onychodystrophy with hypoplasia or absence of distal phalanges

Major Clinical Findings
Cooks syndrome is a brachydactyly with absent or hypoplastic nails affecting all digits. Absent flexion creases can be noted in the digits. There is distal tapering of the phalanges, and the finger pads are prominent. Radiographic examination shows only two phalanges in digits II–V. The nail tufts are small, and there may be a distal elongation corresponding to a rudimentary phalanx. The distal phalanges appear elongated, indicating a developmental fusion between the distal and middle phalanges; however, the phenotype may also be interpreted as absent distal phalanges with partial conversion of the middle phalanx into a distal element. The middle phalanx of the thumb is usually present but may be absent in the hallux. Some individuals have a distinctive facial appearance with a high nasal bridge, prominent bulbous tip, and hypoplastic alae nasi.

Genetic Transmission
Autosomal dominant.

Differential Diagnosis
Other conditions with nail hypoplasia have to be considered. Brachydactyly type V (brachydactyly with nail hypoplasia) is probably the same condition. Individuals with brachydactyly type B show hypoplasia of the distal phalanges with variable degrees of nail hypoplasia. In this condition, however, nail hypoplasia is coupled to the degree of bone hypoplasia of the distal phalanges. The middle phalanges may also be affected, but only if the distal phalanges are absent. Adams–Oliver syndrome is characterized by hypoplasia of the distal phalanges and hypoplastic/aplastic nails. Other types of nonsyndromic congenital nail disorders (NDNC1–10) should be considered. However, the characteristic radiographic appearance with missing middle phalanges and elongated distal phalanges clearly distinguishes Cooks syndrome from other phenotypically related conditions.

Molecular Pathology
Cooks syndrome is caused by genomic duplications that cover approximately 1 Mb of noncoding DNA upstream of *SOX9*. This region has been shown to be involved in the regulation of *SOX9* gene expression and contains many highly conserved sequences, many of which have enhancer activity. SOX9 is a transcription factor involved in several developmental processes. Most importantly, SOX9 regulates the differentiation of precursor cells into cartilage-producing chondrocytes and also regulates development of the male gonad. Accordingly, SOX9 inactivation results in severe, lethal chondrodysplasia with sex reversal in the male, a condition called campomelic dysplasia.

References

Kurth I, Klopocki E, Stricker S, van Oosterwijk J, Vanek S, Altmann J et al (2009) Duplications of noncoding elements 5' of SOX9 are associated with brachydactyly-anonychia. Nat Genet 41(8):862–863

S. Mundlos, D. Horn, *Limb Malformations*,
DOI 10.1007/978-3-540-95928-1_37, © Springer-Verlag Berlin Heidelberg 2014

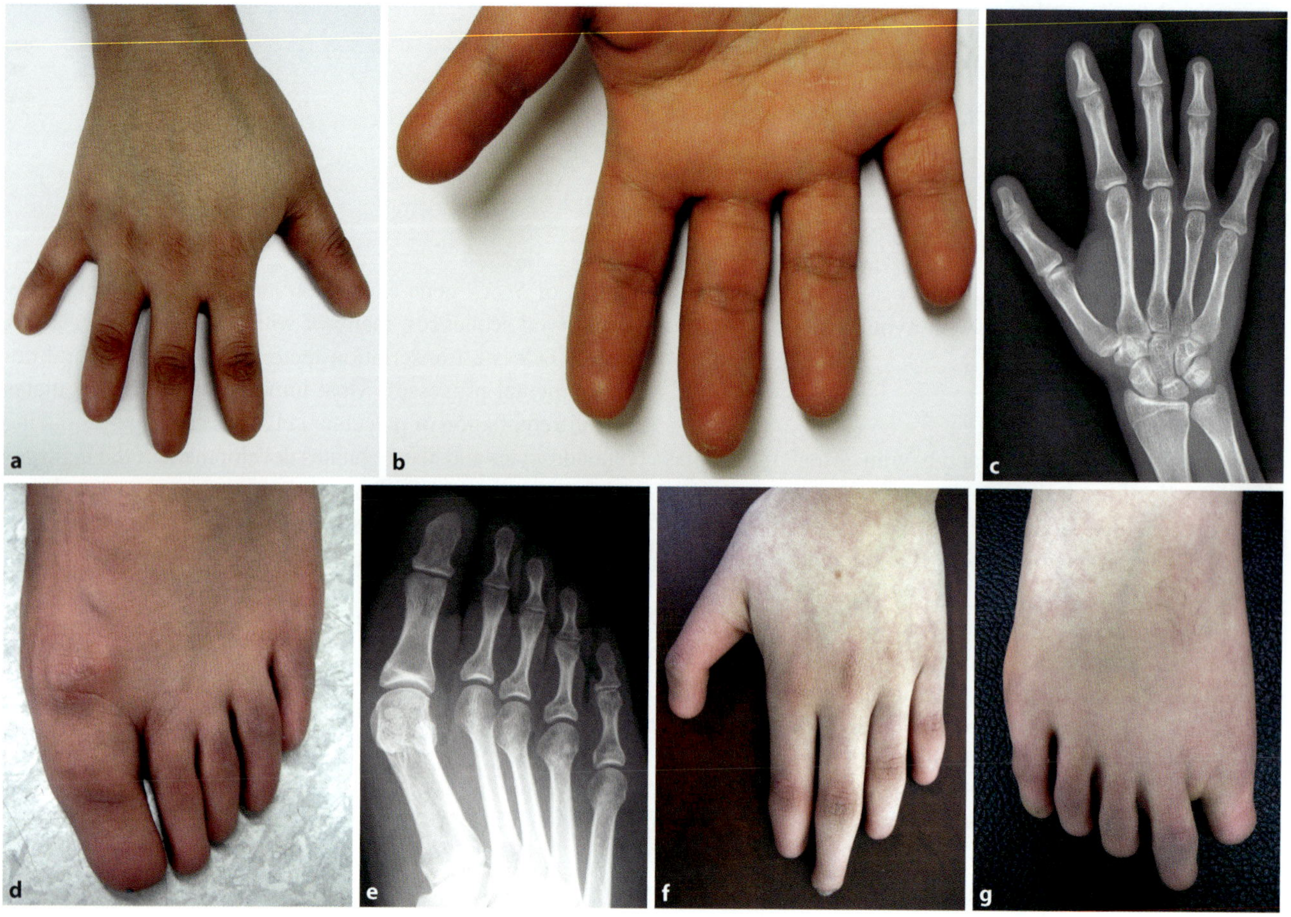

Fig. 37.1 Dorsal (**a**) and palmar (**b**) view of Cooks syndrome hands showing absent nails in all digits, short digits, and missing distal interphalangeal creases. **c** Corresponding radiograph shows missing middle phalanges, elongated proximal phalanges, and missing nail tufts at the distal phalanges. **d** Absent nails and relatively long toes. **e** Corresponding radiograph shows absent middle phalanges, elongated proximal phalanges, and missing nail beds. **f** Variability in Cooks syndrome. Note absent nails but rudimentary nail of digit III. **g** Corresponding foot. (Courtesy of Ingo Kurth, University of Jena, Germany)

Part VII

Disorders: Brachydactyly Associated

38 Adams–Oliver Syndrome

MIM 100300, MIM 614219, MIM 614814

Synonyms
Congenital scalp defects with distal limb reduction anomalies
Aplasia cutis congenita with terminal transverse limb defects

Major Clinical Findings
Adams–Oliver syndrome is characterized by congenital aplasia of the skin (aplasia cutis congenita) and distal limb defects. The skin defects can occur anywhere on the body but are most frequently found on the posterior head affecting the scalp and, in more severe cases, the underlying parietal bones. As a minimal finding, single to multiple round or oval areas of alopecia may be identified in the parietal area. The limb defects are distal truncations affecting the distal phalanges or entire digits. Further proximal elements such as the metacarpals are rarely involved. Hypoplasia of the nails and distal phalanges is at the milder end of the clinical spectrum. Syndactyly of the 2nd and 3rd toes is also observed. Involvement of the limbs may be asymmetric and is more severe in the feet. The clinical features can also include cutis marmorata, dilated scalp veins, vascular defects, congenital cardiac malformations, and brain malformations. Overall, the phenotype is extremely variable even within families. Severity may vary from II/III toe syndactyly, which is a common finding, to hypoplasia of all toes or even absence of a hand or foot. The severity and frequency of the skin defects vary but occur in approximately 75 % of patients. This is a potentially life-threatening condition, and large skin defects that cannot be closed primarily may require skin grafting, flaps, or both.

Occasional Findings
Microcephaly, encephalocele, mental retardation, seizures, hypotonia, enlarged ventricles, pachygyria, polymicrogyria, accessory nipples, microphthalmia.

Genetic Transmission
Autosomal dominant, autosomal recessive.

Differential Diagnosis
Other conditions with nail hypoplasia and distal truncating limb defects must be considered. Individuals with brachydactyly type B show hypoplasia of the distal phalanges with variable degrees of nail hypoplasia; however, only digits II–V are involved (with the exception of thumb duplications in severe cases), and skin defects are not part of the spectrum. Cooks syndrome shows aplasia of the nails and hypoplastic terminal phalanges but never transverse defects. Other types of nonsyndromic congenital nail disorders (NDNC1–10) have to be considered. However, the most important and challenging differentiation concerns transverse limb defects due to amniotic bands. The two conditions may be impossible to distinguish on a single limb, but detailed inspection of the entire picture will lead the way. The involvement of one or few digits in one limb and signs of asymmetry in one limb argue for a nongenetic cause.

Molecular Pathology
Adams–Oliver syndrome is genetically heterogenous. A dominant form is caused by mutations in *ARHGAP31 (AOS1; 100300)*. The gene encodes a Cdc42/Rac1 GTPase regulator that is part of a pathway regulating cell proliferation and motility. The mutations result in premature truncations that confer an activating effect on the protein. Another autosomal dominant form of Adams–Oliver syndrome (AOS3; 614814) is caused by mutation in the *RBPJ* gene. The corresponding protein is a primary regulator for the notch pathway, which is known to be important for boundary formation in developmental processes. An autosomal recessive form of Adams–Oliver syndrome (AOS2; 614219) is caused by mutation in the *DOCK6* gene, which encodes an atypical guanidine exchange factor known to activate the Rho GTPAses Cdc42 and Rac1.

References

Hassed SJ, Wiley GB, Wang S, Lee JY, Li S, Xu W et al (2012) RBPJ mutations identified in two families affected by Adams–Oliver syndrome. Am J Hum Genet 91(2):391–395

Shaheen R, Faqeih E, Sunker A, Morsy H, Al-Sheddi T, Shamseldin HE et al (2011) Recessive mutations in DOCK6, encoding the guanidine nucleotide exchange factor DOCK6, lead to abnormal actin cytoskeleton organization and Adams–Oliver syndrome. Am J Hum Genet 89(2):328–333

Snape KM, Ruddy D, Zenker M, Wuyts W, Whiteford M, Johnson D et al (2009) The spectra of clinical phenotypes in aplasia cutis congenita and terminal transverse limb defects. Am J Med Genet A 149A(8):1860–1881

Southgate L, Machado RD, Snape KM, Primeau M, Dafou D, Ruddy DM et al (2011) Gain-of-function mutations of ARHGAP31, a Cdc42/Rac1 GTPase regulator, cause syndromic cutis aplasia and limb anomalies. Am J Hum Genet 88(5):574–585

S. Mundlos, D. Horn, *Limb Malformations*,
DOI 10.1007/978-3-540-95928-1_38, © Springer-Verlag Berlin Heidelberg 2014

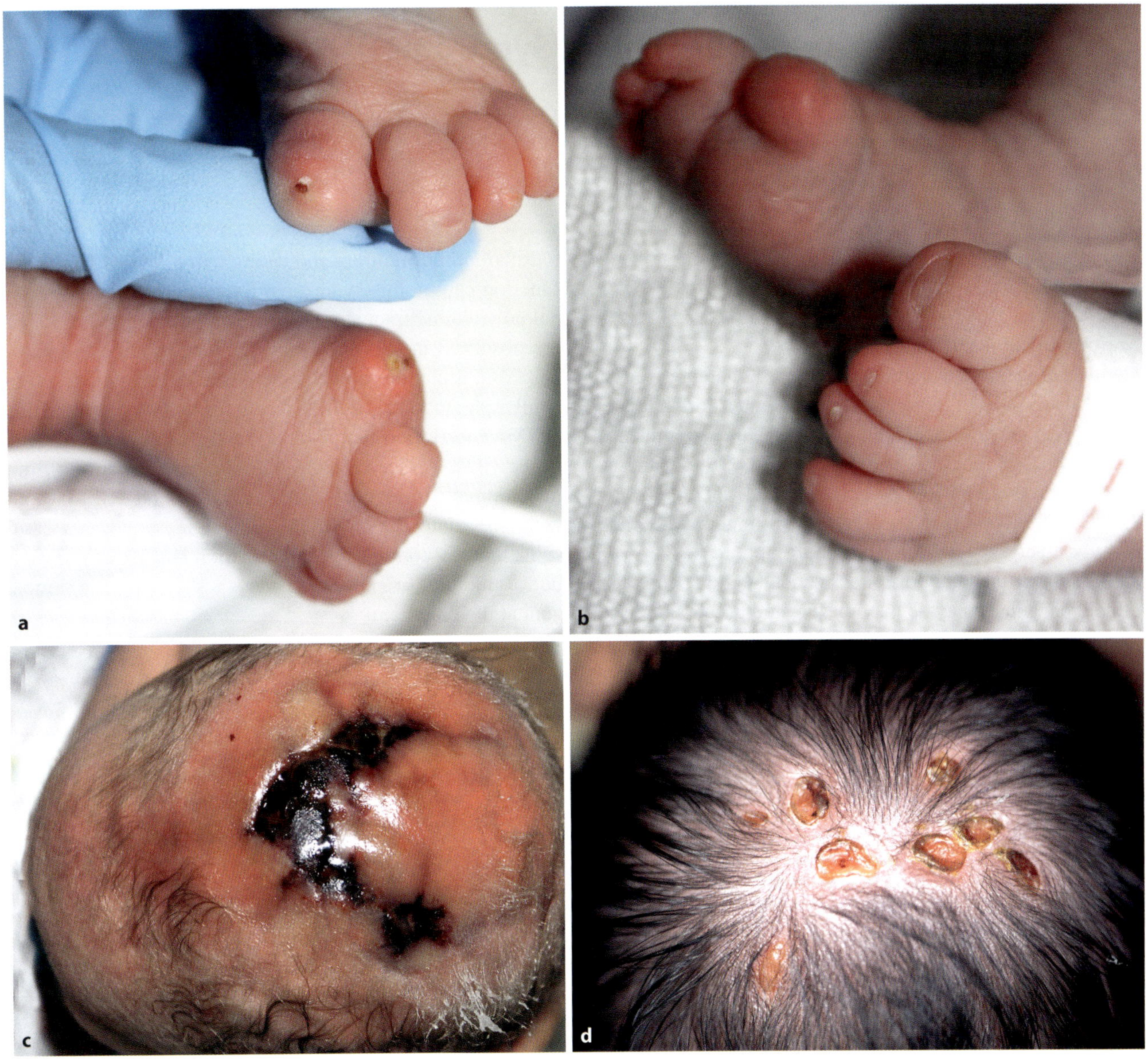

Fig. 38.1 **a** Distal hypoplasia/aplasia of the great toes and absence of nails. **b** Hypoplasia of the distal phalanges and nails of toes II–V. **c, d** Variability in scalp defects

39 Hand-Foot-Genital Syndrome

MIM 140000

Synonyms
Hand–foot–uterus syndrome

Major clinical findings
Hand–foot–genital syndrome (HGS) is characterized by brachydactyly with abnormal thumbs and short halluces. The thumbs are proximally placed, and the thenar eminences are hypoplastic. There is medial deviation of the distal halluces (hallux varus). Radiographic changes include a short 1st metacarpal and metatarsal, short 5th fingers with clinodactyly, fusion of the trapezoid and scaphoid in the wrist, and fusion of the cuneiform and navicular in the foot. The middle phalanges may be hypoplastic, and pseudoepiphyses may be present. Occasionally, symphalangism of the middle and distal phalanges of the 2nd, 3rd, 4th, or 5th toes is seen. There is delayed carpal or tarsal maturation.

Females have duplications of the urogenital tract, including uterus bicornis and longitudinal vaginal septum. Affected males may have penile hypospadias of variable severity with or without chordee, short penis, or bifid scrotum. Ureterovesical reflux, ectopic accessory ureteral orifice, and subsequent recurrent urinary tract infections are common features in both sexes. The limb abnormalities are reported to be fully penetrant, bilateral, and symmetrical, whereas the genitourinary abnormalities are incompletely penetrant and variably severe.

Genetic transmission
Autosomal dominant.

Differential diagnosis
Thumb hypoplasia also occurs in Fanconi anemia syndrome, Holt–Oram syndrome, Duane–radial ray syndrome, Nager syndrome, Townes–Brocks syndrome, and lacrimo-auriculo-dento-digital (LADD) syndrome. Incomplete Müllerian fusion and longitudinal vaginal septum are features of several conditions, including acro-renal-mandibular syndrome, Bardet–Biedl syndrome, Fraser syndrome, Fryns syndrome, and Meckel syndrome.

Molecular pathology
HFGS is caused by mutations in *HOXD13*. Nonsense mutations truncating the encoded protein N-terminal or within the homeodomain as well as missense mutations in the DNA-binding homeodomain produce typical limb and genitourinary abnormalities, indicating that a loss of HOXD13 function causes this syndrome. Expansions of an N-terminal polyalanine tract similar to those observed in HOXD13 are observed in approximately 50% of affected individuals. Point mutations and alanine repeat expansions result in similar phenotypes. HOXA13 belongs to the large family of HOX transcription factors and is the most 5' located gene in the HOX-A cluster. HOXA13 is expressed during limb development in a very similar pattern as HOXD13. Both genes regulate the differentiation of mesenchymal stem cells, thereby controlling the formation and growth of digit bones. In addition, HOXA13 plays a major role in female genital development

References

Goodman FR (2002) Limb malformations and the human HOX genes. Am J Med Genet 112(3):256–265

Goodman FR, Bacchelli C, Brady AF, Brueton LA, Fryns JP, Mortlock DP et al (2000) Novel HOXA13 mutations and the phenotypic spectrum of hand–foot–genital syndrome. Am J Hum Genet 67(1):197–202

Innis JW, Mortlock D, Chen Z, Ludwig M, Williams ME, Williams TM et al (2004) Polyalanine expansion in HOXA13: three new affected families and the molecular consequences in a mouse model. Hum Mol Genet 13(22):2841–2851

Mortlock DP, Innis JW (1997) Mutation of HOXA13 in hand–foot–genital syndrome. Nat Genet 15(2):179–180

S. Mundlos, D. Horn, *Limb Malformations*,
DOI 10.1007/978-3-540-95928-1_39, © Springer-Verlag Berlin Heidelberg 2014

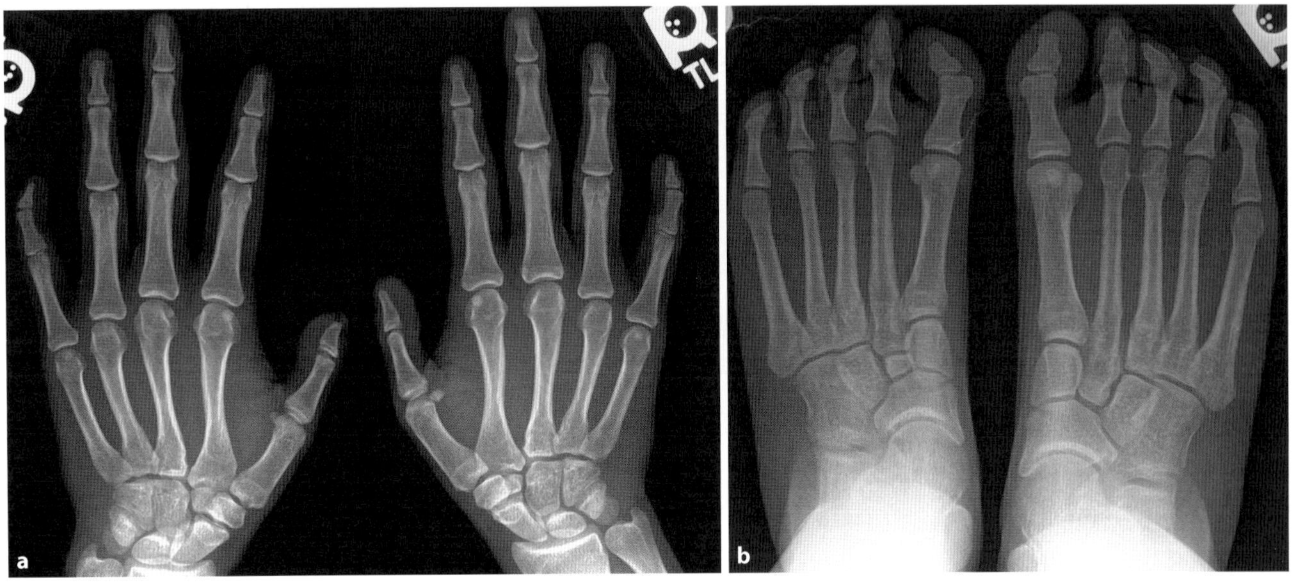

Fig. 39.1 **a** Radiograph of hands showing asymmetric stub thumb, hypoplasia of the distal phalanx of digit V, and clinodactyly. **b** Feet of the same individual. Note lateral deviation of the distal phalanx of the hallux, fused 2nd metatarsal to the tarsal bone on the right, a hypoplastic unfused comparable tarsal on the left, and missing/fused middle phalanges of toes II–V. (Courtesy of Jeffrey Innis, University of Michigan, Ann Arbor, USA)

40 Catel–Manzke Syndrome

MIM 302380

Synonyms
Hyperphalangy–clinodactyly of index finger with Pierre-Robin syndrome
Palatodigital syndrome, Catel–Manzke type
Micrognathia digital syndrome

Major Clinical Findings
Catel–Manzke syndrome is characterized by the combination of clinodactyly of the index finger in combination with Pierre Robin syndrome (microretrognathia and glossoptosis with or without cleft palate). The hallmark of this condition is shortening and radial deviation of the index finger due to an extra ossification at the metacarpophalangeal joint. Radiographic examination shows that this bone is often triangular with an asymmetric growth plate. It is located at the ulnar side between the shortened 2nd metacarpal and a slightly shortened proximal phalanx. The findings are bilateral. Thus, there are four instead of three phalangeal ossifications, a finding that has also been termed hyperphalangism. With age, the accessory bone fuses with the proximal phalanx, resulting in an enlarged and deformed epiphysis. Postnatal failure to thrive has been noted, but this may be due to the feeding problems and the airway obstruction caused by the glossoptosis. Some cases have been described that show only the hand anomalies without the Pierre Robin syndrome.

Occasional Findings
The full spectrum of this condition may include cardiac defects such as atrial septal defect, ventricular septal defect, or transposition of the large vessels. Pectus carinatum and pectus excavatum, joint laxity and dislocations, and developmental delay are other described features.

Genetic Transmission
Autosomal recessive.

Differential Diagnosis
Hyperphalangism is a typical feature of brachydactyly type C; however, in this condition the extra ossifications occur between the phalanges and not in the typical "Manzke" location. There is some clinical overlap with Desbuquois dysplasia (OMIM 251450), a severe skeletal dysplasia that also features extra bones between the metacarpals and proximal phalanges. However, the lack of a generalized skeletal dysplasia in Catel–Manzke syndrome differentiates these conditions.

References

Molecular Pathology. Homozygous and Compound Heterezygous Mutations in TGDS coding for dTDP-D-glucose 4,6-dehydrogenase cause Catel-Manzke Syndrome. TGDS is a conserved protein belonging to the SDR family and likely to play a role in nucleotide sugar metabolism.

Ehmke E, Caliebe A, Koenig R, Kant SG, Cormier-Daire V (2014) Homozygous and Compound Heterozygous Mutations in TGDS Cause Cantel-Manzke Syndrome. AJHG

Manzke H, Lehmann K, Klopocki E, Caliebe A (2008) Catel–Manzke syndrome: two new patients and a critical review of the literature. Eur J Med Genet 51(5):452–465

Sundaram V, Taysi K, Hartmann AF Jr, Shackelford GD, Keating JP (1982) Hyperphalangy and clinodactyly of the index finger with Pierre Robin anomaly: Catel–Manzke syndrome. A case report and review of the literature. Clin Genet 21(6):407–410

S. Mundlos, D. Horn, *Limb Malformations*,
DOI 10.1007/978-3-540-95928-1_40, © Springer-Verlag Berlin Heidelberg 2014

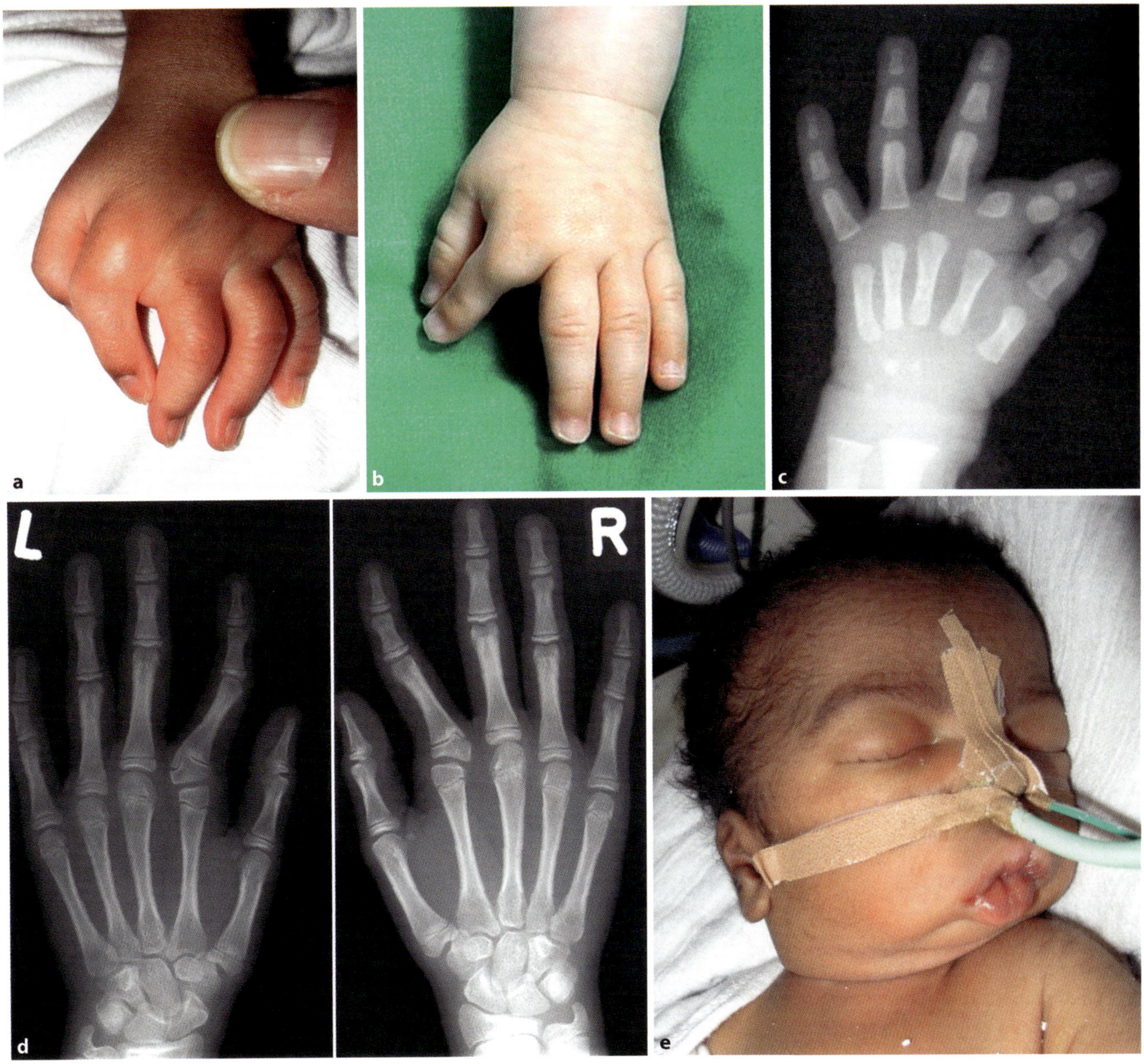

Fig. 40.1 **a** Ulnar deviation of digit II with abnormally shaped knuckle. **b** Hand phenotype in a second individual showing radial deviation of digit II and abnormally shaped knuckle. **c** Corresponding radiograph shows an extra polygonal ossification center medial to the proximal phalanx of digit II and a hypoplastic middle and proximal phalanx of digit II. **d** Radiograph at age 10.5 years shows subluxation and radial deviation of the 2nd fingers bilaterally at the metacarpophalangeal joint and fusion of the extra ossification to the epiphysis of the proximal phalanx, forming a cone-shaped epiphysis. The epiphyses of the 2nd metacarpals are shortened and flattened. **e** Severe micrognathia requiring ventilation. (**a,e** Courtesy of Rainer König, University of Frankfurt, Germany. **d** From Manzke et al. 2008)

41 Feingold Syndrome

MIM 164280

Synonyms
Oculodigitoesophagoduodenal syndrome
Microcephaly-oculo-digito-esophageal-duodenal syndrome
Microcephaly and digital abnormalities with normal intelligence

Major Clinical Findings
Feingold syndrome is characterized by variable combinations of limb malformations, esophageal and duodenal atresias, microcephaly, and mental retardation. Other features include short and/or narrow palpebral fissures, a broad nasal bridge, anteverted nostrils, ear abnormalities, micrognathia, cardiac and renal anomalies, supernumerary spleen, asplenia, hearing loss, and imperforate anus. Hands and feet show hypoplastic thumbs, toes with symphalangism, clinodactyly of the 2nd and 5th fingers, and syndactyly, especially between the 2nd and 3rd as well as the 4th and 5th toes. The middle phalanges, in particular the 2nd and 5th, may be short or absent as in brachydactyly type A. The digital anomalies appear to be the most consistent features of this condition.

Genetic Transmission
Autosomal dominant.

Differential Diagnosis
As differential diagnoses, conditions with hypoplastic thumbs and brachydactyly type A should be considered. These conditions include Fanconi anemia, Rubinstein–Taybi syndrome, Tsukahara syndrome, and Filippi syndrome. VACTERL association (vertebral defects, anal atresia, cardiac defects, tracheoesophageal fistula with esophageal atresia, renal and limb abnormalities) shows considerable overlap, but the two should be distinguishable by the presence of microcephaly, brachymesophalangy, and toe syndactyly in Feingold syndrome. Esophageal atresia, heart defects, and renal abnormalities can be seen in CHARGE syndrome.

Molecular Pathology
Feingold syndrome is caused by mutations in the *MYCN* gene. *MYCN* is an oncogene encoding a transcription factor that plays a role in various developmental processes. *MYCN* amplification is found in neuroblastoma tumors, the most frequent extracranial solid tumors of childhood. *MYCN* has been shown to be activated by hedgehog signaling, giving a link to digit and joint development. Another subtype of Feingold syndrome is caused by hemizygous deletions of chromosome 13q31.3, including MIR17HG. The phenotype is very similar to those of individuals with mutations in *MYCN*; however, they lack gastrointestinal abnormalities and short palpebral fissures.

References

de Pontual L, Yao E, Callier P, Faivre L, Drouin V, Cariou S et al (2011) Germline deletion of the miR-17-92 cluster causes skeletal and growth defects in humans. Nature Genet 43:1026–10

Tészás A, Meijer R, Scheffer H, Gyuris P, Kosztolányi G, van Bokhoven H et al (2006) Expanding the clinical spectrum of MYCN-related Feingold syndrome. Am J Med Genet A 140(20):2254–2256

van Bokhoven H, Celli J, van Reeuwijk J, Rinne T, Glaudemans B, van Beusekom E et al (2005) MYCN haploinsufficiency is associated with reduced brain size and intestinal atresias in Feingold syndrome. Nat Genet 37(5):465–467

S. Mundlos, D. Horn, *Limb Malformations*,
DOI 10.1007/978-3-540-95928-1_41, © Springer-Verlag Berlin Heidelberg 2014

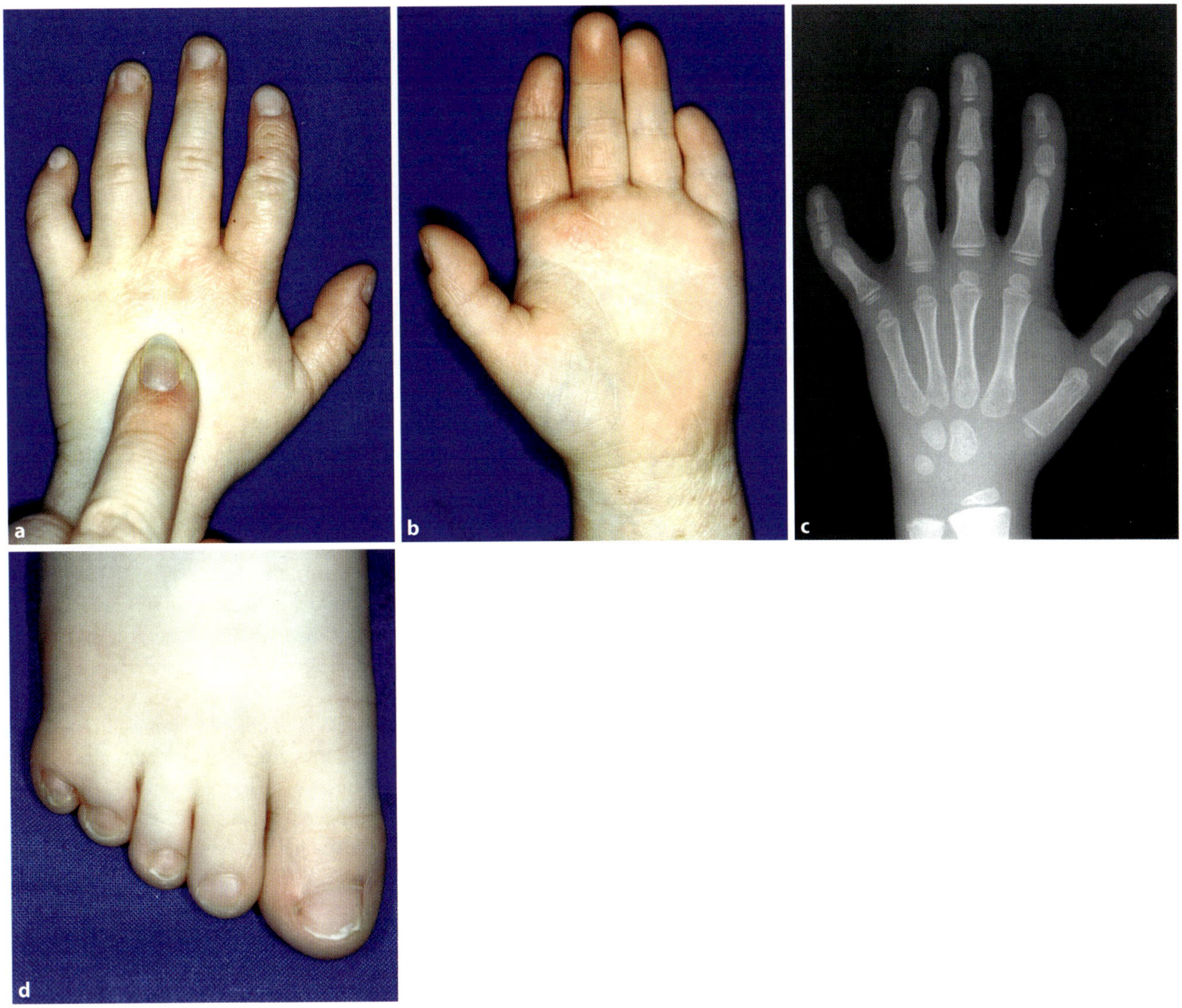

Fig. 41.1 **a** Brachydactyly type A2 in Feingold syndrome. **b** Palmar view. Note the short distance between the interphalangeal creases in digit II and the missing creases in digit V. **c** Corresponding radiograph shows short and dysplastic middle phalanges of digits II and V. **d** Syndactyly of toes IV/V

42 Albright Hereditary Osteodystrophy

MIM 103580, MIM 612463

Includes

Pseudohypoparathyroidism, type Ia
Pseudopseudohypoparathyroidism
Albright hereditary osteodystrophy with multiple hormone resistance
Albright hereditary osteodystrophy without multiple hormone resistance

Major Clinical Findings

The term Albright hereditary osteodystrophy (AHO) refers to a genetically heterogenous clinical entity encompassing brachydactyly type E (BDE), round face, short stature, central obesity, heterotopic subcutaneous ossifications, and variable degrees of mental retardation. The hands and feet are small, and radiographically a shortening of the metacarpals and/or metatarsals III, IV, and V is seen, together with variable shortening of phalanges, in particular the distal 1st, consistent with a BDE phenotype. The clinical manifestation may be mild and variable. For the identification of distinct abnormalities, a metacarpophalangeal pattern profile can be generated from anteroposterior radiographs of the left hand. Together with heterotopic ossification, BDE is the most specific feature of the AHO phenotype. Calcified nodules can often be identified on physical examination. They are usually confined to subcutaneous tissues, but in a subset of patients they can progress to deeper tissues, thus mimicking progressive osseous heteroplasia. Hypocalcemic tetany and seizures may occur. Calcification of the basal ganglion and choroid plexus has been reported.

Occasional Findings

Cataract, nystagmus, delayed tooth eruption, enamel dysplasia, osteoporosis.

Genetic Transmission

Autosomal dominant, imprinting.

Differential Diagnosis

AHO-related BDE and other forms of BDE cannot be differentiated on clinical grounds. Therefore, pseudohypoparathyroidism has to be considered in all BDE cases. Heterotopic ossifications are also features of progressive osseous heteroplasia and fibrodysplasia ossificans progressiva.

Molecular Pathology

Biochemical abnormalities are characteristically detected in AHO that suggest end-organ failure to respond to the actions of parathyroid hormone (PTH). Several subgroups of this condition, collectively termed pseudohypoparathyroidism (PHP), have been defined based on the absence or presence of AHO, with or without hormone resistance. The most frequent variants of PHP include PHP type Ia (PHP1A), pseudopseudohypoparathyroidism (PPHP), and PHP type Ib (PHP1B). Patients with PHP1A have features of AHO and present with hypocalcemia and hyperphosphatemia despite elevated serum PTH levels. Hormone resistance is usually not limited to PTH but includes resistance to thyroid stimulating hormone and gonadotropins, growth hormone releasing hormone, and calcitonin. Patients with PPHP have the typical features of AHO but do not show evidence for resistance to PTH or other hormones. In contrast, patients with PHP1B present with signs and symptoms of PTH resistance but lack the features of AHO, and hormone resistance seems to be confined to the renal actions of PTH. The common factors in these conditions are heterozygous inactivating mutations in the Gs alpha gene (*GNAS*). GNAS gives rise to several transcripts derived from the sense or antisense strand. Transcripts encoding XLαs, a large variant of Gsα, show exclusive paternal expression and are derived through the use of an alternative promoter and a unique first exon. The encoded protein, the α-subunit of the stimulatory GTP binding protein Gsα, is a ubiquitously expressed signaling protein that mediates cellular actions of numerous hormones, paracrine/autocrine factors, and neurotransmitters. The phenotypic differences among the three PHP subgroups appear to depend on the mode of inheritance. In fact, PHP1A and PPHP can be found in the same kindred, and the type of disorder is determined by the gender of the parent transmitting the genetic defect. Inheritance from a male affected by either PHP1A or PPHP leads to AHO without hormone resistance (PPHP) and expression of the mutant variant only from the maternal allele, whereas inheritance of the same Gsα mutation from a female affected by either disorder leads to both AHO and hormone resistance (that is, PHP1A) and expression of the Gs-alpha protein only from the paternal allele. PHP1B has been associated with a maternally inherited deletion in the differentially methylated region of the *GNAS* gene. Laboratory abnormalities include hypocalcemia, hyperphosphatemia, elevated serum PTH, low urinary cyclic adenosine 3′,5′-monophosphate response to PTH administration (PHP1A, PHP1B), and reduced erythrocyte Gs activity (PPHP and PHP1A).

S. Mundlos, D. Horn, *Limb Malformations*,
DOI 10.1007/978-3-540-95928-1_42, © Springer-Verlag Berlin Heidelberg 2014

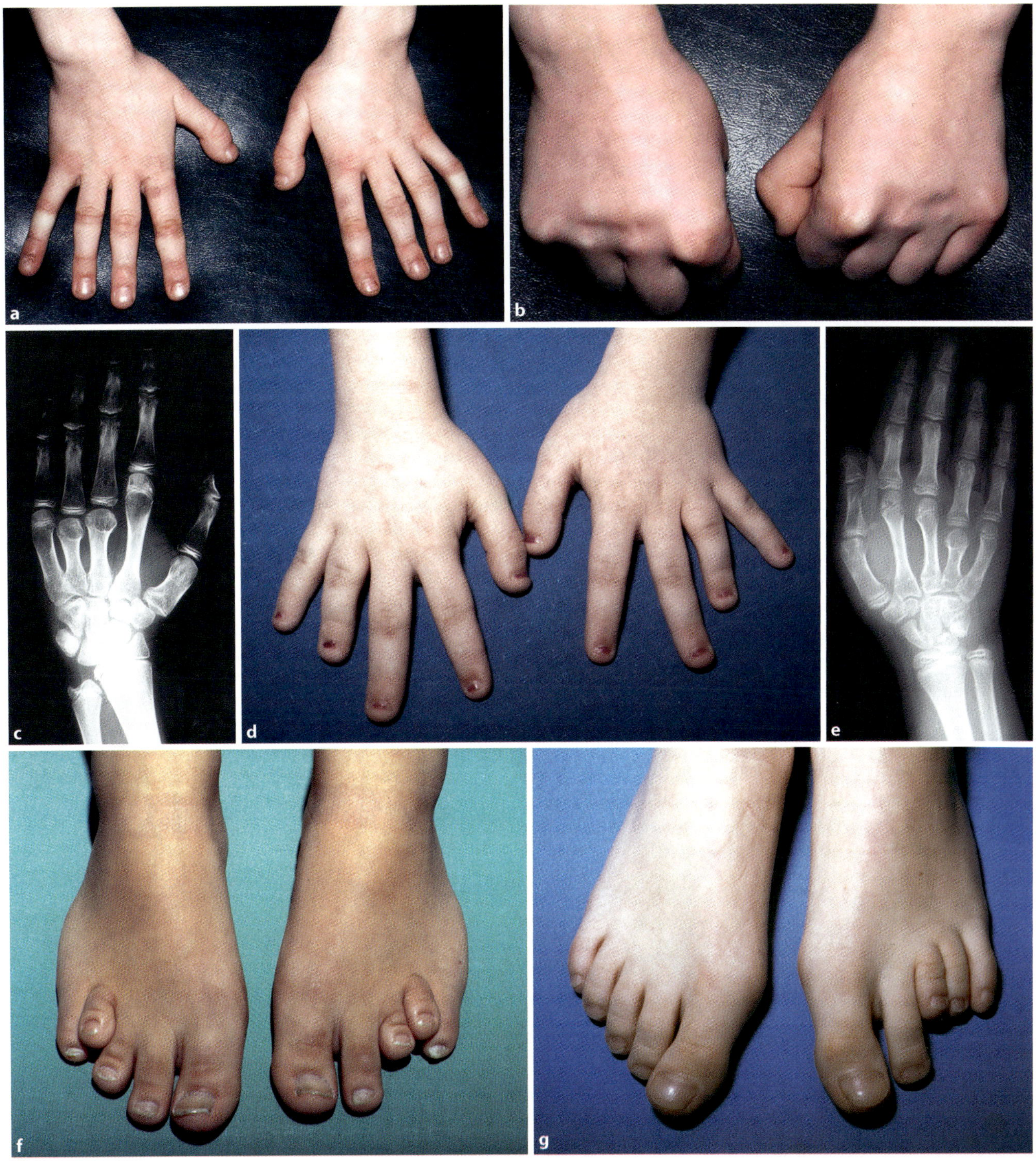

Fig. 42.1 **a, b** Individual with pseudopseudohypoparathyroidism. Note small palm and retraction of knuckles (**b**). **c** Corresponding radiograph shows normal phalanges but short metacarpals I and III–V. **d** Pseudohypoparathyroidism-associated Albright hereditary osteodystrophy in a 12.5-year-old. Note short digits IV and V bilaterally due to very short metacarpals, in particular metacarpal IV. **e** Anteroposterior hand radiograph showing short 4th metacarpal with precociously fused growth plate. **f** Foot phenotype. **g** Brachydactyly may occur unilaterally

References

Bastepe M, Jüppner H (2003) Pseudohypoparathyroidism and mechanisms of resistance toward multiple hormones: molecular evidence to clinical presentation. (Editorial). J Clin Endocrinol Metab 88(9):4055–4058

Levine MA, Germain-Lee E, Jan de Beur SG, Jüppner H, Bastepe M (2006) Different mutations within or upstream of the GNAS locus cause distinct forms of pseudohypoparathyroidism. J Pediatr Endocrinol Metab 19(2):641–646

Mantovani G (2011) Clinical review: pseudohypoparathyroidism: diagnosis and treatment. J Clin Endocrinol Metab 96(10):3020–3030

Poznanski AK, Garn SM et al (1972) Metacarpophalangeal pattern profiles in the evaluation of skeletal malformation. Radiology 104:1–11

43 Brachydactyly-Hypertension Syndrome

MIM 112410

Synonyms

Brachydactyly with hypertension
Brachydactyly type E with short stature and hypertension
Bilginturan syndrome

Major Clinical Findings

This condition is characterized by the combination of brachydactyly type E (BDE) with essential hypertension. The hands are short, showing variable phenotypes ranging from mild to severe BDE. The metacarpals III and IV are most frequently affected just like the distal phalanx of the thumb. In more severe cases, the entire hand is affected, with short and thickened metacarpals and phalanges. Cone-shaped epiphyses may be present. Affected adults are 10–15 cm shorter than unaffected family members. Blood pressure is elevated, ranging from systolic 170–250 mmHg to diastolic 100–150 mmHg. Endocrine function, electrolyte and acid–base status, and calcium and phosphate homeostasis are normal. The blood pressure is not salt sensitive, and renin, aldosterone, and catecholamines react appropriately to volume expansion and contraction. Hypertension is present in early childhood and worsens with age. If left untreated, affected individuals will develop stroke by age 50 years.

Genetic Transmission

Autosomal dominant.

Differential Diagnosis

Other forms of BDE.

References

Schuster H, Wienker TE, Bähring S, Bilginturan N, Toka HR, Neitzel H et al (1996) Severe autosomal dominant hypertension and brachydactyly in a unique Turkish kindred maps to human chromosome 12. Nat Genet 13(1):98–100

Toka O, Maass PG, Aydin A, Toka H, Hübner N et al (2010) Childhood hypertension in autosomal-dominant hypertension with brachydactyly. Hypertension 56(5):988–994

S. Mundlos, D. Horn, *Limb Malformations*,
DOI 10.1007/978-3-540-95928-1_43, © Springer-Verlag Berlin Heidelberg 2014

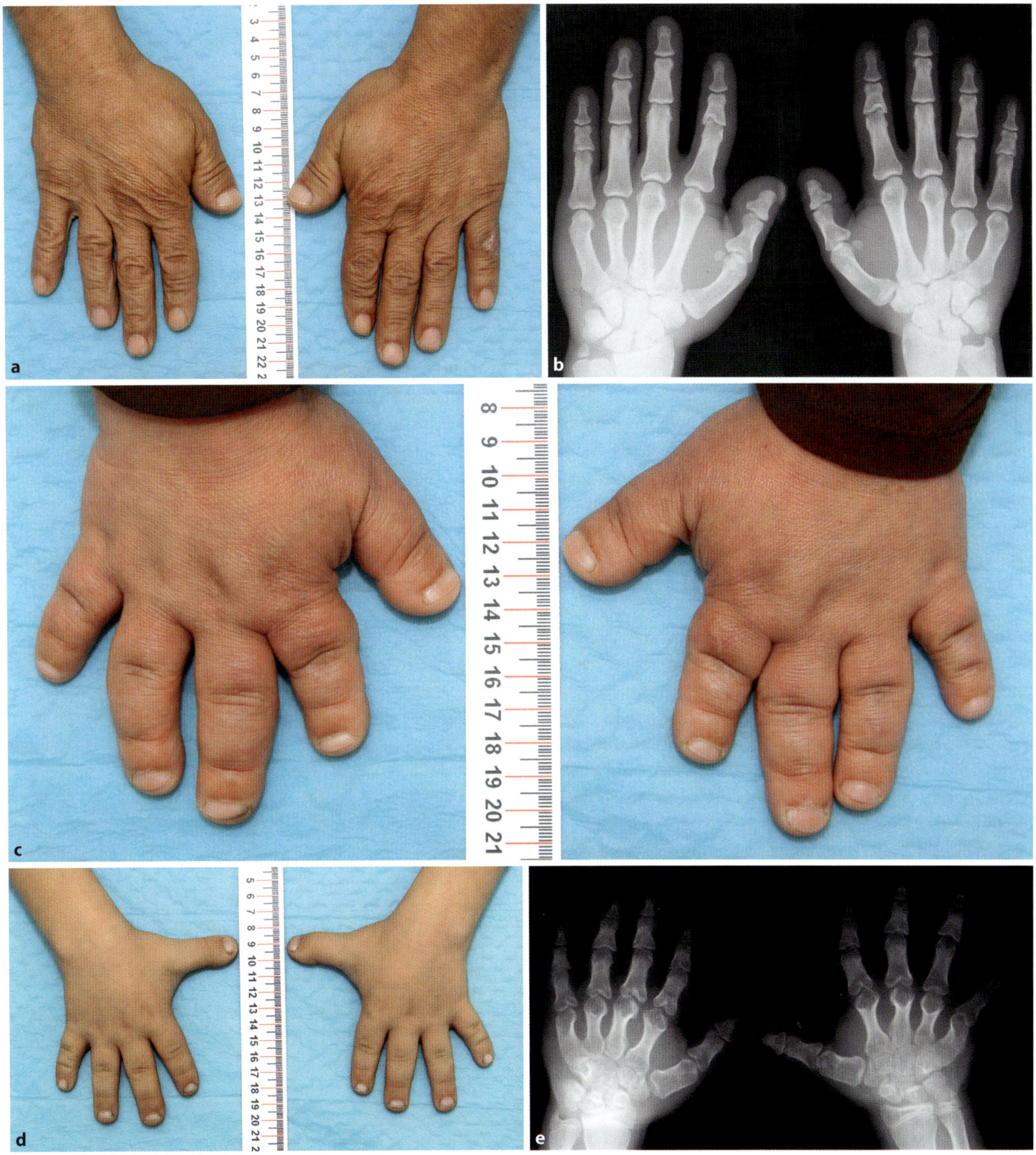

Fig. 43.1 Phenotypic variability in brachydactyly type E (BDE) hypertension syndrome. **a** Moderate severity with proportionately short hands and broad thumbs. **b** Corresponding radiographs. Asymmetrical findings with short metacarpals IV and V on the right, residual of cone epiphyses of the middle phalanx of digit II, hypoplastic middle phalanx of digits II and V, and brachydactyly type D (BDD) bilaterally. **c** Severe type with very short hands. **d** BDE hypertension in a 13-year-old. Note the short digits. **e** Corresponding radiograph. Symmetrical findings with cone-shaped epiphyses residua resulting in metacarpal shortening II–V and proximal and middle phalanges II–V. The distal phalanges are also shortened. BDD. (Courtesy of Silvia Bähring, Max Delbrück Center for Molecular Medicine, Berlin, Germany)

44 Rubinstein–Taybi Syndrome

MIM 180849, MIM 613684

Synonyms

Rubinstein syndrome
Broad thumbs and great toes, characteristic facies, and mental retardation
Broad thumb/hallux syndrome

Major Clinical Findings

Rubinstein–Taybi syndrome (RSTS) is a complex congenital malformation syndrome characterized by typical dysmorphic facial features, broad thumbs and halluces, mental retardation (average IQ of 50), postnatal growth deficiency (75 %), microcephaly, abnormal teeth (80 %), congenital heart disease (30 %), abnormalities of the eyes (80 %), hearing loss (25 %), keloid formation (25 %), and various skeletal manifestations. The facial appearance is quite specific, with a broad nasal bridge, beaked nose, highly arched eyebrows, long eyelashes, low anterior hairline, downward slanting palpebral fissures, microretrognathia, and an abnormal smile (grimacing with almost closure of the eyes). A high, slitlike palate is present. The thumbs are broad and show radial angulation (in approximately 40 %) secondary to a delta proximal phalanx of the thumb, clinodactyly 5. The halluces are broad. On radiographic examination, partial duplication of the 1st ray may be present on either the hands or feet as well as terminal broadening of the phalanges. Persistent fetal fingertip pads have been observed. Skeletal changes include delayed skeletal maturation, joint hypermobility, parietal foramina, scoliosis, small and flared iliac wings, and patellar dislocation. The average height in men has been reported be around 150 cm and in women, 146 cm. About 5 % of RSTS patients develop a neoplasm that tends to occur before 15 years of age, mainly meningioma, other brain tumors, or leukemia.

Occasional Findings

Agenesis of the corpus callosum, iris coloboma, megacolon, hypoplastic kidney, primary immune deficiency, bifid uterus, premature thelarche, café au lait spots.

Genetic Transmission

Autosomal dominant. Practically all cases occur sporadically, resulting from de novo heterozygous mutations.

Differential Diagnosis

Floating–Harbor syndrome, which is caused by mutations in the *SRCAP* gene, a coactivator for CREBBP, shows phenotypic overlap with RSTS.

Molecular Pathology

RSTS has been associated with deletions on chromosome 16p13.3, resulting in a severe form of the condition due to a contiguous gene deletion involving the *CREBBP* gene as well as other neighboring genes. Mutation analysis identified *CREBBP* as the gene responsible for RSTS in approximately 50 %. CREBBP is a nuclear protein participating as a coactivator in cAMP-regulated gene expression. CREBBP-dependent gene transcription has been shown to underlie long-term memory formation. Another rare form of RSTS is caused by mutations in EP300, which also functions as a transcriptional coactivator. Like CREBBP, it functions as potent histone acetyltransferase, suggesting that RSTS is caused by aberrant chromatin regulation.

References

Hennekam RC (2006) Rubinstein–Taybi syndrome. Eur J Hum Genet 14(9):981–985

Petrij F, Giles RH, Dauwerse HG, Saris JJ, Hennekam RC, Masuno M et al (1995) Rubinstein–Taybi syndrome caused by mutations in the transcriptional co-activator CBP. Nature 376(6538):348–351

Roelfsema JH, White SJ, Ariyürek Y, Bartholdi D, Niedrist D, Papadia F et al (2005) Genetic heterogeneity in Rubinstein–Taybi syndrome: mutations in both the CBP and EP300 genes cause disease. Am J Hum Genet 76(4):572–580

Wiley S, Swayne S, Rubinstein JH, Lanphear NE, Stevens CA (2003) Rubinstein–Taybi syndrome medical guidelines. Am J Med Genet A 119A(2):101–110

S. Mundlos, D. Horn, *Limb Malformations*,
DOI 10.1007/978-3-540-95928-1_44, © Springer-Verlag Berlin Heidelberg 2014

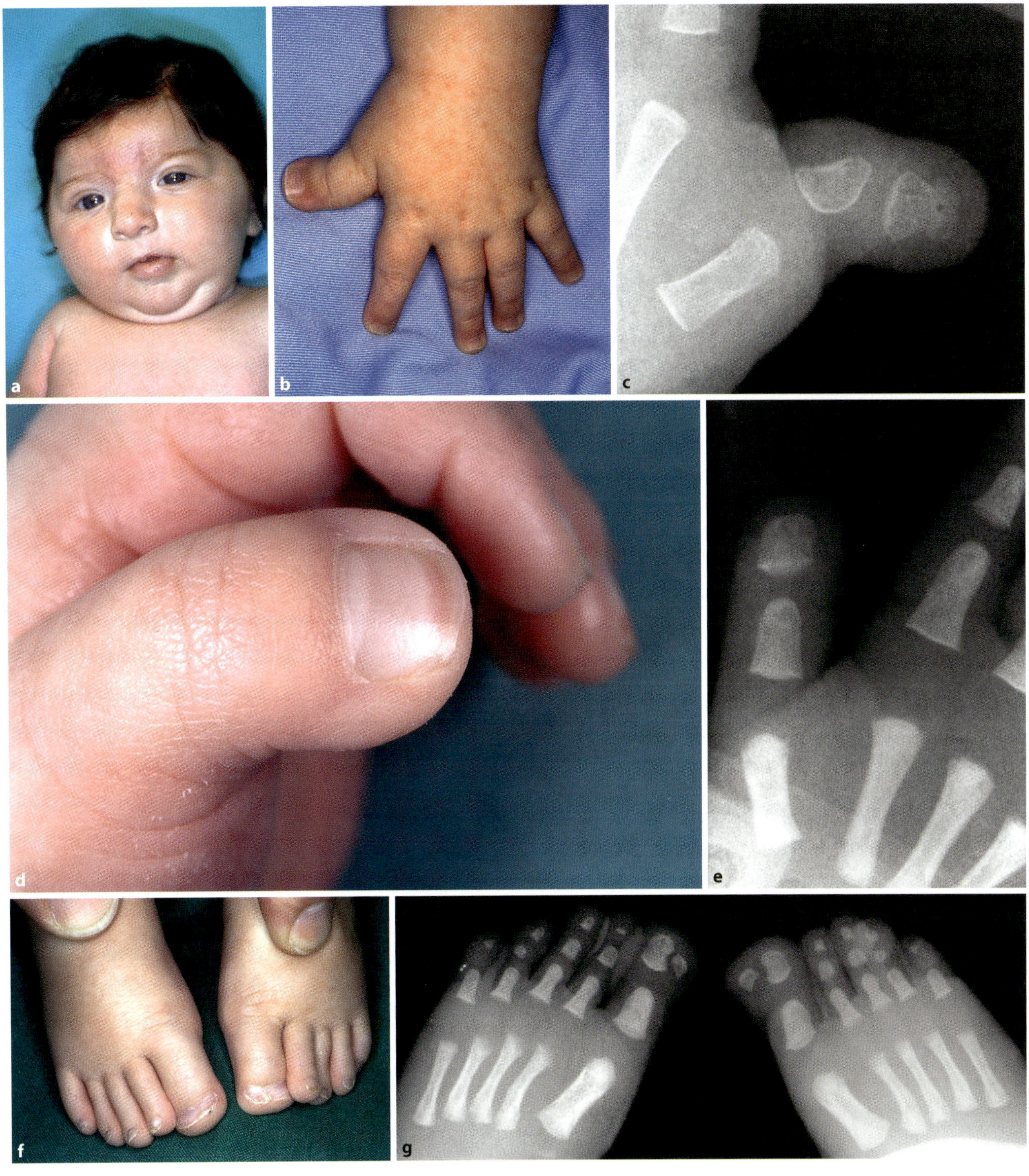

Fig. 44.1 **a** Typical facial appearance: broad nasal bridge, prominent columella, retrognathia. **b** Broad thumb with radial angulation. **c** Corresponding radiograph of thumb shows delta-shaped proximal phalanx and broad partially duplicated distal phalanx. **d** Broad thumb without angulation. **e** Corresponding radiograph shows broad distal phalanx. **f** Broad 1st toes with duplication of nails. **g** Corresponding radiograph shows duplication of distal phalanx of halluces and nonossified middle phalanx V

45 Cranioectodermal Dysplasia

MIM 218330

Synonyms
Sensenbrenner syndrome
Levin syndrome 1

Major Clinical Findings
Cranioectodermal dysplasia (CED) is a disorder characterized by craniosynostosis (mainly sagittal) and facial, ectodermal, and skeletal anomalies. Craniofacial features include dolichocephaly; sparse, fine, slow-growing hair; epicanthal folds; hypodontia and/or microdontia; and taurodontism. Frontal bossing and hypertelorism are further features. Retinal photoreceptor dystrophy has been described in childhood. Skeletal anomalies include rhizomelic shortening of the limbs, most pronounced in the upper limbs; brachydactyly with stubby digits; 5th-finger clinodactyly; symphalangism; soft tissue syndactyly of the fingers; joint laxity; narrow thorax; and pectus excavatum. Radiographic findings of the hand show short phalanges, in particular hypoplasia of the distal phalanges with large corresponding epiphyses. Radiographic abnormalities of the long bones involve metaphyseal widening with flattened epiphyses. The capital femoral epiphysis ossifies late. The fibula is short, and the semilunar notches of the ulna are small. Height is between the 3rd and 10th percentiles. Chronic renal failure may occur as a result of tubulointerstitial nephropathy.

Occasional Findings
Prenatal and postnatal growth retardation, delayed psychomotor development, microcephaly, abnormal nails, inguinal hernia, thoracic hypoplasia, seizures, heart defects, hepatic cysts, liver fibrosis, cutis laxa, abnormalities of the ears.

Genetic Transmission
Autosomal recessive.

Differential Diagnosis
CED should be distinguished from other syndromes with ectodermal abnormalities by the presence of the typical craniofacial appearance and by the skeletal anomalies. In some cases, differential diagnoses may include skeletal dysplasias or syndromes with prominent rhizomelic shortening of the limbs.

Molecular Pathology
CED is a genetically heterogenous ciliopathy. CED1 can be caused by homozygous or compound heterozygous mutations in the *IFT122* gene, which plays an important role in the assembly and maintenance of eukaryotic cilia. Compared with controls, significantly reduced frequency and length of primary cilia have been found in the fibroblasts of patients. CED2 is caused by mutations in the *WDR35* gene; CED3 is caused by mutations in the *IFT43* gene; and CED4 is caused by mutations in the *WDR19* gene.

References

Walczak-Sztulpa J, Eggenschwiler J, Osborn D, Brown DA, Emma F, Klingenberg C et al (2010) Cranioectodermal dysplasia, Sensenbrenner syndrome, is a ciliopathy caused by mutations in the IFT122 gene. Am J Hum Genet 86:949–956

Young ID (1989) Cranioectodermal dysplasia (Sensenbrenner's syndrome). J Med Genet 26:393–396

Zaffanello M, Diomedi-Camassei F, Melzi ML, Torre G, Callea F, Emma F (2006) Sensenbrenner syndrome: a new member of the hepatorenal fibrocystic family. Am J Med Genet 140A:2336–2340

S. Mundlos, D. Horn, *Limb Malformations*,
DOI 10.1007/978-3-540-95928-1_45, © Springer-Verlag Berlin Heidelberg 2014

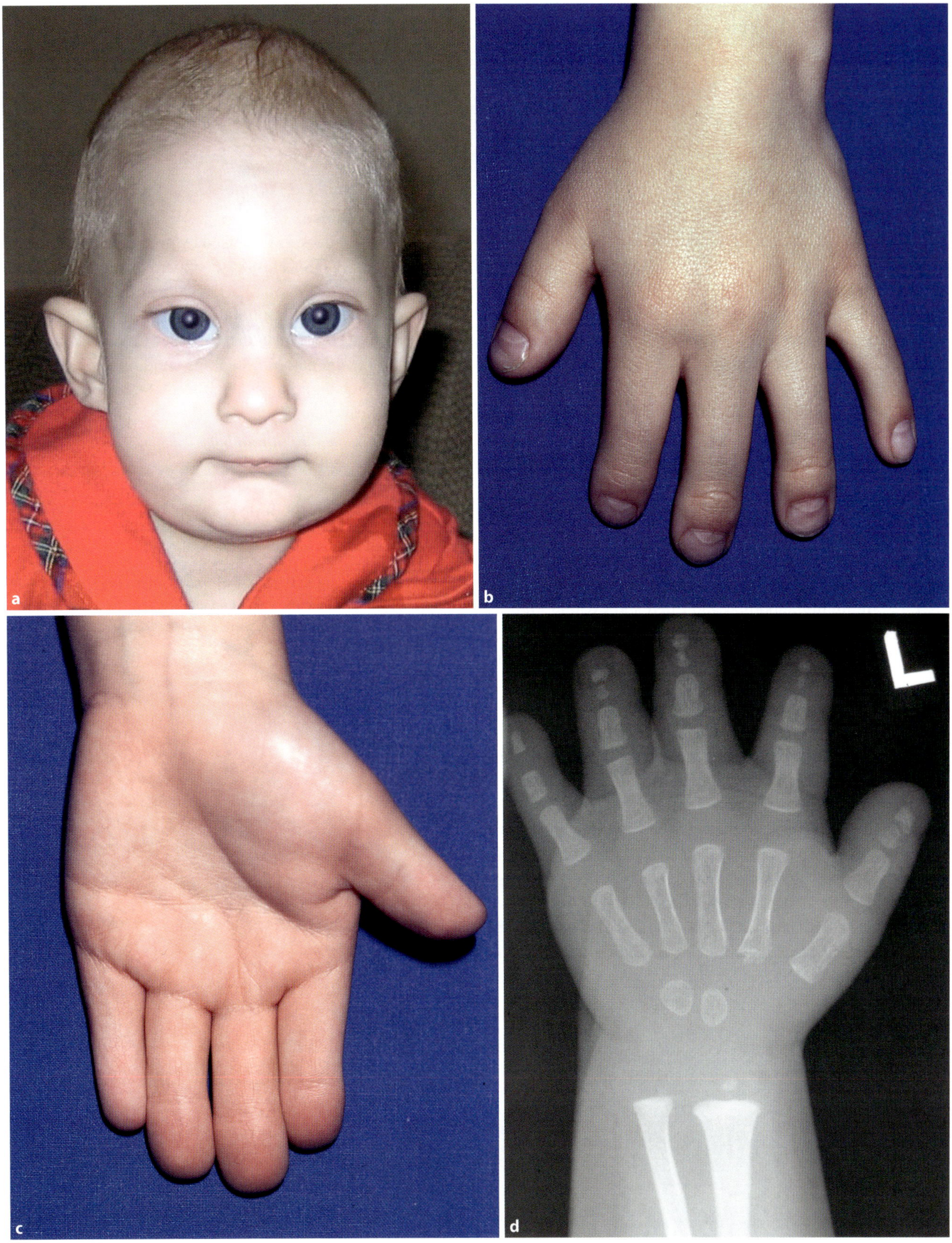

Fig. 45.1 **a** A 3-year-old boy with cranioectodermal dysplasia. Note dolichocephalus (with sagittal suture synostosis) and sparse, fine hair. **b, c** Hand showing brachydactyly, missing middle flexion creases of digits II–V. Digit V has no flexion creases. **d** Corresponding radiograph shows short metacarpal and phalangeal bones, flattened distal portions of proximal phalanges II–IV, and duplicated primary ossification centers of the distal phalanges I–IV

46 Temtamy Preaxial Brachydactyly Syndrome

MIM 605282

Synonyms
Preaxial brachydactyly syndrome, Temtamy type

Major Clinical Findings
Temtamy-type brachydactyly is characterized by brachydactyly of the hands and feet, dental anomalies, and mild facial dysmorphism. The involvement of the hands is characteristically more severe on the radial side (preaxial), resulting in very short thumbs and small, radially deviated digits II and III. The thumb is deviated and may point in a proximal direction. The metacarpophalangeal joints can be dislocated, resulting in an abnormal position of the digits. The interphalangeal joints often show contractures with functional symphalangism. Digits IV and V are usually less severely affected. Radiographically, the metacarpals are short, in particular those of digits I–III. The proximal phalanges of digits I–IV are highly abnormal and often show a longitudinal split because of abnormally positioned epiphyses. This results in abnormal metacarpophalangeal joints and partial joint dislocation. The middle phalanges of digits II–III are often relatively long and slender and show incomplete formation of joints in their distal third, resulting in hyperphalangism. Digit V is the least affected. The feet are short with short, laterally deviated great toes. Radiographs show broad, longitudinally duplicated 1st metatarsals and proximal phalanges. As in the hands, there are abnormally shaped proximal phalanges of digits II and III with joint dislocations. Fusion of tarsal and carpal bones and radioulnar synostosis are other less frequently observed features. Other skeletal abnormalities include kyphoscoliosis, pectus excavatum, and generalized osteoporosis. Dental anomalies include microdontia, talon cusps, midline diastema, and a narrow lower alveolar ridge.

Occasional Findings
Eye abnormalities including optic atrophy, macrophthalmia, blue sclerae, and tilted optic discs. Cleft palate.

Genetic Transmission
Autosomal recessive.

Differential Diagnosis
The combination of findings is very specific. The hand phenotype overlaps somewhat with Catel–Manzke brachydactyly in milder cases.

Molecular Pathology
Temtamy brachydactyly is caused by mutations in chondroitin synthase 1 (CHSY1), a key enzyme in the synthesis of chondroitin sulfate. The latter is synthesized in a multistep process as covalently bound side chains of proteoglycans. Mutations in CHSY1 result in a partial loss of chondroitin sulfate. Part of the pathology in this condition appears to be increased Notch signaling, which leads to enhanced or premature ossification.

References

Li Y, Laue K, Temtamy S, Aglan M, Kotan LD, Yigit G et al (2010) Temtamy preaxial brachydactyly syndrome is caused by loss-of-function mutations in chondroitin synthase 1, a potential target of BMP signaling. Am J Hum Genet 87(6):757–767

Temtamy SA, Meguid NA, Ismail SI, Ramzy MI (1998) A new multiple congenital anomaly, mental retardation syndrome with preaxial brachydactyly, hyperphalangism, deafness and orodental anomalies. Clin Dysmorph 7:249–255

S. Mundlos, D. Horn, *Limb Malformations*,
DOI 10.1007/978-3-540-95928-1_46,

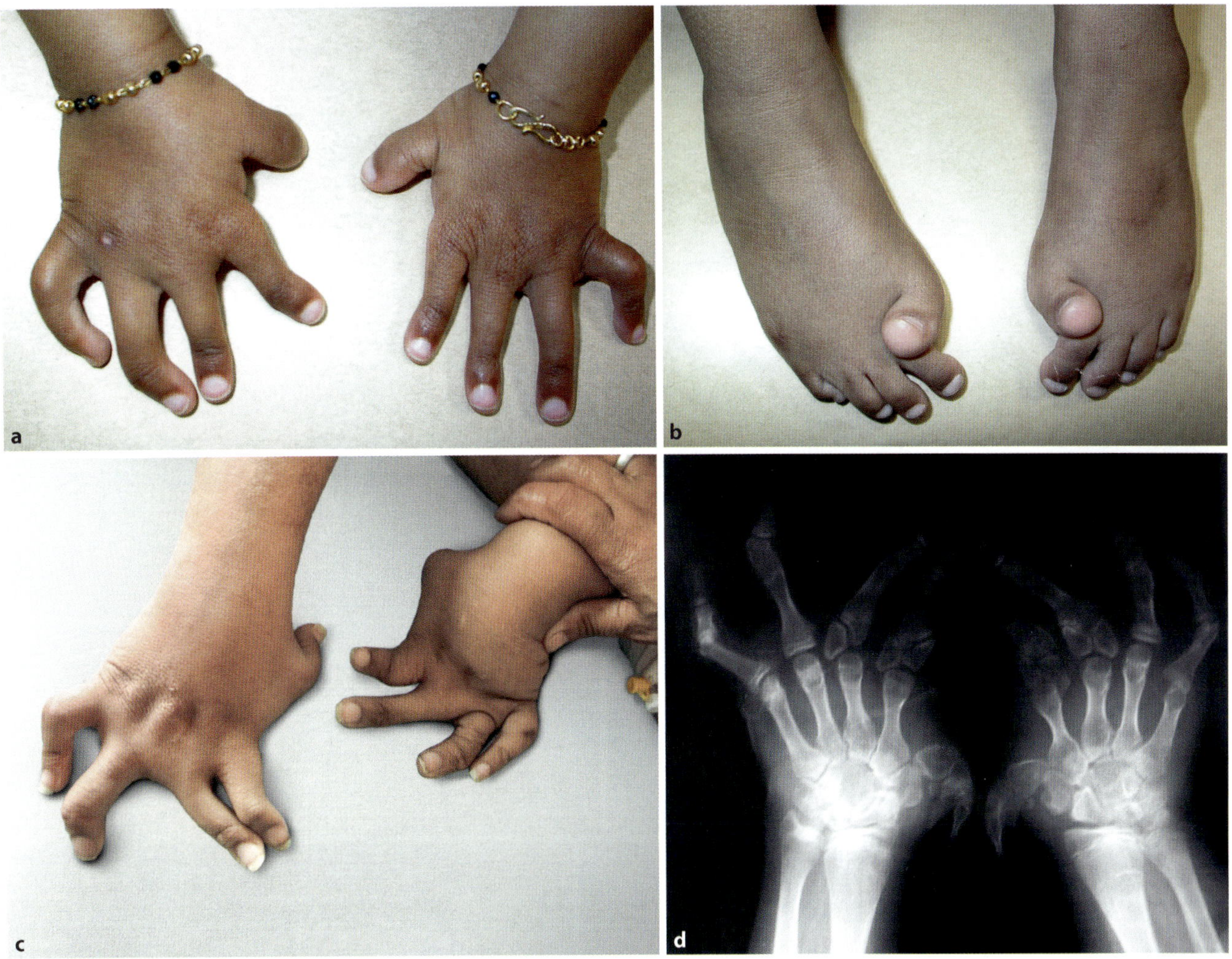

Fig. 46.1 **a** Generalized brachydactyly most pronounced in digits I–III (preaxial). Note the very short, proximally deviated thumb; small, hypoplastic digits II and III; and contracture deformity of digits V on the left and IV and V on the right. **b** Feet of the same individual. Laterally deviated, upturned halluces. **c** More severe case with very short, proximally pointing thumbs, short digits, camptodactyly, phalangeal synostoses, and/or missing phalanges. **d** Corresponding radiograph. Note the very short 1st metacarpals, hypoplastic thumb including phalanges, and short metacarpals II and III. The epiphyses of the proximal phalanges of digits II and III show two enlarged duplicated ossification centers. Synostoses of the distal interphalangeal joints are present in several digits

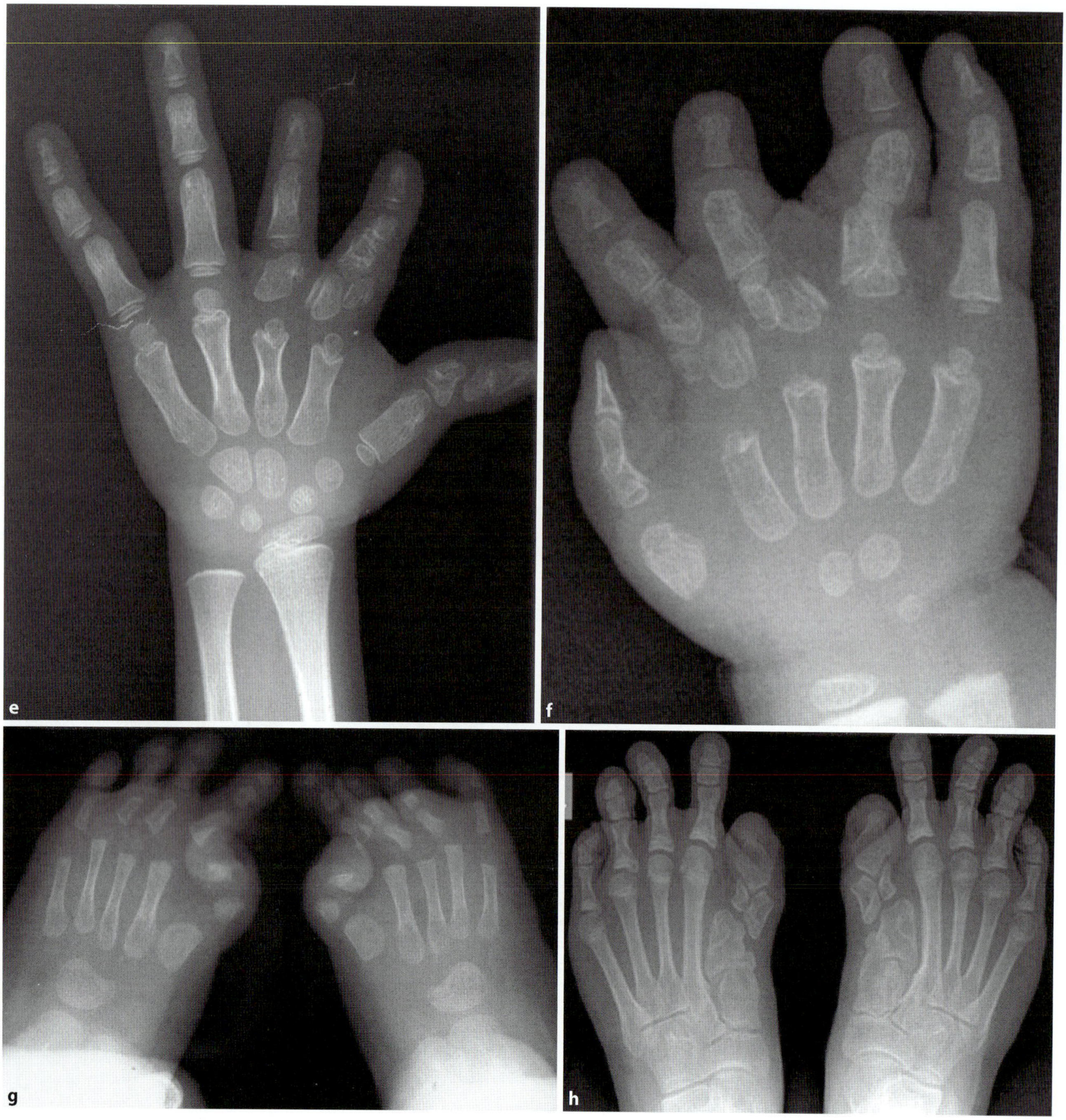

Fig. 46.1 (*continued*) **e** Radiograph of hand showing a short, proximally deviated thumb with abnormal proximal and distal phalanges and very short digits II and III with bizarre phalangeal development and relatively normal digits IV and V. Note short metacarpals II and III with cone-shaped epiphyses. Abnormal shapes of proximal phalanges I–III appear partially split due to delta-shaped phalangeal epiphyses. **f** Radiograph of hand showing short metacarpals, hypoplastic phalanges of thumb, double ossification centers of proximal phalanges II–IV, and fusion of interphalangeal joints. **g** Radiograph of feet in **b** showing broad and short 1st metatarsal, short proximal/distal phalanges, and deviated 1st phalanx. **h** More severe case showing short hallux with major abnormalities. There is a very short and broad 1st metatarsal, laterally split phalanges with two ossification centers, broad distal phalanges, and tarsal fusions. (Courtesy of Bernd Wollnik, University of Cologne, Germany)

Fibrodysplasia Ossificans Progressiva

MIM 135100

47

Major Clinical Findings

Fibrodysplasia ossificans progressiva (FOP) is characterized by heterotopic ossification and abnormalities of the halluces. At birth, individuals with FOP are normal except for short great toes, which can be medially deviated and monophalangic. Other more variable but common congenital abnormalities include cervical spine malformations (80%); a short, broad femoral neck (70%); conductive hearing impairment; short thumb with short 1st metacarpal and/or monophalangism (50%); and 5th-finger clinodactyly. However, the major problem for these individuals is progressive heterotopic ossifications that follow a characteristic anatomical pattern. They start with swellings, sometimes accompanied by pain and fever, located in muscles, tendons, aponeuroses, and fasciae. The most common sites of early heterotopic ossification are the neck, spine, and shoulder girdle extending over the entire thorax. The age of onset varies between the 1st year of life and the mid-20s, with an average age of 5 years. Ossification generally proceeds in an axial to appendicular direction and from cranial to caudal and proximal to distal. With increasing ossification, movement becomes restricted and eventually results in complete immobility, thoracic insufficiency, and death. Ossification events appear to be often triggered by trauma, including medical intervention such as intramuscular injections, tooth extractions, and diagnostic biopsies. Due to the initial lack of symptoms and the only moderate changes of the great toe, there is usually a major delay in correct diagnosis even after the onset of ectopic ossification.

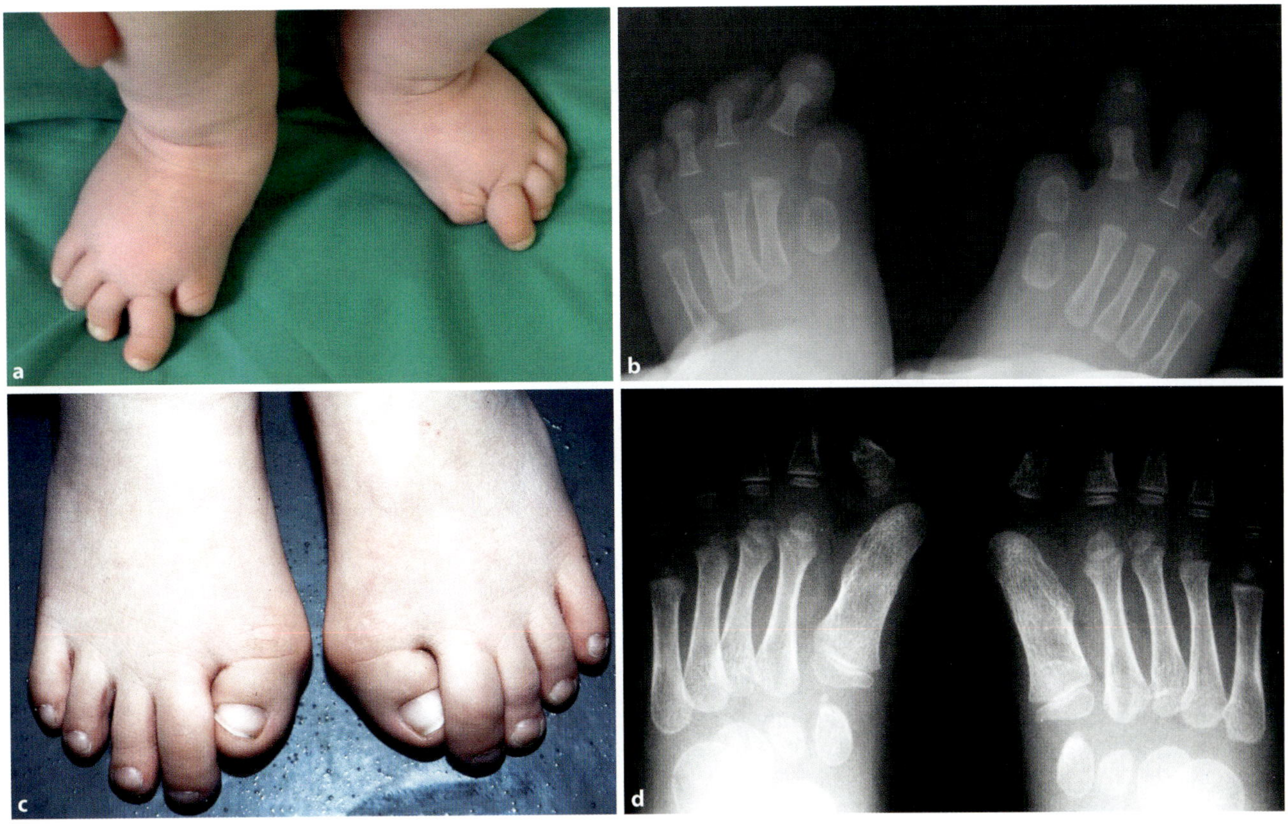

Fig. 47.1 **a** Variability of foot phenotype in fibrodysplasia ossificans progressive (FOP). **b** Radiograph corresponding to **a**. The halluces show hypoplastic round 1st metatarsals, abnormally round middle phalanges, and absence of distal phalanges bilaterally. **c** Milder FOP foot phenotype. **d** Corresponding radiograph. Note broad, medially deviated metatarsal I, proximal phalanx fused to the metatarsal, and laterally deviated distal phalanx

S. Mundlos, D. Horn, *Limb Malformations*,
DOI 10.1007/978-3-540-95928-1_47, © Springer-Verlag Berlin Heidelberg 2014

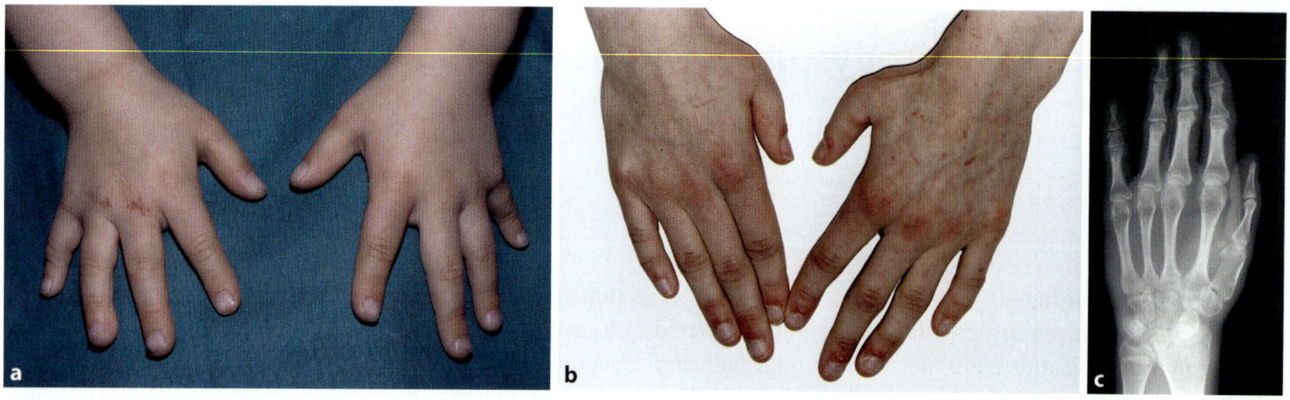

Fig. 47.2 The hand phenotype is usually less pronounced shows considerable variability. **a** Short thumb and mild digit V clinodactyly. **b** Short, distally placed thumb. **c** Corresponding radiograph shows short and slightly broad metacarpal I, small proximal phalanx I, and hypoplastic middle phalanx of digit V

Occasional Findings

Patients with classic FOP and the most common mutation (p.R206H) have a highly penetrant condition with typical findings as described above. However, other less typical forms exist that are usually due to other mutations in the same gene. These include severe variable reduction deficits of the digits, absence of nails in affected digits, intraarticular synovial osteochondromatosis, sparse and thin scalp hair, mild cognitive impairment, growth retardation, and childhood glaucoma. Some individuals may have normal toes.

Genetic Transmission

Autosomal dominant.

Differential Diagnosis

Other less well-defined conditions with heterotopic ossification exist. Progressive osseous heteroplasia is a rare autosomal dominant disorder characterized by dermal ossification beginning in infancy but with normal toes, followed by increasing and extensive bone formation in deep muscle and fascia. The condition is caused by heterozygous inactivating mutations in the *GNAS1* gene, with the mutant allele being inherited exclusively from the father, indicating imprinting. Hypoplasia of the halluces also occurs also in brachydactyly type A2 (BDA2) and hand–foot–genital syndrome.

Molecular Pathology

FOP is caused by mutations in the bone morphogenetic protein (BMP) receptor ACVR1. BMPs were identified for their ability to produce ectopic bone after implantation in, for example, muscle. ACVR1 belongs to a family of BMP receptors with similar structure. They consist of an extracellular domain for ligand binding and intracellular domains for signal transduction. The intracellular part consists of a so-called GS domain, which is important for protein binding and activation, and a protein kinase domain. The mutations are all located with either the GS domain or the kinase domain and result in aberrant activation of the receptor. This causes increased levels of BMP signaling in cells. Other triggers such as inflammation may increase this level to eventually result in ectopic bone formation. The short toes/thumbs are developmental effects of the mutations. The BMP pathway is essential for digit development and is particularly important for joint formation. See also mutations in the BMP receptor 1B that cause brachydactyly type A2.

The great majority of FOP patients carry the canonical R206H mutation. However, other changes in ACVR1 have been described that result in similar or less severe phenotypes.

References

Cohen RB, Hahn GV, Tabas JA, Peeper J, Levitz CL, Sando A et al (1993) The natural history of heterotopic ossification in patients who have fibrodysplasia ossificans progressiva: a study of forty-four patients. J Bone Joint Surg 75A:215–219

Kaplan FS, Xu M, Seemann P, Connor JM, Glaser DL, Carroll L, Delai P et al (2009) Classic and atypical fibrodysplasia ossificans progressiva (FOP) phenotypes are caused by mutations in the bone morphogenetic protein (BMP) type I receptor ACVR1. Hum Mutat 30(3):379–390

Shen Q, Little SC, Xu M, Haupt J, Ast C, Katagiri T et al (2009) The fibrodysplasia ossificans progressiva R206H ACVR1 mutation activates BMP-independent chondrogenesis and zebrafish embryo ventralization. J Clin Invest 119(11):3462–3472

Shore EM, Kaplan FS (2010) Inherited human diseases of heterotopic bone formation. Nat Rev Rheumatol 6(9):518–527

Shore EM, Xu M, Feldman GJ, Fenstermacher DA, Cho T-J, Choi IH et al (2006) A recurrent mutation in the BMP type I receptor ACVR1 causes inherited and sporadic fibrodysplasia ossificans progressiva. Nature Genet 38:525–527

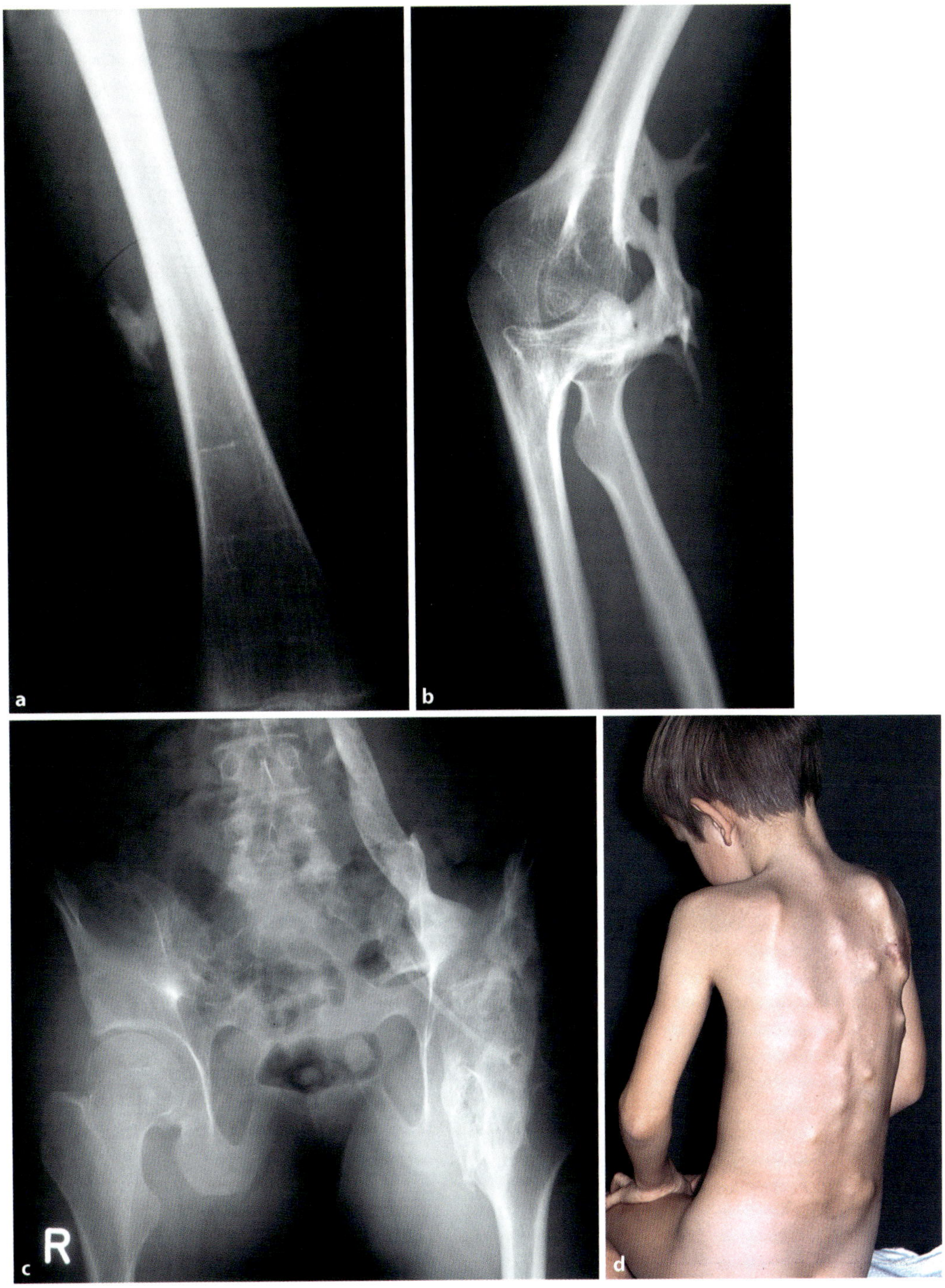

Fig. 47.3 Ectopic ossification and progression in fibrodysplasia ossificans progressiva. **a** Single ectopic calcification close to femur after minor injury. **b** Extensive bony bridges around elbow. **c** Complete ossification of left hip joint and into the lumbar spine region. **d** Clinical appearance: progressive ossification along the spine extending into the pelvis and hip region

48 Enchondromatosis, Ollier Type

MIM 166000

Included
Maffucci Syndrome
MIM 614569

Synonyms
Osteochondromatosis
Dyschondroplasia

Major Clinical Findings
Enchondromas are benign cartilage tumors that usually appear between the 1st and 5th years of age. These lesions are most numerous in the phalangeal bones of the hands and feet. Clinical findings include asymmetric limb shortening, swelling of the fingers and toes, and disturbed movements of the interphalangeal joints. They may occur unilaterally, but frequently they are bilateral. After puberty no new enchondromas develop, and tumor growth in adulthood is considered to be malignant degeneration of these tumors. Pathological fractures in the affected bones may occur. Radiographs show oval or linear radiolucent defects in the metaphyseal regions of tubular bones. These lesions are frequently associated with expansion of the affected bone and cortical thinning of this area.

The combination of enchondromas with hemangiomas is called Maffucci syndrome. Patients with Maffucci syndrome may develop chondrosarcomas. Hemangiomas in Maffucci syndrome, most commonly located on the skin, may be present at birth or develop later. Phlebolithiasis has been noted. A diverse spectrum of neoplasms other than chondrosarcomas has been reported in Maffucci syndrome, but rarely in enchondromatosis.

Occasional Findings
Short stature, oral hemangiomas, hemangiomas of the meninges.

Genetic Transmission
Most cases of Ollier disease and Maffucci syndrome are sporadic. Few instances of familial occurrence have been reported.

Differential Diagnosis
The differential diagnosis includes other disorders with multiple enchondromas. In metachondromatosis (the combination of exostoses and enchondromas), the enchondromatous lesions affect the long and short tubular bones as well as the iliac crest. These lesions may regress. In genochondromatosis, the lesions predominantly affect the hands and feet, the upper end of the humerus, the knee, and the clavicles. In contrast to enchondromatosis type Ollier and Maffucci syndrome, both conditions are autosomal dominantly inherited. Multiple cartilaginous exostoses are easy to distinguish from enchondromas by different radiographic findings. In the case of Maffucci syndrome, other conditions with multiple hemangiomas such as Klippel–Trénaunay syndrome and Proteus syndrome should be excluded.

Molecular Pathology
Specific mutations in *IDH1* and *IDH2* have been identified in tumors of individuals with Ollier disease as well as in those with Maffucci syndrome. *IDH1* mutations in cartilage tumors are associated with hypermethylation and downregulated expression of several genes. Mutations were absent in DNA isolated from the blood, muscle, and saliva of the affected subjects. Thus, the mutations are likely to be early postzygotic events, implying that the mutations are required for tumorigenesis.

Furthermore, heterozygous missense mutations in *PTHR1* have been described in patients with Ollier disease. Two mutations were present only in enchondromas, and one mutation was present in both enchondroma and leukocyte DNA of the affected individual. These mutations activate hedgehog signaling that may induce enchondromatous growth.

References

Amary MF, Damato S, Halai D, Eskandarpour M, Berisha F, Bonar F et al (2011) Ollier disease and Maffucci syndrome are caused by somatic mosaic mutations of IDH1 and IDH2. Nature Genet 43:1262–1265
Couvineau A, Wouters V, Bertrand G, Rouyer C, Gerard B, Boon LM et al (2008) PTHR1 mutations associated with Ollier disease result in receptor loss of function. Hum Molec Genet 17:2766–2775
Pansuriya TC, Kroon HM, Bovee JVMG (2010) Enchondromatosis: insights on the different subtypes. Int J Clin Exp Pathol 3:557–569
Sun T-C, Swee RG, Shives TC, Unni KK (1985) Chondrosarcoma in Maffucci's syndrome. J Bone Joint Surg Am 67:1214–1219

S. Mundlos, D. Horn, *Limb Malformations*,
DOI 10.1007/978-3-540-95928-1_48, © Springer-Verlag Berlin Heidelberg 2014

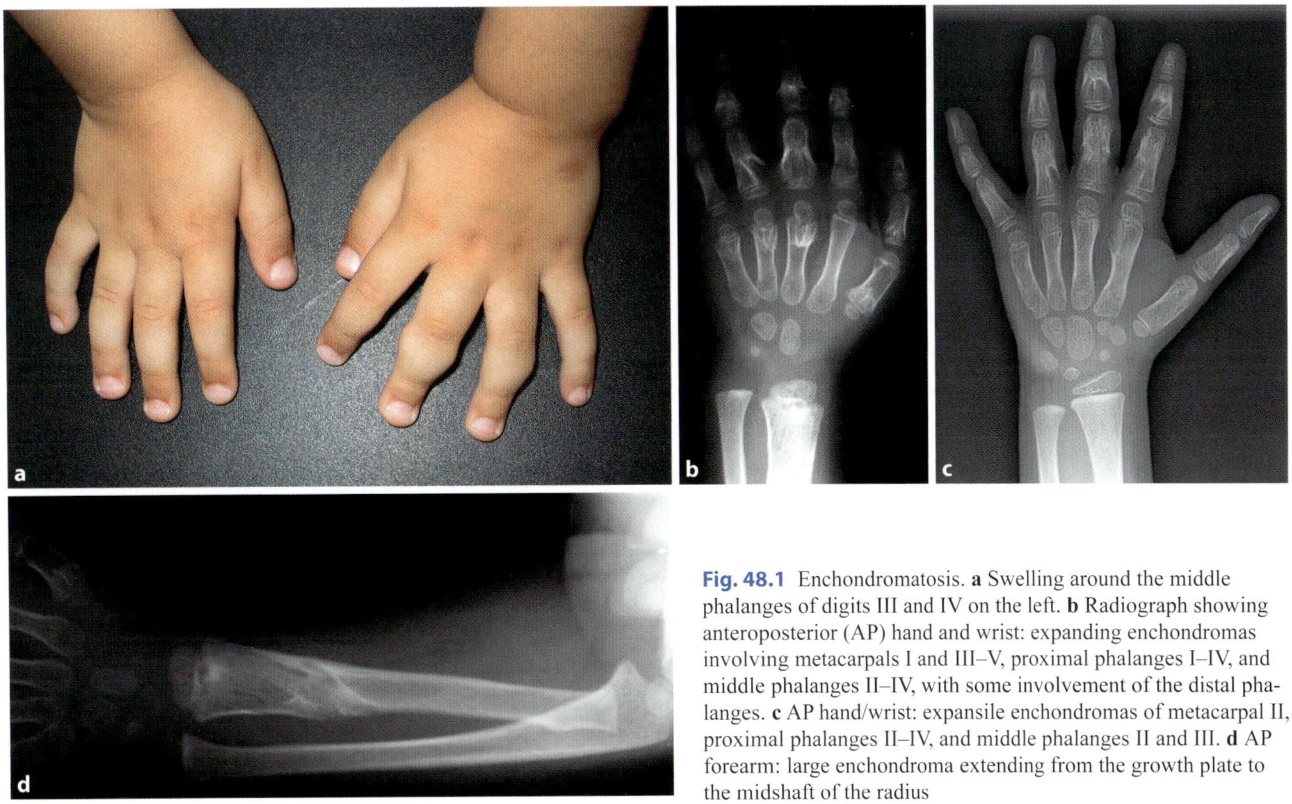

Fig. 48.1 Enchondromatosis. **a** Swelling around the middle phalanges of digits III and IV on the left. **b** Radiograph showing anteroposterior (AP) hand and wrist: expanding enchondromas involving metacarpals I and III–V, proximal phalanges I–IV, and middle phalanges II–IV, with some involvement of the distal phalanges. **c** AP hand/wrist: expansile enchondromas of metacarpal II, proximal phalanges II–IV, and middle phalanges II and III. **d** AP forearm: large enchondroma extending from the growth plate to the midshaft of the radius

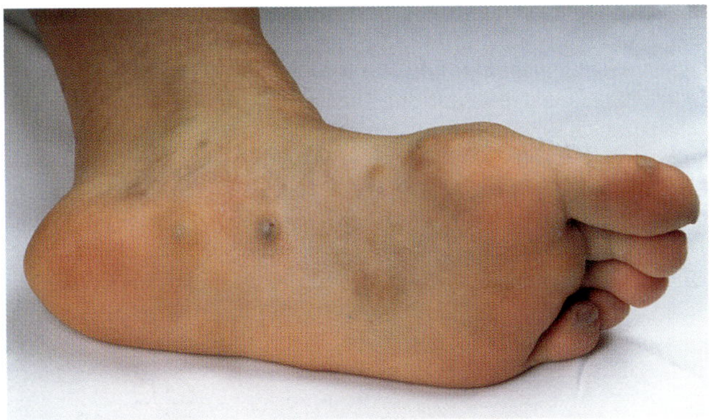

Fig. 48.2 Maffucci syndrome. Multiple hemangiomas at the toes and sole of foot

49 Trichorhinophalangeal Syndrome

MIM 190350

Synonyms

Trichorhinophalangeal dysplasia

Major Clinical Findings

Trichorhinophalangeal syndrome (TRPS) features distinctive craniofacial and skeletal abnormalities. Affected individuals show sparse and slowly growing scalp hair as well as sparse eyebrows. Facial features include nose with a bulbous tip and hypoplastic alae nasi, a long philtrum, a thin upper vermilion border, and prominent ears. The fingers are short with prominent interphalangeal joints and axial deviation. Hand radiographs show shortening of phalangeal bones, typical cone-shaped epiphyses (Giedion type 12), and premature epiphyseal fusion. Cone-shaped epiphyses are most frequently present in the middle and less often in the proximal phalanges of the 2nd, 3rd, and 4th fingers. Multiple cone-shaped epiphyses may also be noted in the toes. The capital femoral epiphyses may be flattened and deformed. Adult-onset chronic joint pain, particularly in the hips, may occur. The adult height is usually below the 10th percentile.

TRPS is subdivided into two types. Type 1 features only the signs described above, whereas type 2 is a contiguous gene syndrome combining the manifestations of TRPS type 1 and multiple exostoses type 1. In addition, mild intellectual disability is a feature in the majority of affected individuals. Exostoses appear in the first years of life, mainly in the long and short tubular bones, and especially near the metaphyses. They increase in size and number with growth. Postnatal growth retardation is a constant feature. Small capital epiphyses with deformities may be present. Hypermobility of joints and redundant skin in infancy have been documented.

Occasional Findings

Flat distal femoral epiphyses, pectus carinatum, scoliosis, delayed bone age, supernumerary teeth, intellectual disability.

Genetic Transmission

Autosomal dominant.

Differential Diagnosis

TRPS type 1 can be distinguished from TRPS type 2 by the presence of multiple cartilaginous exostoses and intellectual disability in the latter. The severe end of the TRPS spectrum has been classified as TRPS type 3, characterized by severe brachydactyly with short metacarpals and severe short stature as well as the presence of specific missense mutations of the GATA DNA-binding motif of the gene. Other brachydactyly syndromes, such as acrodysostosis, differ by the absence of the specific facial and hair anomalies. Cone-shaped epiphyses may also occur as an isolated finding.

Molecular Pathology

TRPS type 1 is caused by haploinsufficiency of the *TRPS1* gene, which encodes a zinc-finger transcription factor involved in chondrocyte and perichondrium development. TRPS type 2 is a contiguous gene syndrome on chromosome 8q24.1 caused by haploinsufficiency of the *TRPS1* and *EXT1* genes.

References

Giedion A (1966) Das Tricho-rhino-phalangeale Syndrom. Helv Paediat Acta 21:475–482

Ludecke H-J, Schaper J, Meinecke P, Momeni P, Gross S, von Holtum D et al (2001) Genotypic and phenotypic spectrum in tricho-rhino-phalangeal syndrome types I and III. Am J Hum Genet 68:81–91

Ludecke H-J, Wagner MJ, Nardmann J, La Pillo B, Parrish JE, Willems PJ et al (1995) Molecular dissection of a contiguous gene syndrome: localization of the genes involved in the Langer–Giedion syndrome. Hum Mol Genet 4:31–36

Momeni P, Glockner G, Schmidt O, von Holtum D, Albrecht B, Gillessen-Kaesbach G et al (2000) Mutations in a new gene, encoding a zinc-finger protein, cause tricho-rhino-phalangeal syndrome type I. Nature Genet 24:71–74

S. Mundlos, D. Horn, *Limb Malformations*,
DOI 10.1007/978-3-540-95928-1_49, © Springer-Verlag Berlin Heidelberg 2014

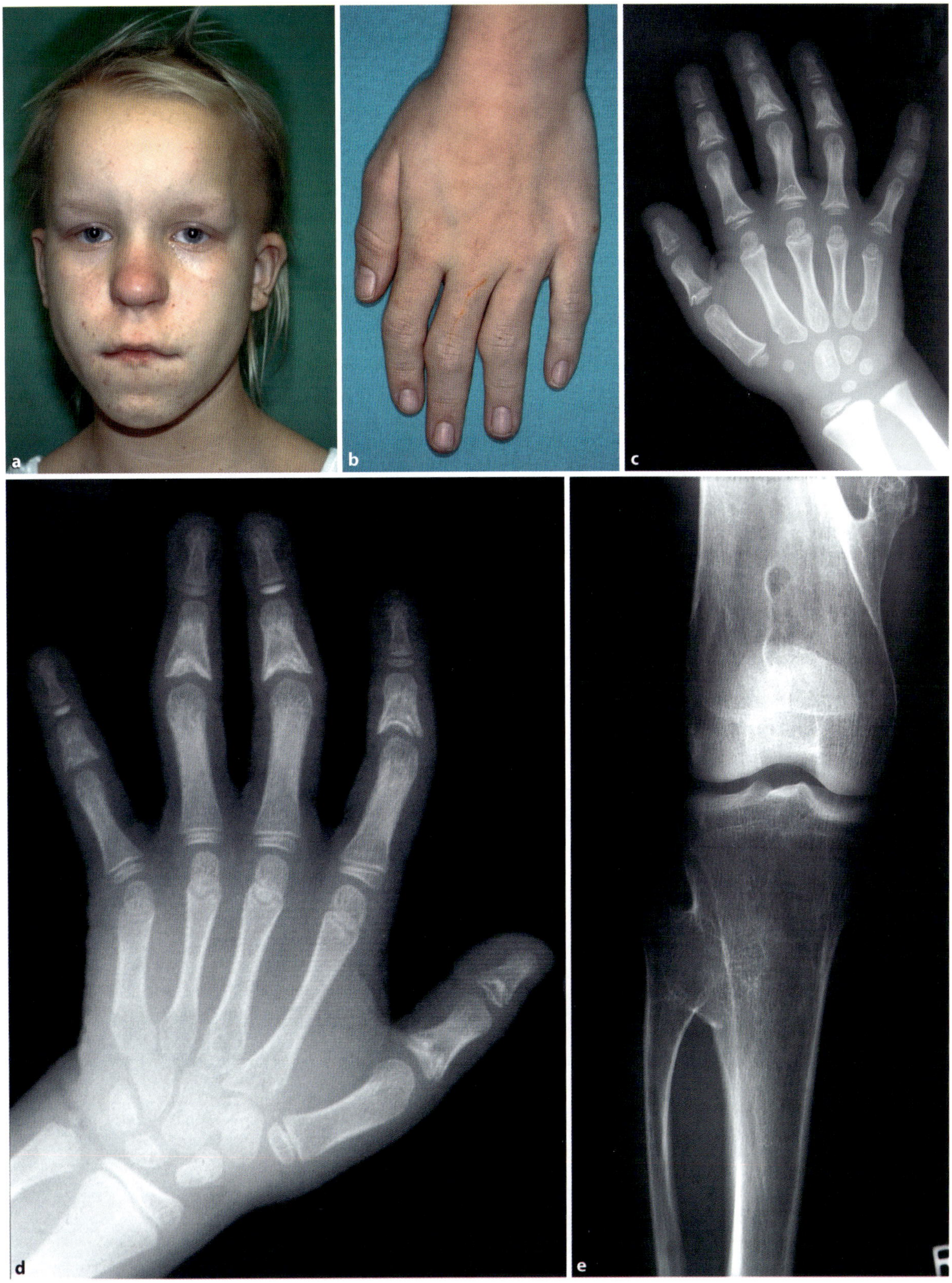

Fig. 49.1 **a** Typical facial appearance with sparse hair and bulbous nose with a high and long philtrum. **b** Small hand with radial deviation of digits II–IV in the metacarpophalangeal joints and ulnar deviation in the proximal interphalangeal joints. **c** Corresponding radiograph (age 5 years) shows mild brachydactyly of the middle phalanges and cone-shaped epiphyses of the proximal phalanges of digits I–V, middle phalanges of digits II–IV, and distal phalanx of digit I. **d** Anteroposterior hand radiograph shows cone epiphyses of the proximal/distal phalanges of the thumb and middle phalanges of digits II–V and ivory epiphyses of the distal phalanges of digits III and V. **e** Exostoses around the knee in trichorhinophalangeal syndrome type 2. Note the bony protrusion at the distal femur and secondary fusion of the proximal fibula with the tibia

50 Acrodysostosis, With or Without Hormone Resistance

MIM 101800

Major Clinical Findings

Acrodysostosis is characterized by facial abnormalities, brachydactyly, and short stature of variable degree. Besides nasal hypoplasia, facial features include a round face, midface hypoplasia, short nose, maxillary hypoplasia, and prognathism. Peripheral dysostosis with short hands and feet is characteristic. Radiologically, the phalanges and metacarpals are short and broad, and cone-shaped epiphyses of the proximal and middle phalanges are present. Advanced bone age with premature epiphyseal fusion is frequent. Epiphyseal stippling is a consistent radiological sign during infancy. Spinal stenosis occurs in the majority of affected individuals. Laboratory studies show resistance to multiple hormones, including parathyroid, thyrotropin, calcitonin, growth hormone releasing hormone, and gonadotropins. Delayed speech development and intellectual disability are frequent. The clinical findings are variable. Some patients have hormone resistance with skeletal and other changes, whereas others have only the skeletal changes.

Occasional Findings

Impaired hearing, neurological signs of spinal claudication, cervical stenosis, disproportionately broad hallux, obesity.

Genetic Transmission

Autosomal dominant.

Differential Diagnosis

It is difficult to distinguish clinically between patients with *PRKAR1A* mutations and those with mutations in *PDE4D*. Both groups have mild short stature with brachydactyly, facial dysostosis, spinal stenosis, variable endocrine abnormalities, and variable degrees of developmental disability. Characteristic facial features, namely midface hypoplasia with the nasal hypoplasia, may be more pronounced in individuals with *PDE4D* mutations.

The skeletal findings of hands, feet, and face in acrodysostosis may resemble those of severe manifestations of Albright hereditary osteodystrophy. Abnormal results of laboratory studies, namely hormone resistance, can distinguish between them. Spinal stenosis is not a feature of Albright hereditary osteodystrophy.

Molecular Pathology

Acrodysostosis is a heterogenous condition; acrodysostosis 1 is caused by heterozygous mutations in the *PRKAR1A* gene. PRKAR1A encodes an AMP-dependent regulatory subunit of protein kinase A (PKA), the main mediator of cAMP signaling in mammals. Phosphorylation mediated by the cAMP/PKA signaling pathway is involved in regulating cell proliferation, differentiation, and apoptosis. Inactivation of PRKAR1A has been suggested to result in reduced cAMP binding, reduced PKA activation, and decreased downstream signaling. PKA has been shown to regulate Smo, the cell surface coreceptor for hedgehog signaling. Interestingly, inactivation of hedgehog signaling in bones also results in brachydactyly. Acrodysostosis 2 is caused by mutations in the *PDE4D* gene. PDE4D is a class IV cAMP-specific cyclic nucleotide phosphodiesterase that regulates cellular concentrations of cyclic nucleotides and thereby plays a role in signal transduction. Like mutations in *PRKAR1A*, mutations in *PDE4D* result in deregulation of cAMP levels and alterations in the cAMP signaling pathway.

References

Graham JM Jr., Krakow D, Tolo VT, Smith AK, Lachman RS (2001) Radiographic findings and Gs-alpha bioactivity studies and mutation screening in acrodysostosis indicate a different etiology from pseudohypoparathyroidism. Pediat Radiol 31:2–9

Lee H, Graham JM Jr., Rimoin DL, Lachman RS, Krejci P, Tompson SW et al (2012) Exome sequencing identifies PDE4D mutations in acrodysostosis. Am J Hum Genet 90:746–751

Linglart A, Menguy C, Couvineau A, Auzan C, Gunes Y, Cancel M et al (2011) Recurrent PRKAR1A mutation in acrodysostosis with hormone resistance. New Eng J Med 364:2218–2226

Maroteaux P, Malamut G (1968) L'acrodysostose. Presse Med 76:2189–2192

Michot C, Le Goff C, Goldenberg A, Abhyankar A, Klein C, Kinning E et al (2012) Exome sequencing identifies PDE4D mutations as another cause of acrodysostosis. Am J Hum Genet 90:740–745

S. Mundlos, D. Horn, *Limb Malformations*,
DOI 10.1007/978-3-540-95928-1_50, © Springer-Verlag Berlin Heidelberg 2014

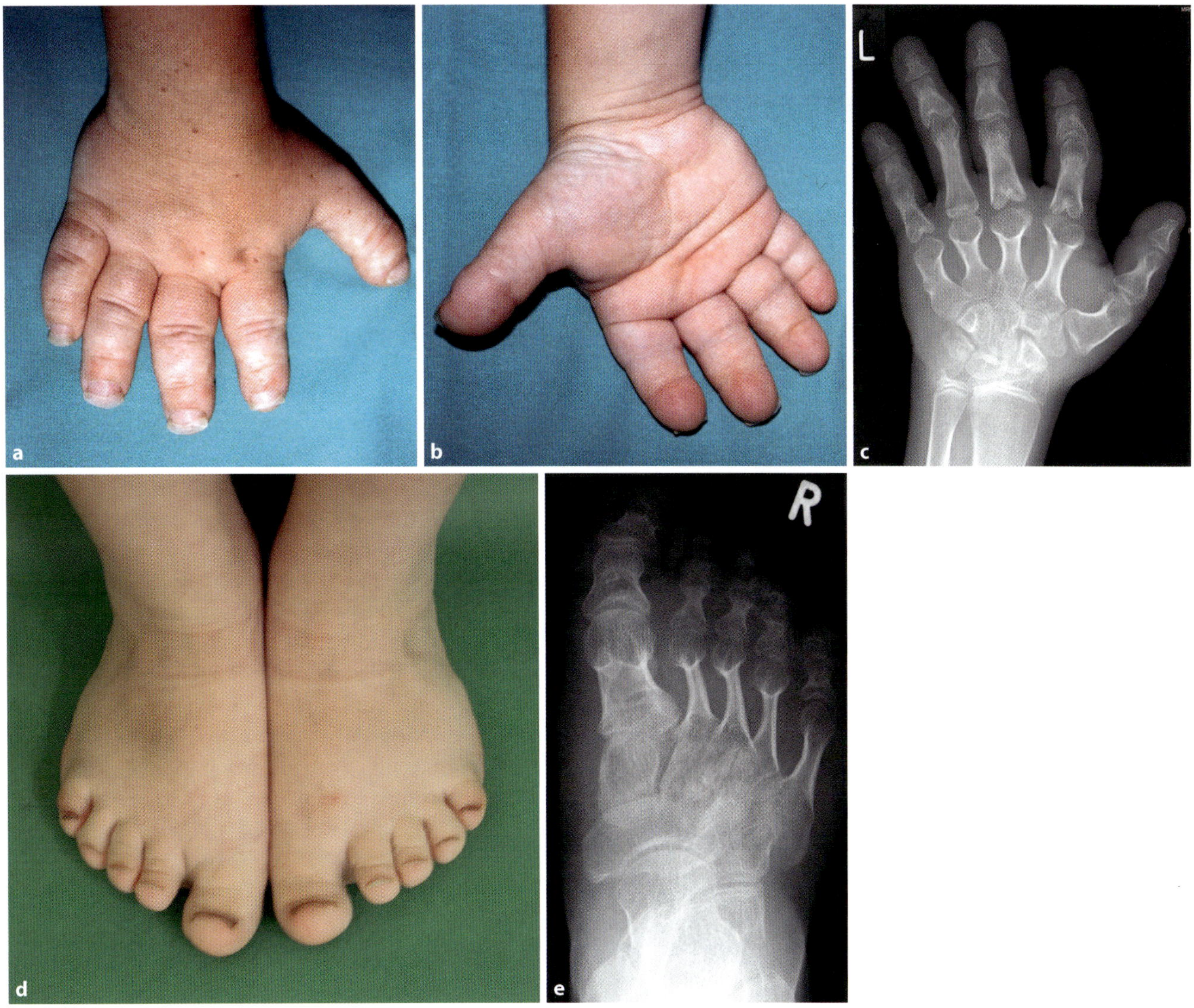

Fig. 50.1 **a, b** Dorsal and palmar views of the hand showing small hands with markedly short fingers. **c** Anteroposterior radiograph of the hand showing very short metacarpals, short/broad proximal and middle phalanges, and short distal phalanges. The distal and middle phalanges are the most severely affected. Premature closure of the epiphyses and cone-shaped epiphyses are most pronounced at the proximal phalanges II, III, and IV as well as middle phalanges II and IV. **d** Short feet with broad first toes. **e** Corresponding radiograph reveals toes II–V with findings similar to the hands, with hallux enlargement

51 Acromicric Dysplasia

MIM 102370

Major Clinical Findings

Acromicric dysplasia is characterized by severe short stature, brachydactyly, limited joint mobility, and facial anomalies. Birth length is normal, and short stature becomes evident in infancy or early childhood. The limbs are short with disproportionally short hands and feet.

Affected individuals have distinct facial features, including a round face with narrow palpebral fissures, a bulbous nose with anteverted nostrils, and thick upper lips with a small mouth. A hoarse voice and pseudomuscular build are often noted. Radiologic features include short metacarpal and phalangeal bones, cone-shaped epiphyses, delayed bone age, short long tubular bones, small proximal femoral epiphyses, and ovoid vertebral bodies. The metacarpals show proximal pointing with an internal notch of the 2nd metacarpal and an external notch of the 5th metacarpal. The femoral head has an internal notch. The final height of affected individuals varies between 115 cm and 140 cm. Carpal tunnel syndrome is present in older patients.

Occasional Findings

Repeated infections of the upper respiratory tract, myopia, hyperopia, congenital heart defect.

Genetic Transmission

Autosomal dominant. Most cases are sporadic.

Differential Diagnosis

Allelic disorders with overlapping skeletal and joint features include geleophysic dysplasia type 2 and the autosomal dominant form of Weill–Marchesani syndrome. The geleophysic dysplasia differs by progressive cardiac valve thickening, hepatosplenomegaly, thickening of the skin, and different facial features. In Weill–Marchesani syndrome, microspherophakia and additional ocular findings are present.

Molecular Pathology

Acromicric dysplasia is caused by specific heterozygous mutations in *FBN1*, the gene commonly associated with Marfan syndrome. All mutations that have been identified were located in exons 41 and 42 that encode the TGFβ-binding protein-like domain 5 of *FBN1*. The specific effects of these mutations are likely to be linked to a specific function of this domain in TGFß signaling. Accordingly, enhanced TGFβ signaling is a consistent feature in fibroblasts of affected individuals. Geleophysic dysplasia 2 and Weill–Marchesani syndrome are phenotypically different, but they are allelic conditions also caused by mutations in *FBN1*.

References

Faivre L, Le Merrer M, Baumann C, Polak M, Chatelain P, Sulmont V et al (2001) Acromicric dysplasia: long term outcome and evidence of autosomal dominant inheritance. J Med Genet 38:745–749

Hennekam RC, van Bever Y, Oorthuys JW (1996) Acromicric dysplasia and geleophysic dysplasia: similarities and differences. Eur J Pediatr 155:311–314

Le Goff C, Mahaut C, Wang LW, Allali S, Abhyankar A, Jensen S et al (2011) Mutations in the TGF-beta binding-protein-like domain 5 of FBN1 are responsible for acromicric and geleophysic dysplasias. Am J Hum Genet 89:7–14

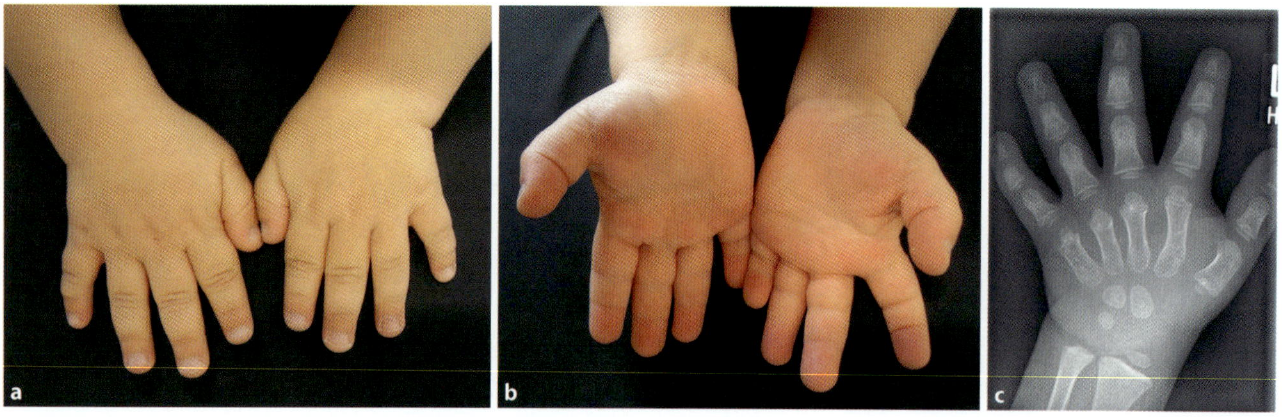

Fig. 51.1 **a b**, Dorsal and palmar views of hands, respectively. **c** Anteroposterior hand radiograph shows generalized brachydactyly, tiny cone-shaped epiphyses of the middle phalanx of finger II, and proximal phalanx of finger V

S. Mundlos, D. Horn, *Limb Malformations*,
DOI 10.1007/978-3-540-95928-1_51, © Springer-Verlag Berlin Heidelberg 2014

Part VIII
Abnormal Joint Formation/ Synostosis

52 Symphalangism; Multiple Synostoses Syndrome; Tarsal/Carpal Coalition Syndrome; Teunissen–Cremers Syndrome

MIM 185800; MIM 186500; MIM 186570; MIM 184460

Major Clinical Findings

Symphalangism (SYM) is characterized by variable fusion of the proximal interphalangeal joints. Occasionally the distal joints are affected. Clinically, there is inability to flex the affected joints, loss of the interphalangeal creases, and fusion of carpal and tarsal bones. Conductive hearing loss due to stapes ankylosis is frequently present.

Multiple synostoses syndrome (SYNS, including more than one form) refers to the more severe variant of this condition, with additional joint fusion in the elbow and/or other large joints.

Tarsal/carpal coalition may appear as an isolated trait in conjunction with SYM.

Teunissen–Cremers syndrome refers to stapes ankylosis, hyperopia, broad thumbs, broad 1st toes, and syndactyly. The stapedial ankylosis is bilateral, resulting in conductive hearing loss. Fusion of cervical vertebrae may occur. However, in contrast to SYM, carpal and tarsal fusion and symphalangism are not present.

The four conditions can be considered part of one mutational spectrum that shows considerable overlap.

Genetic Transmission

Autosomal dominant.

Differential Diagnosis

Other conditions with joint fusions or joint dysfunction must be considered. Fusion of the interphalangeal joints occurs in various types of brachydactyly, in particular BDA1, BDA2, BDC, and BDB, as well as in Cooks syndrome.

Molecular Pathology

SYM, SYNS1, tarsal/carpal coalition, and Teunissen–Cremers syndrome are caused by heterozygous mutations in the gene *NOG* encoding for Noggin, a bone morphogenetic protein (BMP) antagonist. The mutations are likely to result in a loss of function. Noggin is essential for the development of digits and joints, as Nog knockout mice have massively enlarged cartilage elements and fused joints. As a BMP inhibitor, Nog is important in orchestrating the prochondrogenic effect of the BMPs. SYM and SYNS2 can also be caused by mutations in *GDF5*. These mutations have been shown to result in an activation of GDF5 and thus an increase in BMP signaling. Apparently, the fine-tuning of BMP signaling is particularly important in the developing digits and joints.

References

Brown DJ, Kim TB, Petty EM, Downs CA, Martin DM, Strouse PJ, et al. Autosomal dominant stapes ankylosis with broad thumbs and toes, hyperopia, and skeletal anomalies is caused by heterozygous nonsense and frameshift mutations in NOG, the gene encoding noggin. Am J Hum Genet. 2002 Sep;71(3):618–24.

Dawson K, Seeman P, Sebald E, King L, Edwards M, Williams J 3rd, et al. GDF5 is a second locus for multiple-synostosis syndrome. Am J Hum Genet. 2006 Apr;78(4):708–12.

Dixon ME, Armstrong P, Stevens DB, Bamshad M. Identical mutations in NOG can cause either tarsal/carpal coalition syndrome or proximal symphalangism. Genet Med. 2001 Sep–Oct;3(5):349–53.

Gong Y, Krakow D, Marcelino J, Wilkin D, Chitayat D, Babul-Hirji R, et al. Heterozygous mutations in the gene encoding noggin affect human joint morphogenesis. Nat Genet. 1999 Mar;21(3):302–4.

Seemann P, Schwappacher R, Kjaer KW, Krakow D, Lehmann K, Dawson K, et al. Activating and deactivating mutations in the receptor interaction site of GDF5 cause symphalangism or brachydactyly type A2. J Clin Invest. 2005;115:2373–81.

S. Mundlos, D. Horn, *Limb Malformations*,
DOI 10.1007/978-3-540-95928-1_52, © Springer-Verlag Berlin Heidelberg 2014

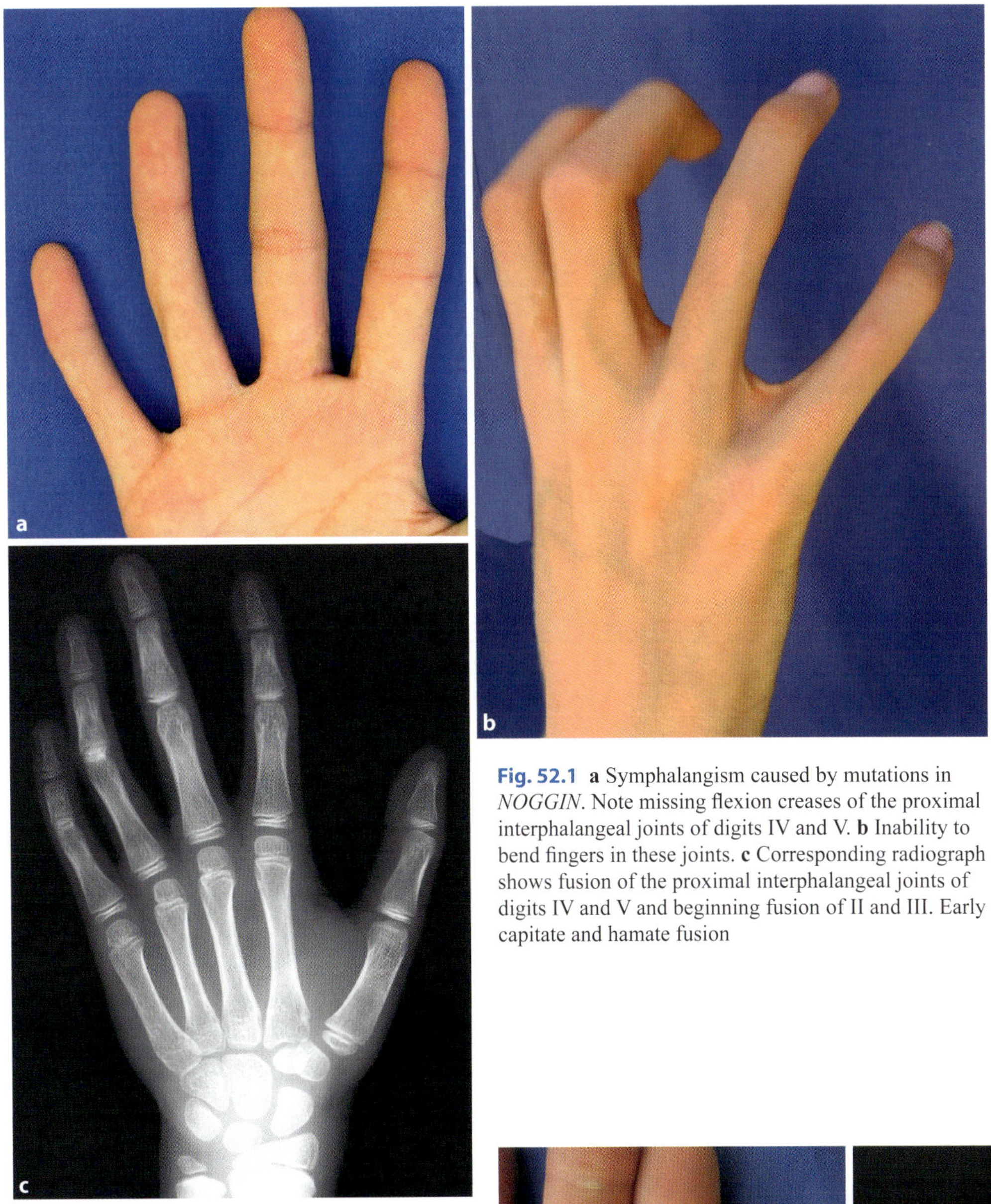

Fig. 52.1 **a** Symphalangism caused by mutations in *NOGGIN*. Note missing flexion creases of the proximal interphalangeal joints of digits IV and V. **b** Inability to bend fingers in these joints. **c** Corresponding radiograph shows fusion of the proximal interphalangeal joints of digits IV and V and beginning fusion of II and III. Early capitate and hamate fusion

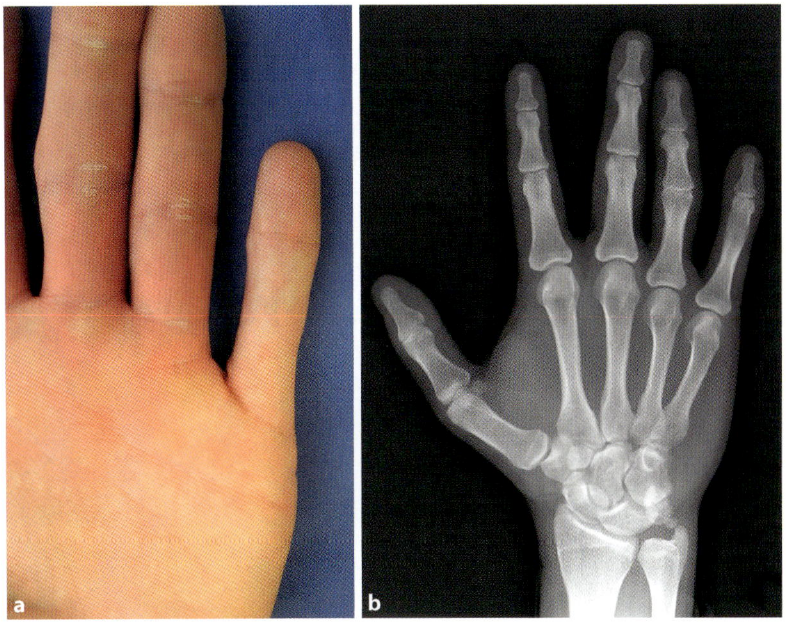

Fig. 52.2 **a** Symphalangism caused by mutation in *GDF5* (R438L). Note missing flexion crease of the interphalangeal joint in digit V. **b** Corresponding radiograph shows complete fusion of the proximal with the middle phalanx of digit V. In addition, note the narrowed joint space of the proximal interphalangeal joint of digits II–IV and incomplete fusion across the distal interphalangeal space of the thumb

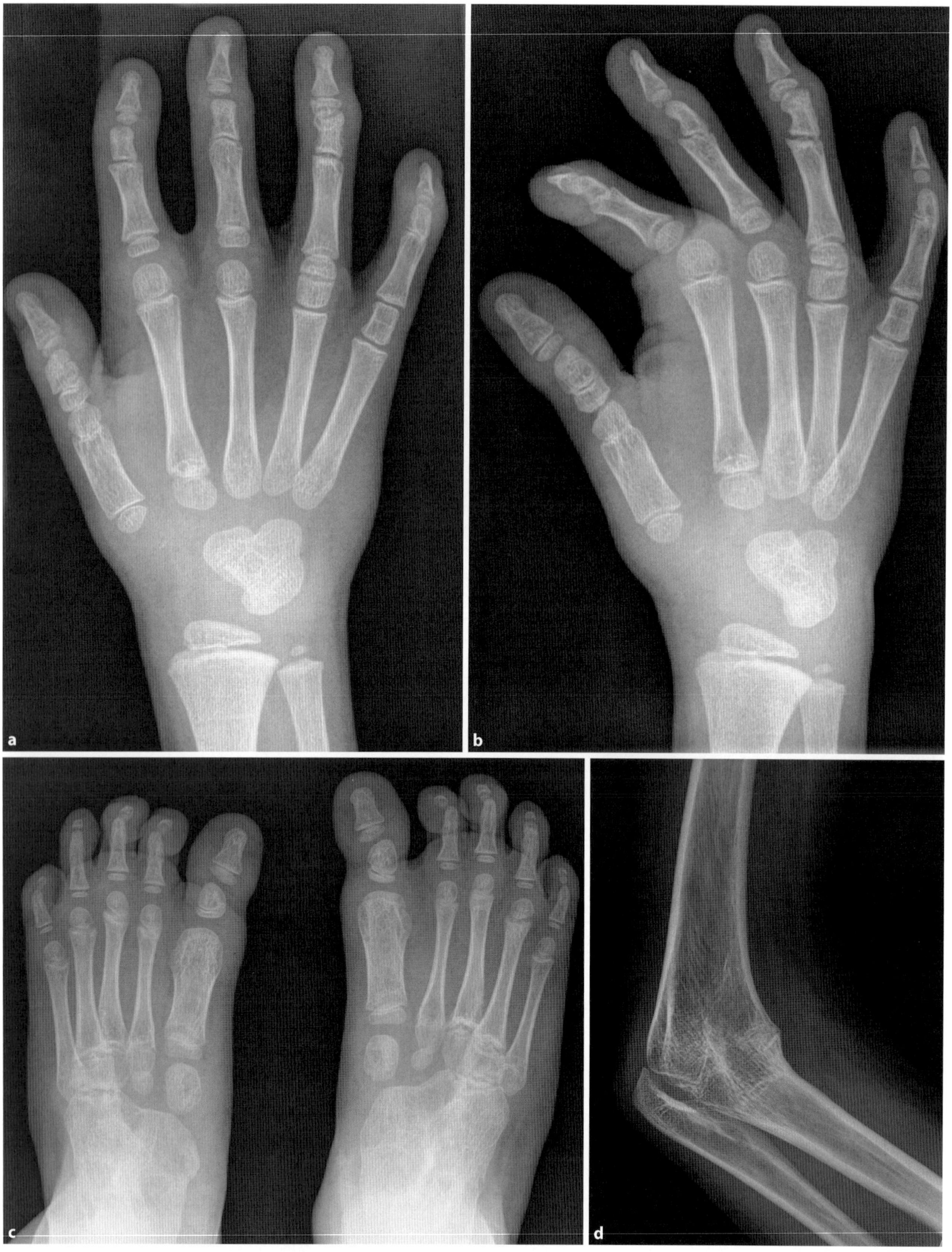
a
b
c
d

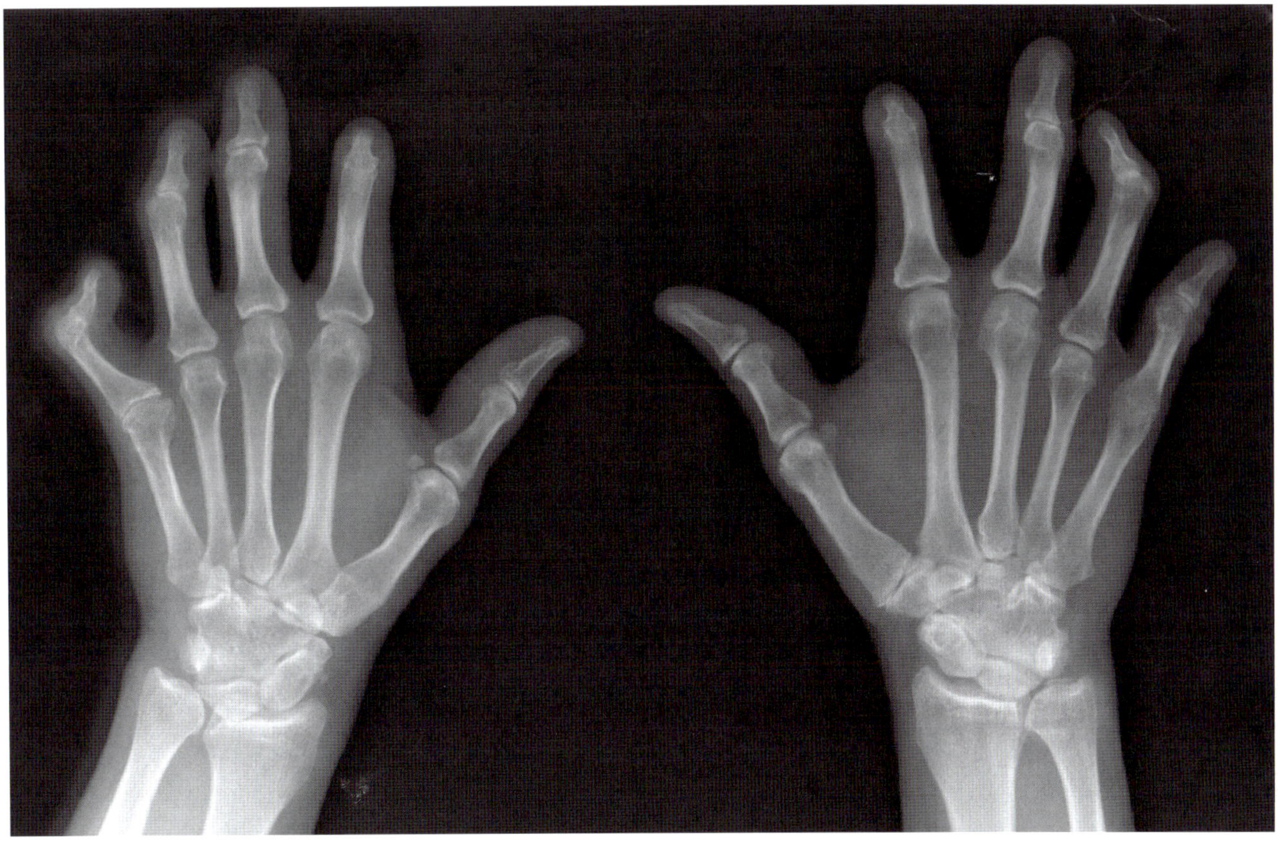

Fig. 52.4 Severe symphalangism. Radiograph of both hands of an individual with mutation in *GDF5* (W414R). There is fusion of the carpal bones, complete and incomplete fusion of the metacarpophalangeal joints of fingers V, elongated proximal phalanges that have probably fused with the middle phalanges, and partial fusion/dislocation of several distal interphalangeal joints

Fig. 52.3 Anteroposterior (AP) (**a**) and oblique (**b**) radiographic views of multiple synostosis syndrome (SYN) hand caused by mutation in *GDF5* (N445K). Note fusion of carpal bones, fusion of both epiphyses through the joint space in the metacarpophalangeal joints of digits IV and V, pseudoepiphyses of metacarpals I and II (normal variants), and small and partially fused middle phalanges of digits II–V with synostosis developing between the middle phalanx and distal phalanx of digits IV and V. **c** AP view of feet of the same individual, showing abnormally shaped broad metatarsal I, small round proximal phalanx I, fusion of proximal interphalangeal joints of toes II–V, and diffuse tarsal fusion. **d** Lateral view of elbow showing humeroradial fusion and dislocation of the ulna

53 Antley–Bixler Syndrome With/Without Genital Anomalies or Disordered Steroidogenesis

MIM 201750, MIM 207410

Synonyms
Trapezoidocephaly–synostosis syndrome
Multisynostotic osteodysgenesis with long bone fractures

Major Clinical Findings
Antley–Bixler syndrome is a craniosynostosis syndrome mainly affecting the coronal and lambdoid sutures, with a specific congenital type of radio-ulnar-humeral synostosis. Typical facial appearance includes brachycephaly, midface hypoplasia, large anterior fontanel, frontal bossing, a depressed nasal bridge, proptosis of the eyes, and a long philtrum. There may be choanal atresia/stenosis, dysplastic ears, and stenosis of the auditory canals. A characteristic finding is the synostosis between radius, humerus, and ulna. Bowing of the femur and ulna and neonatal fractures of the bowed femur are seen. The hands may show arachnodactyly and camptodactyly as well as fusion of the carpal and tarsal bones. The pelvis is narrow. Various foot abnormalities including rocker-bottom feet. There is a wide spectrum of associated anomalies, including atrial septal defect, upper airway obstruction, a narrow chest, and kidney abnormalities. In cases with P450 oxidoreductase (POR) deficiency, disorders of sex development – such as vaginal atresia, clitoromegaly, sinus urogenitalis, fused labia minora, and hypoplastic labia majora in females and micropenis, hypospadias, and hypoplastic scrotum in males – are characteristic features. Mortality is high in the neonatal period, primarily due to airway compromise.

Prognosis improves with increasing age. If craniectomy is performed to treat sutural synostosis and if secondary factors, such as apnea, are avoided, surviving patients appear to have normal intelligence. Patients with *POR* mutations may be at risk for adrenal insufficiency and Addisonian crisis and may require steroid hormone supplementation, especially at times of severe febrile illness or surgery. It is thus important to distinguish patients with disordered steroidogenesis and POR deficiency from those with normal steroidogenesis.

Laboratory abnormalities in individuals with POR deficiency include normal baseline cortisol, blunted cortisol response to adrenocorticotropic hormone (ACTH), elevated 17-hydroxyprogesterone, mildly elevated ACTH, elevated progesterone, elevated pregnenolone, and a specific steroid excretion profile in the urine.

Genetic Transmission
Autosomal dominant (*FGFR2*), autosomal recessive (*POR*).

Differential Diagnosis
The differential diagnosis includes other conditions with bowed femurs, osteogenesis imperfecta (fractures and bowing), and acrocephalosyndactyly syndromes (craniosynostosis). However, the combination of features is rather unique. Some patients with POR deficiency have only ambiguous genitalia or other evidence of disordered steroidogenesis without the skeletal signs of Antley–Bixler syndrome.

Molecular Pathology
Mutations of the P450 oxidoreductase gene (*POR*) have been reported in those patients with genital anomalies, impaired steroidogenesis, or both. POR is the obligatory flavoprotein intermediate that transfers electrons from reduced nicotinamide adenine dinucleotide phosphate (NADPH) to all microsomal cytochrome P450 enzymes. The malformations observed are thought to reflect the impaired activities of POR-related enzymes in cholesterol synthesis and retinoic acid metabolism. Individuals with Antley–Bixler syndrome and POR deficiency appear to have a characteristic profile of steroid excretion, which can be used for diagnostic purposes. Congenital adrenal hyperplasia without Antley–Bixler skeletal anomalies can also result from POR mutations. A specific mutation in *FGFR2* (Ser351-to-Cys) has been reported predominantly in those patients with normal genitalia and steroidogenesis.

References

Antley RM, Bixler D (1975) Trapezoidocephaly, midface hypoplasia and cartilage abnormalities with multiple synostoses and skeletal fractures. Birth Defects Orig Art Ser XI(2):397–401

Fluck CE, Tajima T, Pandey AV, Arlt W, Okuhara K, Verge CF et al (2004) Mutant P450 oxidoreductase causes disordered steroidogenesis with and without Antley–Bixler syndrome. Nature Genet 36:228–230

Huang N, Pandey AV, Agrawal V, Reardon W, Lapunzina PD, Mowat D et al (2005) Diversity and function of mutations in P450 oxidoreductase in patients with Antley–Bixler syndrome and disordered steroidogenesis. Am J Hum Genet 76:729–749

Krone N, Reisch N, Idkowiak J, Dhir V, Ivison HE, Hughes BA et al (2012) Genotype-phenotype analysis in congenital adrenal hyperplasia due to P450 oxidoreductase deficiency. J Clin Endocrinol Metab 97:E257–E267

McGlaughlin KL, Witherow H, Dunaway DJ, David DJ, Anderson PJ (2010) Spectrum of Antley–Bixler syndrome. J Craniofac Surg 21:1560–1564

S. Mundlos, D. Horn, *Limb Malformations*,
DOI 10.1007/978-3-540-95928-1_53,

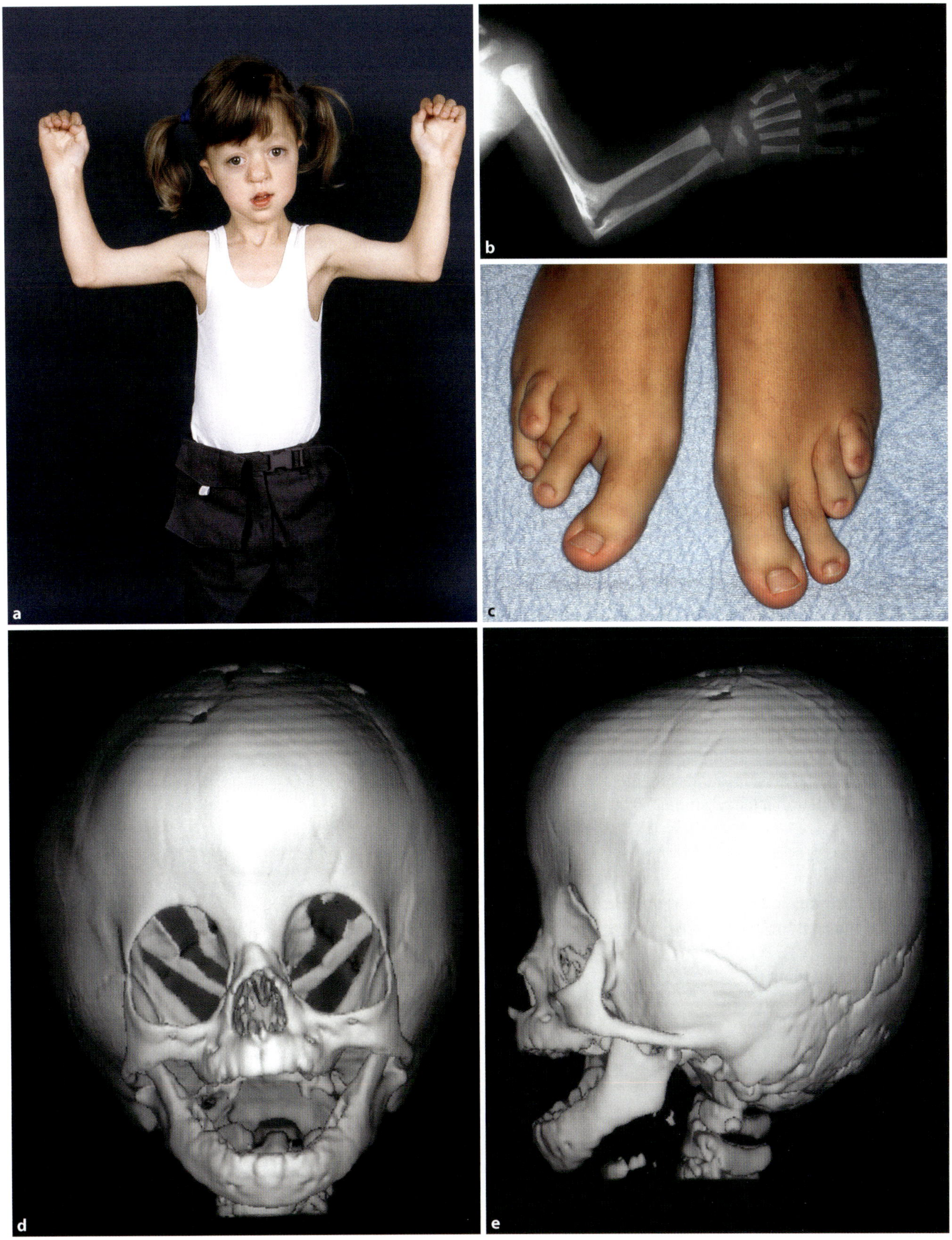

Fig. 53.1 **a** A 7-year-old girl with Antley–Bixler syndrome and P450 oxidoreductase (POR) deficiency. Note inability to extend the elbows. **b** Fusion of humerus with the ulna and radius bilaterally. Note dislocation of the ulna with fusion of the humerus to the olecranon process, fusion of carpal bones, and thin metacarpals. **c** Feet of same individual at age 16. Note short metatarsals III–V and missing 5th toe on the left. **d** Three-dimensional computed tomography scan of skull revealing diffuse craniosynostosis. Note fused metopic suture. **e** Lateral view showing fusion of the coronal/lambdoid/squamosal sutures; midface hypoplasia with small maxilla. (Courtesy of N. Adolphs, Charité, Germany)

54 Liebenberg Syndrome

MIM 186550

Synonyms
Synostosis, carpal, with dysplastic elbow joints and brachydactyly
Brachydactyly with joint dysplasia

Major Clinical Findings
Liebenberg syndrome is characterized by abnormalities of the elbows, wrists, and hands. Affected individuals are unable to fully extend the elbows, and their hands show deviation to the ulnar side. Radiographs show a highly abnormal elbow joint. The olecranon is very small or missing, and the radius and ulna have a flattened joint surface. The distal humerus is broadened and has a medial and lateral condyle separated by an intercondylar fossa. Thus, these elbows show characteristics of a knee joint. Radiographs of the wrist show fusion of the triquetral and pisiform, resulting in a structure similar in shape to the calcaneus of the ankle. Furthermore, the scaphoid and lunate bones are fused and form an element that resembles in shape the talus in the ankle. Radiographs of the hands show relatively long metacarpals and short phalanges. Further changes can be observed in the muscles and tendons. The extensor minimi digiti muscle straightens the little finger and is present only in the hand, not in the foot. This muscle and its tendon are absent in the hands of Liebenberg patients. Similarly, the extensor carpi radialis muscle, a characteristic muscle of the hand, and its two tendons are absent.

Altogether these changes have been interpreted as a homeotic transformation in which the upper extremities have acquired features of the lower limbs.

Genetic Transmission
Autosomal dominant.

Differential Diagnosis
Very specific phenotype; no major differential diagnosis.

Molecular Pathology
Liebenberg syndrome is caused by structural variations involving the *PITX1* locus. PITX1 is a transcription factor with essential function for hindlimb (leg) determination. Together with TBX4 it is specifically expressed in the hindlimb. Misexpression of PITX1 in the forelimb, such as via a transgenic approach in mice, results in forelimbs that adopt hindlimb identity. The latter includes loss of the olecranon and fusion abnormalities of the wrist bones together with abnormalities in muscle and tendon insertion. Thus, the Pitx1-overexpressing mouse closely resembles the human Liebenberg phenotype. The structural changes identified in Liebenberg syndrome are deletions of a nearby gene and in one case a translocation 5' of PITX1. Both changes are believed to activate enhancers nearby that drive PITX1 expression in the forelimb (arm), thus inducing the phenotype.

References

Spielmann M, Brancati F, Krawitz PM, Robinson PN, Ibrahim DM, Franke M et al (2012) Homeotic arm-to-leg transformation associated with genomic rearrangements at the PITX1 locus. Am J Hum Genet 91:629–635

S. Mundlos, D. Horn, *Limb Malformations*,
DOI 10.1007/978-3-540-95928-1_54, © Springer-Verlag Berlin Heidelberg 2014

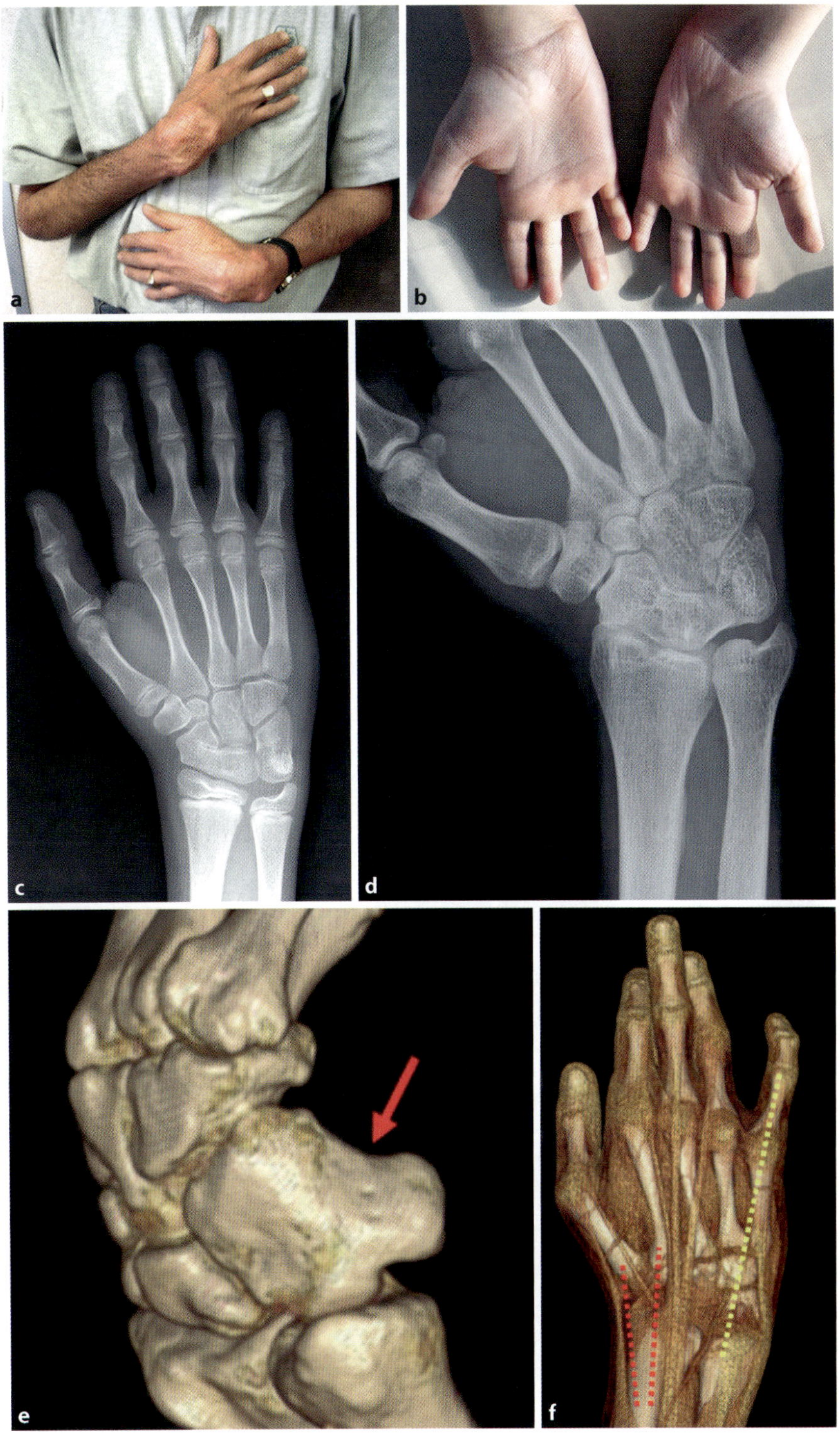

Fig. 54.1 **a** Abnormal wrists in Liebenberg syndrome. **b** Hands are characterized by large palms and relatively short digits. **c** Corresponding radiograph shows fusion of the proximal carpal row (triquetral, pisiform, scaphoid, and lunate). **d** Same finding in adult wrist. **e** Scaphoid and lunate bone fusion form an element similar to the shape of the talus in the ankle (*arrow*), as shown by three-dimensional computed tomography (CT) of the wrist. **f** The extensor minimi digiti muscle straightens digit V and is present only in the hand, not in the foot. This muscle and its tendon (indicated by *yellow line*) are absent in the hands of Liebenberg individuals, as shown in soft tissue technique CT. Similarly, the extensor carpi radialis muscle, a characteristic muscle of the hand, and its two tendons (indicated by *red lines*) are absent in Liebenberg individuals. (From Spielmann et al. 2012)

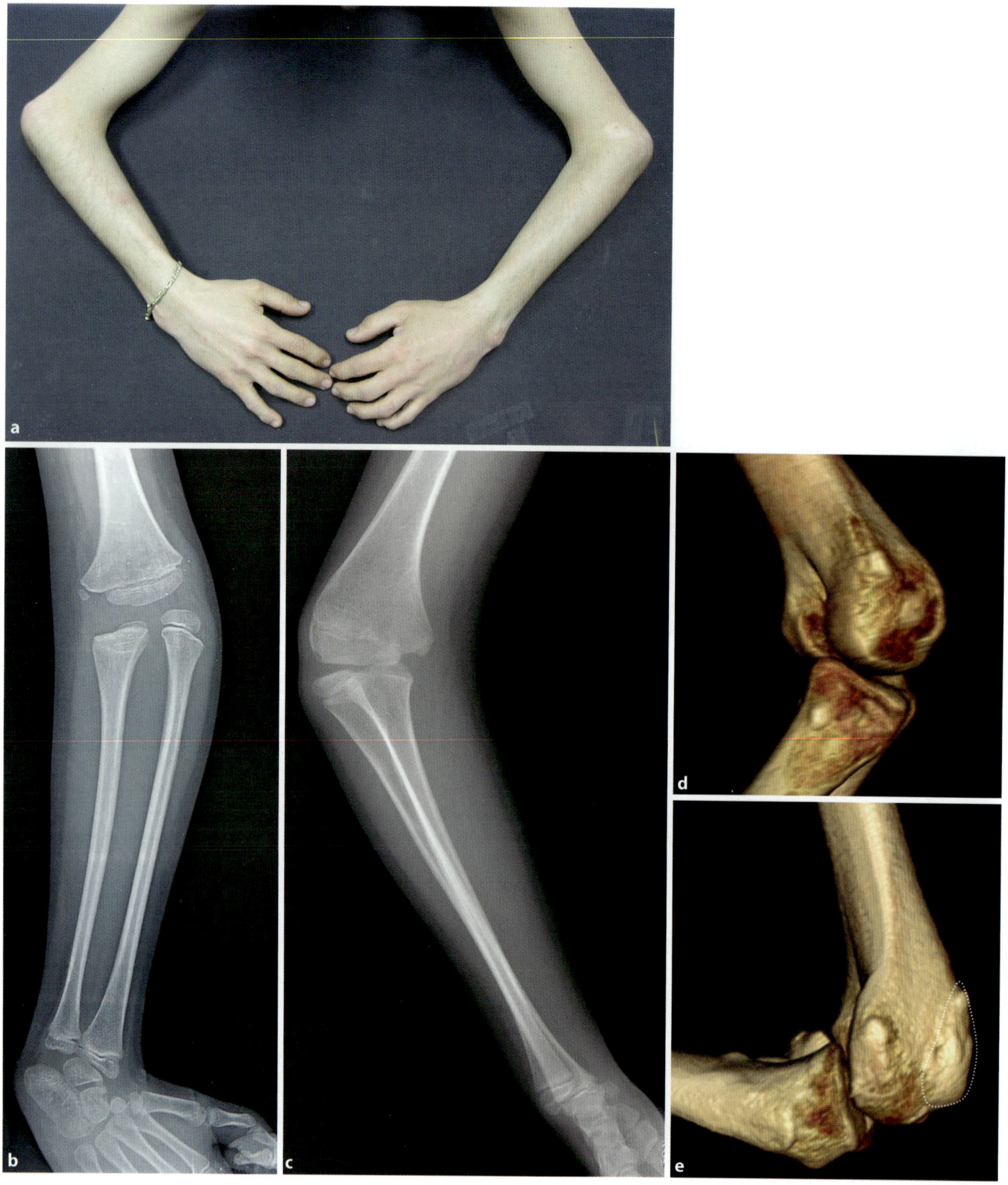

Fig. 54.2 **a** Abnormal elbows with inability to fully extend in an individual with Liebenberg syndrome. **b** Radiograph of arm showing lack of olecranon at the elbow and very large bone in the ulnar side of the wrist, with both proximal and distal carpal rows fusions. **c** Lateral view of elbow showing lack of olecranon, a flat joint surface, and an overall knee-like appearance. **d** Three-dimensional computed tomography scan of elbow shows abnormal shape of distal humerus with a medial and lateral condyle separated by an intercondylar fossa resembling the femoral epicondyles of the knee. **e** Frontal view showing a patella-like structure fused to the distal head of the humerus (outlined in *white*). (From Spielmann et al. 2012)

Nail–Patella Syndrome

MIM 161200

55

Synonyms

Onychoosteodysplasia
Turner–Kieser syndrome

Major Clinical Findings

Nail–patella syndrome (NPS) is characterized by dysplasia of the nails, absent or hypoplastic patellae, iliac horns, abnormality of the elbows, and nephropathy. Abnormalities of the nails are the most characteristic feature. Nails may be absent, hypoplastic, dystrophic, ridged, pitted, or otherwise abnormal. Triangular lunulae are characteristic. Nail changes may be observed at birth and are most often bilateral and symmetrical. There is a radioulnar gradient of severity with a decrease toward digit V. Furthermore, each individual nail is usually more severely affected on its ulnar side. Reduction in flexion of the distal interphalangeal joints and loss of skin creases are common signs. Hyperextension of the proximal interphalangeal joint and flexion of the distal interphalangeal joints result in "swan necking." Abnormalities of the elbows are common, with cubitus valgus and limitation of extension, pronation, and supination seen.

Typical radiologic findings include dysplasia of the radial head, hypoplasia of the lateral epicondyle and capitellum, and prominence of the medial epicondyle. These abnormalities may result in dislocation of the radial head, usually posteriorly. The patellae may be small, irregularly shaped, asymmetric, or absent. Recurrent subluxation or dislocation of the patella is common. Iliac horns are bilateral, conical, bony processes that project posteriorly and laterally from the central part of the iliac bones of the pelvis and are considered pathognomonic of NPS. Back pain is a common problem in individuals with NPS. Renal involvement occurs in approximately a third of affected individuals. The first sign of renal involvement is usually proteinuria, with or without hematuria. It may remit spontaneously, remain as asymptomatic proteinuria, or progress to nephrotic syndrome or nephritis and eventually to renal failure (approximately 5 %).

Occasional Findings

Difficulty putting on weight (particularly muscle) despite adequate dietary intake and exercise. Decrease in muscle mass in the upper arms and upper legs. Glaucoma and ocular hypertension. Peripheral neurological symptoms with intermittent episodes of numbness and tingling. Dental problems with weak, crumbling teeth. Osteoporosis of the femoral neck. Epilepsy.

Genetic Transmission

Autosomal dominant.

Differential Diagnosis

Conditions with abnormal patella must be considered: small patella syndrome, Meier–Gorlin syndrome, genitopatellar syndrome, isolated patella hypoplasia/aplasia, and familial dislocation of the patella. Conditions with hypoplastic/aplastic nails also have to be considered: DOOR syndrome, Coffin–Siris syndrome, and Senior syndrome.

Molecular Pathology

NPS is caused by mutations in *LMX1B*. The LIM-homeodomain protein LMX1B plays a central role in dorsal/ventral patterning of the vertebrate limb. It is a downstream target of Wnt7a and is expressed along the dorsoventral axis during limb development. Inactivation in mice results in an absence of nails and patellae. The kidneys of LMX1B mutant mice exhibit pathological changes similar to those observed in NPS. Lmx1b is expressed in the podocyte and was shown to regulate the expression of both the alpha-3 and alpha-4 chains of type IV collagen, important components of the glomerular basement membrane, suggesting that its deregulation in glomerular basement membrane contributes to the renal pathology and nephrosis in NPS.

References

Chen H, Lun Y, Ovchinnikov D, Kokubo H, Oberg KC, Pepicelli CV et al (1998) Limb and kidney defects in Lmx1b mutant mice suggest an involvement of LMX1B in human nail patella syndrome. Nat Genet 19(1):51–55

Dreyer SD, Zhou G, Baldini A, Winterpacht A, Zabel B, Cole W et al (1998) Mutations in LMX1B cause abnormal skeletal patterning and renal dysplasia in nail patella syndrome. Nat Genet 19(1):47–50

McIntosh I, Dunston JA, Liu L, Hoover-Fong JE, Sweeney E (2005) Nail patella syndrome revisited: 50 years after linkage. Ann Hum Genet 69(4):349–363

Morello R, Zhou G, Dreyer SD, Harvey SJ, Ninomiya Y, Thorner PS et al (2001) Regulation of glomerular basement membrane collagen expression by LMX1B contributes to renal disease in nail patella syndrome. Nat Genet 27(2):205–208

Sweeney E, Fryer A, Mountford R, Green A, McIntosh I (2003) Nail patella syndrome: a review of the phenotype aided by developmental biology. J Med Genet 40(3):153–162

S. Mundlos, D. Horn, *Limb Malformations*,
DOI 10.1007/978-3-540-95928-1_55, © Springer-Verlag Berlin Heidelberg 2014

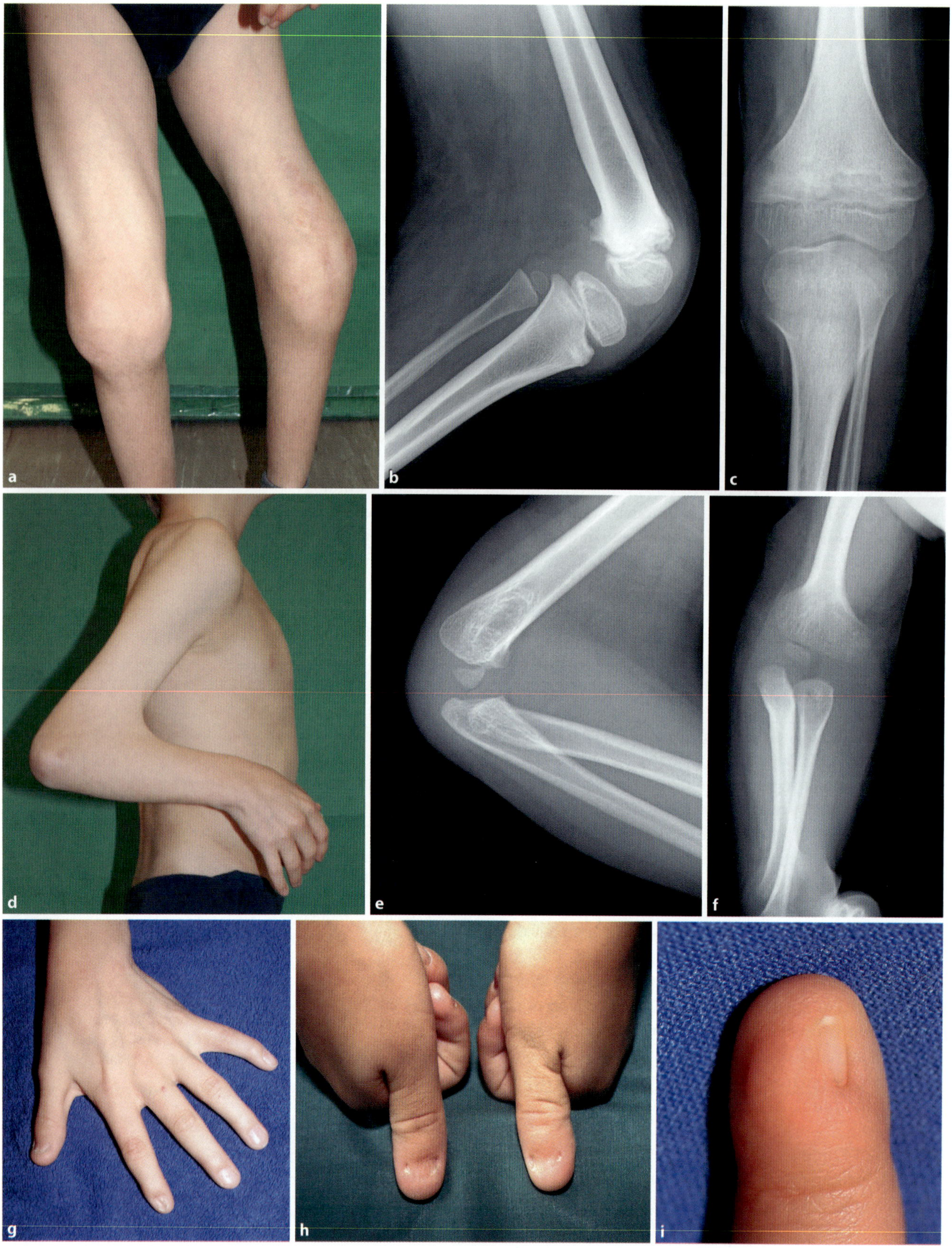
a
b
c
d
e
f
g
h
i

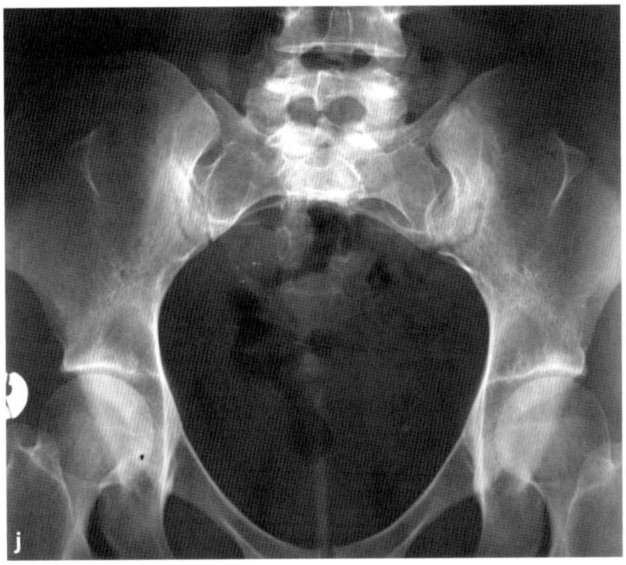

Fig. 55.1 **a** Abnormal knees in nail–patella syndrome. Note absence of patella and hypoplastic quadriceps muscle. **b, c** Corresponding radiographs, lateral (**b**) and anteroposterior (AP; **c**) views, showing the absence of patella and abnormal configuration of the posterior distal femoral metaphysis. **d** Abnormal elbow. Note pterygium, inability to fully extend the elbow, and hypoplastic triceps musculature. **e** Lateral/oblique and (**f**) AP radiographs of elbow in flexion with dislocated radial head. **g** Nail hypoplasia in nail–patella syndrome. Digits I and II are the most affected. **h** Close-up of nail dysplasia. **i** Note laterality. The radial side is more severely affected. **j** Radiograph of pelvis showing iliac horns

56 Small Patella Syndrome

MIM 147891

Synonyms
Ischiopatellar dysplasia
Coxopodo patellar syndrome
Scott–Taor syndrome

Major Clinical Findings
Small or absent patella and abnormalities of the pelvic girdle are the characteristic findings. The patella may show recurrent dislocations and abnormal ossification centers, and the pelvis may show irregular ossification at the ischiopubic junction, hypoplastic ossification of the ischia, or infra-acetabular axe-cut notches. Other skeletal anomalies include elongated femoral necks, flattened and widened proximal femoral epiphyses, hypoplasia of the lesser trochanter, and tarsal anomalies. The feet show a wide gap between the 1st and 2nd toes, short 4th and 5th rays of the feet, and pes planus.

Genetic Transmission
Autosomal dominant.

Differential Diagnosis
Small patella syndrome has overlapping features with nail–patella syndrome. The latter, however, features dysplastic nails, and the pelvic changes are different. Meier–Gorlin syndrome features absent or hypoplastic patellae but shows primordial dwarfism and markedly small ears in addition. Other conditions to be considered are genitopatellar syndrome, isolated patella hypoplasia/aplasia, and familial dislocation of the patella.

Molecular Pathology
Small patella syndrome is caused by loss-of-function mutations in the *TBX4* gene. TBX4 encodes a transcription factor with conserved homology to the classic mouse gene Brachyury (T). TBX4 is expressed throughout the developing hindlimb, but not in forelimb buds. PITX1 (see Liebenberg syndrome Chap. 54) is upstream of TBX4. The gene is involved in initiating limb outgrowth but does not determine limb-specific morphologies. The loss of the patella can be interpreted as a partial loss of hindlimb identity.

References

Bongers EM, Duijf PH, van Beersum SE, Schoots J, Van Kampen A, Burckhardt A et al (2004) Mutations in the human TBX4 gene cause small patella syndrome. Am J Hum Genet 74(6):1239–1248

Bongers EM, van Bokhoven H, van Thienen MN, Kooyman MA, Van Beersum SE, Boetes C et al (2001) The small patella syndrome: description of five cases from three families and examination of possible allelism with familial patella aplasia-hypoplasia and nail–patella syndrome. J Med Genet 38(3):209–214

Bongers EM, van Kampen A, van Bokhoven H, Knoers NV (2005) Human syndromes with congenital patellar anomalies and the underlying gene defects. Clin Genet 68(4):302–19

S. Mundlos, D. Horn, *Limb Malformations*,
DOI 10.1007/978-3-540-95928-1_56, © Springer-Verlag Berlin Heidelberg 2014

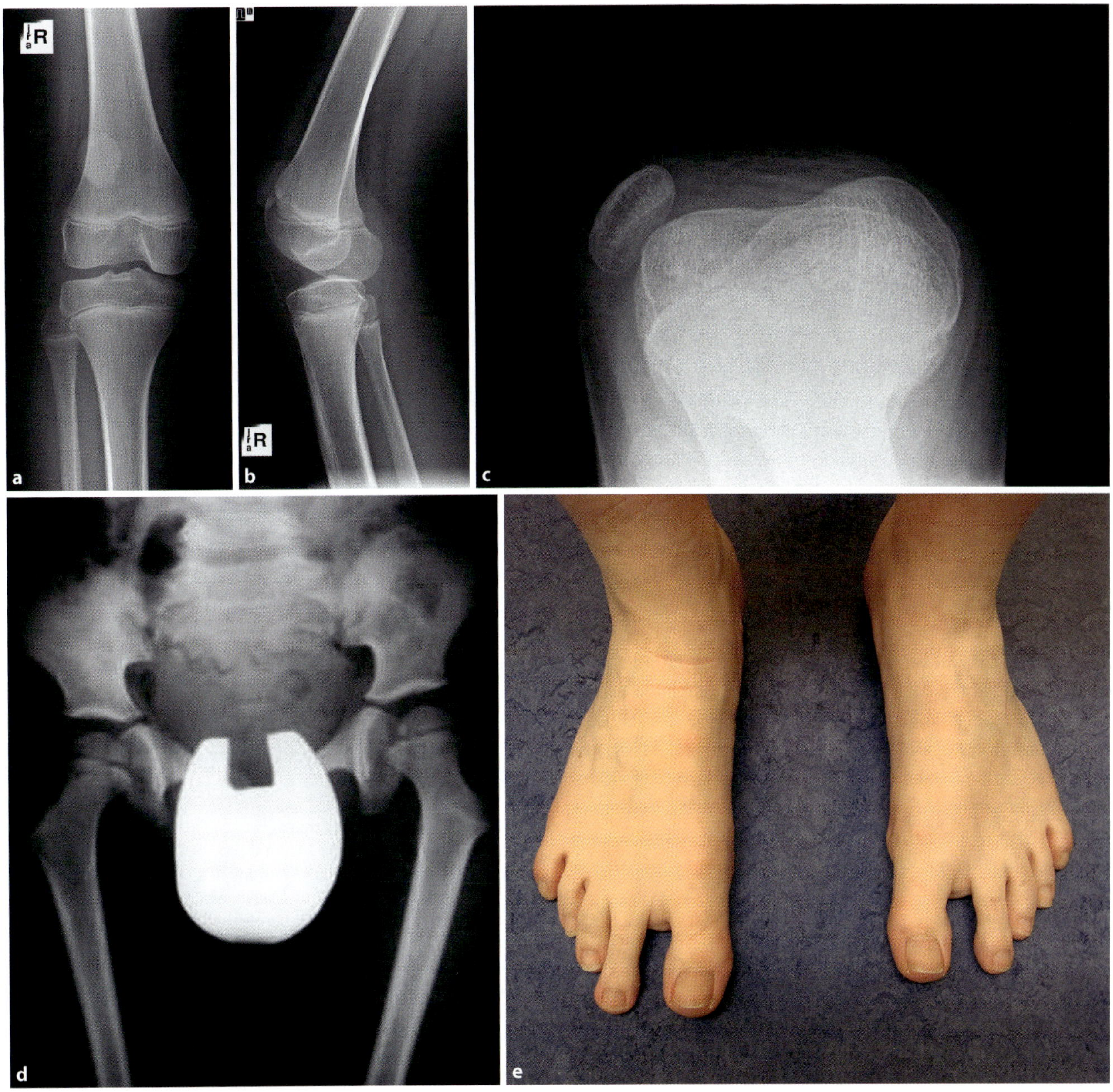

Fig. 56.1 Anteroposterior (AP; **a**) and (**b**) lateral films of knees showing a hypoplastic dislocated patella. **c** Axial view of flexed knee shows small, medially displaced patella. **d** AP film of pelvis and hips reveals marked hypoplasia of both ischia. **e** Wide space between the 1st and 2nd toes; short 4th and 5th rays

57 Larsen Syndrome

MIM 150250

Major Clinical Findings

Larsen syndrome is characterized by multiple congenital joint dislocations, craniofacial abnormalities, and short stature. The skeletal features include dislocations of the hip, knee, elbow joints, and wrists as well as equinovarus or equinovalgus foot deformities. The patella is often dislocated laterally. The fingers have a cylindrical shape, most marked in the thumb. Thoracolumbar scoliosis and cervical kyphosis often become evident during infancy. Radiographic abnormalities of the hands and feet are short distal phalanges (especially the 1st distal phalanx), metacarpals, and metatarsals; supernumerary carpal bones; and irregular carpal maturation. A juxtacalcaneal accessory bone/calcaneal duplication occurs in the first years of life in approximately 40 % of affected individuals. Abnormal segmentation and/or hypoplasia of cervical and thoracic vertebrae can be an additional feature. Craniofacial anomalies include frontal bossing, hypertelorism, a depressed nasal bridge, and a flattened midface. Cleft lip/palate occurs in about 30 %, and hypodontia may be present. Sensorineural, mixed, and conductive hearing loss is a well-recognized complication. Intellectual disability has been noted in about 15 %.

Occasional Findings

Cervical vertebral instability, heart defect, laryngeal stenosis, tracheomalacia, cleft uvula, cryptorchidism.

Genetic Transmission

This syndrome is heterogenous. Autosomal dominant and autosomal recessive forms have been documented. The differentiation of the two forms is not possible in an individual case, but the recessive form may more often be associated with cardiac and respiratory complications.

Differential Diagnosis

Other disorders with multiple joint dislocations such as those associated with *B3GAT3* or *CHST3* mutations show similar features. However, *B3GAT3* mutations are associated with congenital heart defects, and *CHST3* mutations are characterized by severe skeletal dysplasia, especially affecting the joints and spine. Multiple joint dislocations, in particular congenital bilateral hip dislocation, are features of Ehlers–Danlos syndrome type VII.

Molecular Pathology

The autosomal dominant form of Larsen syndrome is caused by heterozygous mutations in the gene encoding filamin B (FLNB). FLNB is expressed in human growth plate chondrocytes and developing vertebral bodies. Furthermore, it plays a role in vertebral segmentation and joint formation. Autosomal recessive mutations in *CHST3* cause a spondyloepiphyseal dysplasia that may also present with joint dislocations in the neonatal period. Another autosomal recessive condition (MIM 245600) with overlapping features, including multiple joint dislocations, short stature, craniofacial dysmorphism, and congenital heart defects, has been shown to be caused by mutations in the beta-1,3-glucuronyltransferase 3 gene (*B3GAT3*). Ehlers–Danlos syndrome type VII is caused by mutations in the procollagen of collagen type 1 (A1 and A2).

References

Baasanjav S, Al-Gazali L, Hashiguchi T, Mizumoto S, Fischer B, Horn D et al (2011) Faulty initiation of proteoglycan synthesis causes cardiac and joint defects. Am J Hum Genet 89:15–27

Becker R, Wegner R-D, Kunze J, Runkel S, Vogel M, Entezami M (2000) Clinical variability of Larsen syndrome: diagnosis in a father after sonographic detection of a severely affected fetus. Clin Genet 57:148–150

Bicknell LS, Farrington-Rock C, Shafeghati Y, Rump P, Alanay Y, Alembik Y et al (2007) A molecular and clinical study of Larsen syndrome caused by mutations in FLNB. J Med Genet 44:89–98

Hermanns P, Unger S, Rossi A, Perez-Aytes A, Cortina H, Bonafe L et al (2008) Congenital joint dislocations caused by carbohydrate sulfotransferase 3 deficiency in recessive Larsen syndrome and humero-spinal dysostosis. Am J Hum Genet 82:1368–1374

Krakow D, Robertson SP, King LM, Morgan T, Sebald ET, Bertolotto C et al (2004) Mutations in the gene encoding filamin B disrupt vertebral segmentation, joint formation and skeletogenesis. Nature Genet 36:405–410

S. Mundlos, D. Horn, *Limb Malformations*,
DOI 10.1007/978-3-540-95928-1_57, © Springer-Verlag Berlin Heidelberg 2014

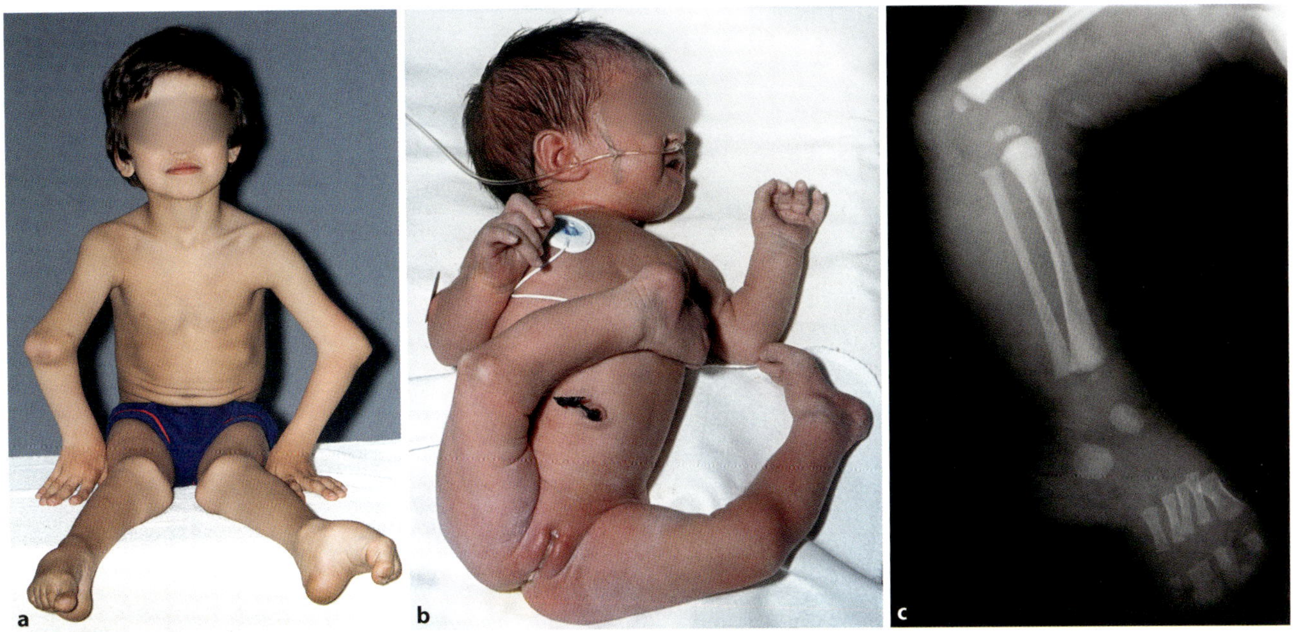

Fig. 57.1 **a** Multiple joint dislocations in a boy with Larsen syndrome. **b** Dislocated hips and knees in newborn. **c** Corresponding lateral radiograph of distal femur to feet showing a markedly dislocated knee (the tibia and fibula are in a reversed position in relation to the femur). Soft tissue density reveals an anterior patella; parallel talus/calcaneus and forefoot angulation indicate a severe clubfoot deformity

Part IX
Contracture Deformities

58 Amyoplasia Congenita

MIM 108110

Synonyms
Arthrogryposis multiplex congenita

Major Clinical Findings
Amyoplasia congenita refers to a heterogeneous group of disorders characterized by congenital nonprogressive joint contractures. The term amyoplasia was chosen by Hall to describe the absence of limb muscles that have been replaced by fibrous and fatty tissue. The main features of amyoplasia congenita are variable contractures of the major joints with a specific pattern. The elbow joints are usually in extension with flexed wrists and hands, and the shoulders are internally rotated. Severe flexion contractures are present at the metacarpophalangeal joints, with milder manifestations of contractures at the interphalangeal joints. The lower limbs are affected with dislocated or flexed hip joints, flexed or dislocated knee joints, and bilateral equinovarus position of the feet. Involvement of all four limbs has been observed in 90 % of patients. Muscle mass and bone growth of the involved limbs are decreased, and skeletal muscle is replaced by dense fibrous tissue and fat. Associated facial anomalies include a round face with micrognathia, an upturned nose, and often a midline capillary hemangioma. Intelligence is usually normal. The majority of patients become ambulatory with early physical therapy.

Occasional Findings
Dimples at contractures sites, congenital scoliosis, gastroschisis, Poland sequence, Moebius sequence, amniotic bands, cryptorchidism, hypoplastic labia, bowel atresia.

Genetic Transmission
This disorder occurs sporadically.

Differential Diagnosis
Amyoplasia congenita can be clinically delineated from other disorders with multiple contractures by the characteristic positioning at the shoulders (internal rotation), extension at the elbows, and flexion at the wrists.

References

Hall JG, Reed SD, Driscoll EP (1983) Amyoplasia: a common, sporadic condition with congenital contractures. Am J Med Genet 15:571–590

Reid COMV, Hall JG, Anderson C et al (1986) Association of amyoplasia with gastroschisis, bowel atresia, and defects of the muscular layer of the trunk. Am J Med Genet 24:701–710

Sells JM, Jaffe KM, Hall JG (1996) Amyoplasia, the most common type of arthrogryposis: the potential for good outcome. Pediatrics 97:225–231

S. Mundlos, D. Horn, *Limb Malformations*,
DOI 10.1007/978-3-540-95928-1_58,

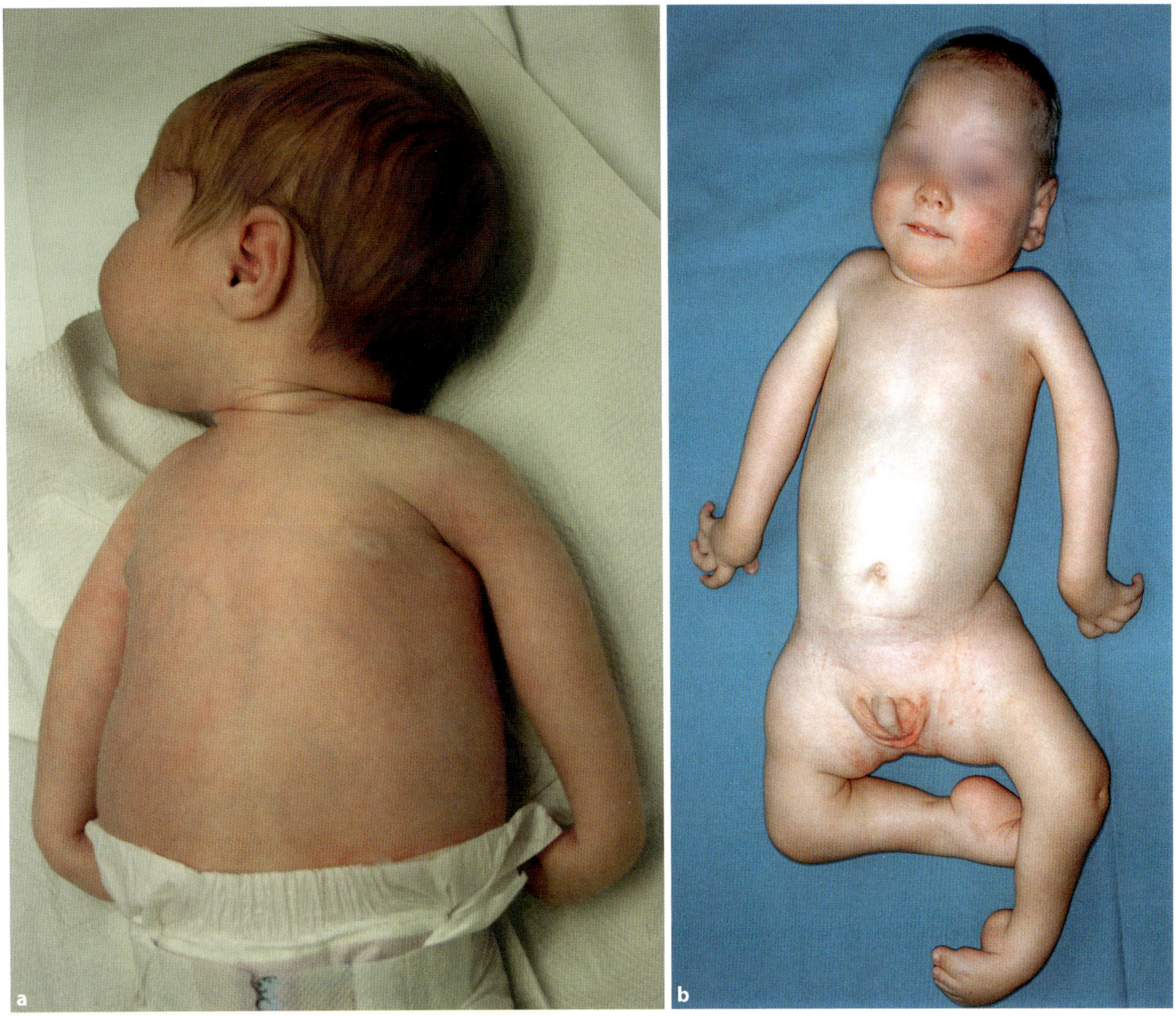

Fig. 58.1 **a** Newborn with contracture deformities of the upper limbs. The shoulders are internally rotated, and the elbow joints are in extension with flexed wrists and hands. Further flexion contractures are present at the metacarpophalangeal joints. **b** Newborn with amyoplasia. Note the dislocated hip joints, flexed or dislocated knee on the left with central dimple, and equinovarus position of the foot

59 Freeman–Sheldon Syndrome

MIM 193700

Synonyms
Arthrogryposis, distal, type 2A
Whistling face syndrome

Major Clinical Findings
Freeman–Sheldon syndrome is characterized by contractures of the hands and feet, oropharyngeal abnormalities, scoliosis, and a distinctive face that includes a very small oral orifice, puckered lips, and an H-shaped dimple of the chin ("whistling face syndrome"). Microstoma and long philtrum are frequently found. Other facial features such as a small nose with bulbous tip and small alae nasi, deep-set eyes, micrognathia, and a short and broad neck are less consistent findings. Strabismus, epicanthal folds, ptosis, downward slanting palpebral fissures, and hypertelorism have been documented. The hard palate is often highly arched, and the mandible and tongue appear to be small. Short stature is usually present. Flexion contractures of the fingers with ulnar deviation and contractures of the metacarpophalangeal joints of the thumbs are characteristic. Talipes equinovarus and kyphoscoliosis have been observed in the majority of affected individuals. Limited movement at the hips, elbows, and other joints as well as the neck has been noted. Hypoplastic muscles of the forearm and shank have been frequently documented. Tube feeding is necessary in most affected infants. Anesthetic problems such as muscle rigidity and malignant hyperthermia have been reported, and 30% of affected individuals have hearing loss.

Occasional Findings
Spina bifida occulta, inguinal hernia, dislocation of the radial heads, steep anterior cerebral fossa, pterygium colli, nasal speech, fixed facial expression.

Genetic Transmission
Most cases are compatible with autosomal dominant inheritance. Reduced penetrance may occur.

Differential Diagnosis
Individuals with Freeman–Sheldon syndrome and distal arthrogryposis type 1 may have similar limb phenotypes, but they can be distinguished by differences in facial morphology. Families in which different affected individuals were diagnosed with Freeman–Sheldon syndrome or with distal arthrogryposis type 1 have been reported. A severe variant of Freeman–Sheldon syndrome with additional brain anomalies, namely cerebellar and brainstem atrophy, has been described. Further differential diagnoses include other forms of arthrogryposis, such as Burton syndrome (characterized by a skeletal dysplasia with similar facial features and additional ectopia lentis), and more severe skeletal abnormalities, such as dumbbell-shaped long bones with flared metaphyses and an autosomal recessive mode of inheritance. Schwartz–Jampel syndrome can be distinguished by myotonia and bowed long bones with metaphyseal widening.

Molecular Pathology
Freeman–Sheldon syndrome is caused by mutations in the *MYH3* gene that encodes a myosin heavy chain. Mutations in this gene also underlie distal arthrogryposis type 2B, also known as Sheldon–Hall syndrome. Mutations detected in patients with Freeman–Sheldon syndrome and mutations found in distal arthrogryposis type 2B affect different myosin residues, demonstrating that the MYH3 genotype is predictive of the phenotype. Nearly all of the *MYH3* mutations are predicted to interfere with myosin's catalytic activity.

References

Bamshad M, Van Heest AE, Pleasure D (2009) Arthrogryposis: a review and update. J Bone Joint Surg Am 91:40–46

Stevenson DA, Carey JC, Palumbos J, Rutherford A, Dolcourt J, Bamshad MJ (2006) Clinical characteristics and natural history of Freeman–Sheldon syndrome. Pediatrics 117:754–762

Toydemir RM, Rutherford A, Whitby FG, Jorde LB, Carey JC, Bamshad MJ (2006) Mutations in embryonic myosin heavy chain (MYH3) cause Freeman–Sheldon syndrome and Sheldon–Hall syndrome. Nature Genet 38:561–565

S. Mundlos, D. Horn, *Limb Malformations*,
DOI 10.1007/978-3-540-95928-1_59,

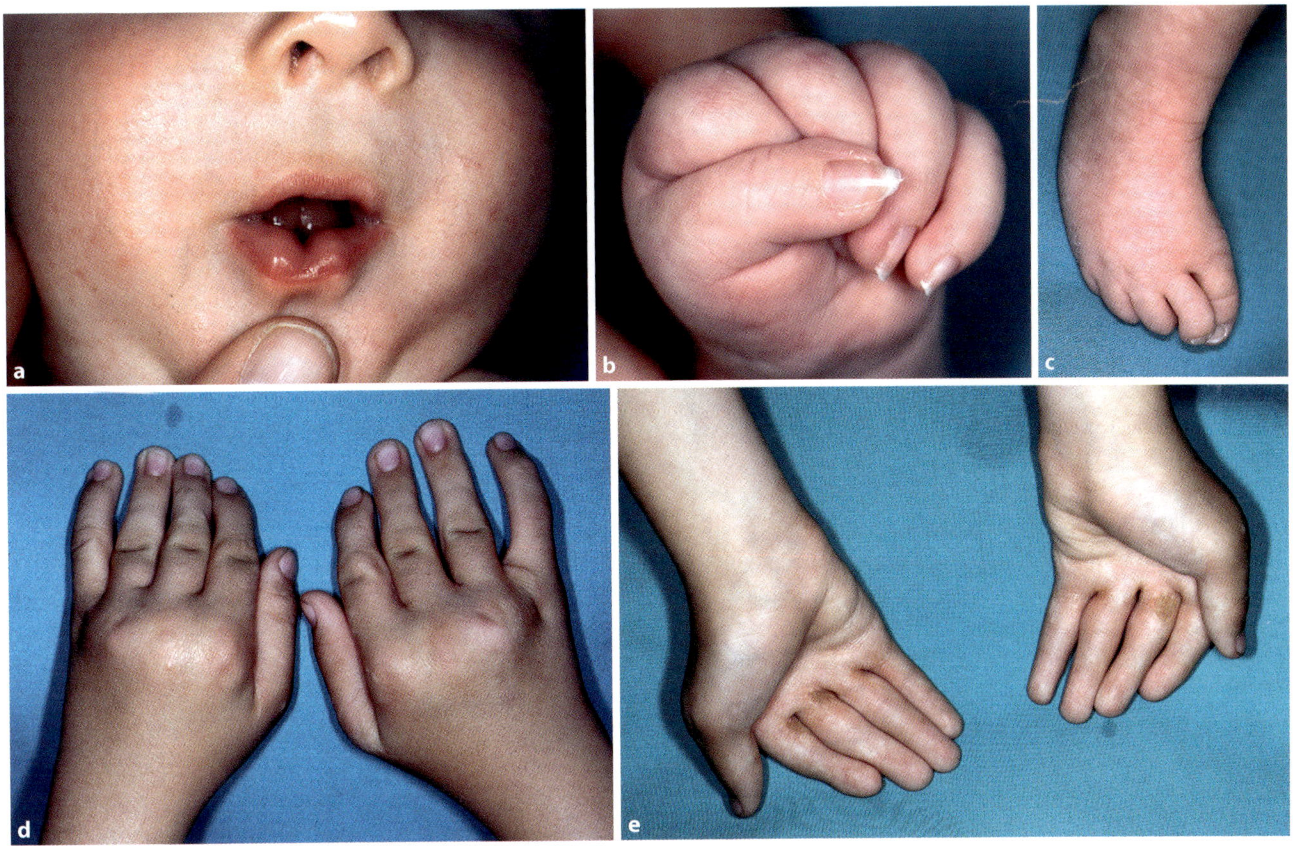

Fig. 59.1 **a** Small ("whistling") mouth and small chin. **b** Contracture deformity in newborn. Note overriding fingers, thumb adduction, and contractures of the proximal interphalangeal and the metacarpophalangeal joints. **c** Mild talipes equinovarus; inverted toes with contractures. **d** Contractures of the metacarpophalangeal joints. **e** Hypoplastic or absent interphalangeal creases and contractures of the interphalangeal joints

60 Multiple Pterygium Syndrome, Escobar Variant

MIM 265000

Synonyms
Escobar syndrome
Multiple pterygium syndrome, nonlethal type

Major Clinical Findings
Escobar syndrome belongs to a group of disorders characterized by joint contractures and variable degrees of webbing (multiple pterygia) mainly affecting the neck and large joints. The multiple pterygium syndromes are phenotypically and genetically heterogeneous. Clinically they have been separated into prenatally lethal and nonlethal (Escobar) types. Clinical features include short stature; pterygia of the neck, axilla, antecubital, popliteal, digital, and intercrural areas; multiple joint contractures (arthrogryposis multiplex congenita); absent or dysplastic patella; mild cutaneous syndactyly; camptodactyly; arachnodactyly; and "rocker-bottom" feet with vertical talus. Other skeletal anomalies such as scoliosis and fusion of the cervical vertebrae may occur.

Reduced fetal movements detected by ultrasound or reported by mothers may be the first clinical sign. Contractures may be noted on ultrasound toward the end of the 2nd trimester of pregnancy. Facial dysmorphism such as a long and expressionless face, high arched palate, small mouth, retrognathia, and cleft lip/palate may be present. Further facial anomalies are downward slanting palpebral fissures, mild ptosis, puffiness around the eyes, epicanthal folds, and decreased facial movements.

In males, cryptorchidism as well as a small penis and scrotum have been observed. In females, small clitoris and aplasia of the labia majora have been documented. Morbidity secondary to respiratory impairment may occur, and dilated aortic root and moderately severe aortic regurgitation present from birth have been documented. Congenital heart defects have been reported in about 25 %. Patients are frequently affected with reduced muscular mass.

Occasional Findings
Pectus excavatum, intercrural webs, dislocated hips, dislocated radial head, hearing deficit, malignant hyperthermia.

Genetic Transmission
Autosomal recessive.

Differential Diagnosis
Milder cases of Escobar syndrome may be confused with Noonan syndrome and other conditions with pterygia of the neck. Popliteal pterygium syndrome can be distinguished by the absence of other pterygia. However, elbow webbing may also occur in this syndrome. An Escobar-like condition with multiple joint contractures, hydramnios, and decreased fetal movements can be caused by maternal autoantibodies against the acetylcholine receptor.

Molecular Pathology
Generally, congenital contractures such as in Escobar syndrome can be caused by reduced fetal movements. In fact, it has been shown in animal models that lack of functional musculature leads to contractures, pterygia, and even joint fusion. Possible causes of decreased fetal mobility include drugs, diminished musculature, metabolic conditions, neuromuscular disorders such as myasthenia gravis that reduce muscle innervation, and space constraints such as oligohydramnios. The Escobar variant of multiple pterygium syndrome is caused by homozygous or compound heterozygous mutations in *CHRNG*, which encodes the gamma subunit of the acetylcholine receptor. Congenital contractures are likely to be caused by the transient inactivation of the neuromuscular end plate, which is followed by reduced fetal movements at sensitive times of development. Gene expression of the gamma subunit (CHRNG) is restricted to early development but is replaced by the epsilon subunit in the late fetal and perinatal period, thereby forming the adult AChR. This explains the lack of myasthenic symptoms later in life. A similar arthrogryposis phenotype can be caused by maternal AChR autoantibodies that cross the placenta and cause transient inactivation of the AChR pathway. Mutations in CHRNG can also cause the lethal variant of this phenotype.

References

Escobar V, Bixler D, Gleiser S, Weaver DD, Gibbs T (1978) Multiple pterygium syndrome. Am J Dis Child 132:609–611
Hall JG, Reed SD, Rosenbaum KN, Gershanik J, Chen H, Wilson KM (1982) Limb pterygium syndromes: a review and report of eleven patients. Am J Med Genet 12:377–409
Hoffmann K, Muller JS, Stricker S, Megarbane A, Rajab A, Lindner TH et al (2006) Escobar syndrome is a prenatal myasthenia caused by disruption of the acetylcholine receptor fetal gamma subunit. Am J Hum Genet 79:303–312
Rajab A, Hoffmann K, Ganesh A, Sethu AU, Mundlos S (2005) Escobar variant with pursed mouth, creased tongue, ophthalmologic features, and scoliosis in 6 children from Oman. Am J Med Genet 134A:151–157

S. Mundlos, D. Horn, *Limb Malformations*,
DOI 10.1007/978-3-540-95928-1_60, © Springer-Verlag Berlin Heidelberg 2014

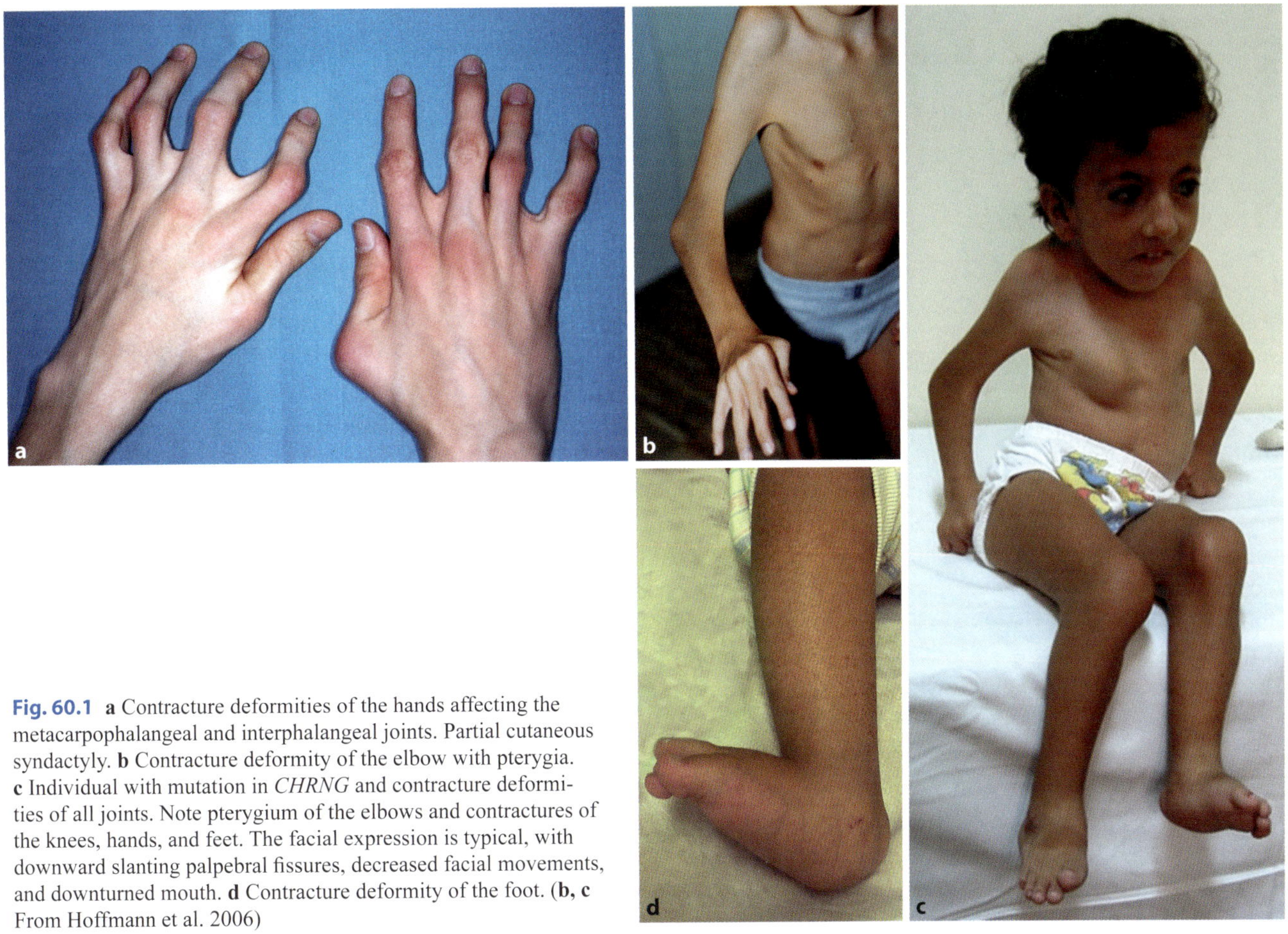

Fig. 60.1 **a** Contracture deformities of the hands affecting the metacarpophalangeal and interphalangeal joints. Partial cutaneous syndactyly. **b** Contracture deformity of the elbow with pterygia. **c** Individual with mutation in *CHRNG* and contracture deformities of all joints. Note pterygium of the elbows and contractures of the knees, hands, and feet. The facial expression is typical, with downward slanting palpebral fissures, decreased facial movements, and downturned mouth. **d** Contracture deformity of the foot. (**b, c** From Hoffmann et al. 2006)

61 Beals Syndrome

MIM 121050

Synonyms

Beals–Hecht syndrome
Congenital contractural arachnodactyly
Arthrogryposis, distal, type 9

Major Clinical Findings

The major features of Beals syndrome are arachnodactyly, joint contractures, and malformed ears. Limb anomalies include dolichostenomelic and slim limbs with arachnodactyly and camptodactyly. Joint contractures are present at the knee, elbow, and hip joints. The proximal interphalangeal joints of the fingers and toes may also have flexion contractures. The joint limitations usually show a gradual improvement. Kyphoscoliosis has been observed in about half of the patients, and talipes equinovarus occurs in a third. "Crumpled" ears present as a distortion of the course of the normal ear folds, with the appearance of supernumerary crura, such as crus tertium, and folds. The majority of affected individuals show muscular hypoplasia, especially of the calf muscles. Progressive enlargement of the ascending aorta and mitral valve prolapse with regurgitation have been documented.

Occasional Findings

Micrognathia, frontal bossing, dolichocephaly, myopia, congenital heart defects.

Genetic Transmission

Autosomal dominant.

Differential Diagnosis

Beals syndrome must be distinguished from other disorders with arachnodactyly, especially Marfan and Loeys–Dietz syndromes. In these conditions, joint contractures as seen in Beals syndrome are not a characteristic feature.

Molecular Pathology

Beals syndrome is associated with mutations in *FBN2*, the gene encoding the extracellular matrix component fibrillin 2. *FBN2* mutations cluster in the region of fibrillin 2 that is homologous to the so-called neonatal Marfan syndrome region of fibrillin 1.

References

Beals RK, Hecht F (1971) Congenital contractural arachnodactyly: a heritable disorder of connective tissue. J Bone Joint Surg Am 53:987–993

Gupta PA, Putnam EA, Carmical SG, Kaitila I, Steinmann B, Child A et al (2002) Ten novel FBN2 mutations in congenital contractural arachnodactyly: delineation of the molecular pathogenesis and clinical phenotype. Hum Mutat 19:39–48

Putnam EA, Zhang H, Ramirez F, Milewicz DM (1995) Fibrillin-2 (FBN2) mutations result in the Marfan-like disorder, congenital contractural arachnodactyly. Nature Genet 11:456–458

S. Mundlos, D. Horn, *Limb Malformations*,
DOI 10.1007/978-3-540-95928-1_61, © Springer-Verlag Berlin Heidelberg 2014

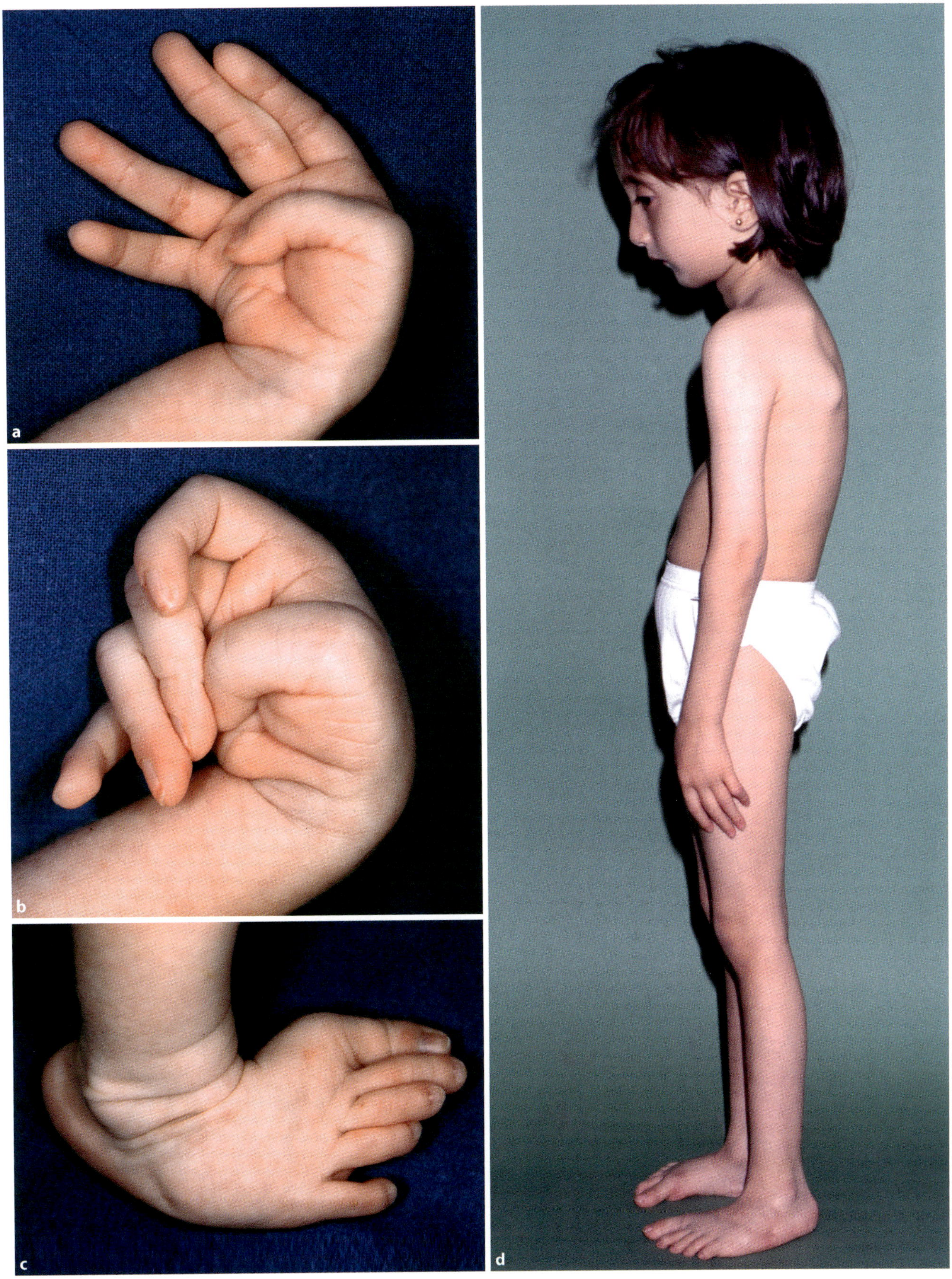

Fig. 61.1 Contracture deformity of hands (**a**,**b**) showing adducted thumb, ulnar deviation of the hand, flexion contracture, and inability to extend the fingers. **c** Malformed foot with metatarsus varus and talipes equinovarus. **d** Dolichostenomelia, Marfanoid habitus, and retrognathia

Part X

Reduction Anomalies: Upper and Lower Limbs

62 Acheiropodia

MIM 200500

Synonyms
Acheiropody

Major Clinical Findings
Acheiropodia is characterized by bilateral congenital truncations of the upper and lower extremities. In the upper limb, the distal part of the humerus is missing, including the entire elbow joint and more distal structures. Distal to the humerus, fingerlike appendage stumps (so-called Bohomoletz bones) may be present. In the lower limb, the knee is present, including the proximal tibia, but the middle and distal tibia and fibula and all more distal structures are absent.

Genetic Transmission
Autosomal recessive.

Differential Diagnosis
Acheiropodia is distinguished from other hemimelias by its specific pattern of malformations. In peromelia with (Hanhart syndrome) or without micrognathism, truncation defects with absence of the hands and feet occur, but the pattern is different. With the exception of two affected siblings in Puerto Rico, all reported cases are of Brazilian origin.

Molecular Pathology
The acheiropodia phenotype strikingly resembles that of Shh-/- mice. Shh-/- limbs consist of a truncated humerus with a small fingerlike appendage and truncation of the hind limb distal to the knee joint (see also Fig. 1.3d). Acheiropodia has been shown to be caused by a deletion of 4–6 kb in the *LMBR1* gene, which removes exon 4 and several kilobases of flanking intronic sequence. The gene itself, however, is not involved in limb development. Based on the similarities of the mouse and human phenotypes, the deletion is expected to interfere with SHH expression, probably via long-range enhancers. However, the reported deletion does not encompass the known limb regulatory region for Shh, the zone of polarizing activity regulatory sequence (ZRS).

References

Fett-Conte AC, Richieri-Costa A (1990) Acheiropodia: report on four new Brazilian patients. Am J Med Genet 36:341–344

Freire-Maia A (1981) Historical note: the extraordinary handless and footless families of Brazil—50 years of acheiropodia. Am J Med Genet 9(1):31–41

Freire-Maia A, Laredo-Filho J, Freire-Maia N (1978) Genetics of acheiropodia ("the handless and footless families of Brazil"): X. roentgenologic study. Am J Med Genet 2:321–330

Grimaldi A, Masiero D, Richieri-Costa A, Freire-Maia A (1983) Variable expressivity of the acheiropodia gene. Am J Med Genet 16(4):631–634

Ianakiev P, van Baren MJ, Daly MJ, Toledo SP, Cavalcanti MG, Neto JC et al (2001) Acheiropodia is caused by a genomic deletion in C7orf2, the human orthologue of the Lmbr1 gene. Am J Hum Genet 68(1):38–45

Silveira EL, Freire-Maia A (1998) Acheiropodia: new cases from Brazil. Clin Genet 54(3):256–257

Fig. 62.1 **a** Loss of distal structures in acheiropodia. Note the amputation-like phenotype at the level of the distal humerus with distal tapering and lower limb truncation distal to the knee with a thin remnant of tibia. **b** Corresponding radiograph shows hypoplastic humerus with a small, dysplastic bone at the distal end. **c, d** Further affected individuals from the same family. **c** A 2-year-old girl with distal truncations of the limbs. At the elbow region, a single ray is present with a single hypoplastic finger. **d** Truncations of the upper and lower limbs in a 7-month-old girl. In contrast to **c**, no distal elements are present in the upper limb. (**a** from Freire-Maia et al. 1978; **c, d** from Fett-Conte and Richieri-Costa 1990)

S. Mundlos, D. Horn, *Limb Malformations*,
DOI 10.1007/978-3-540-95928-1_62, © Springer-Verlag Berlin Heidelberg 2014

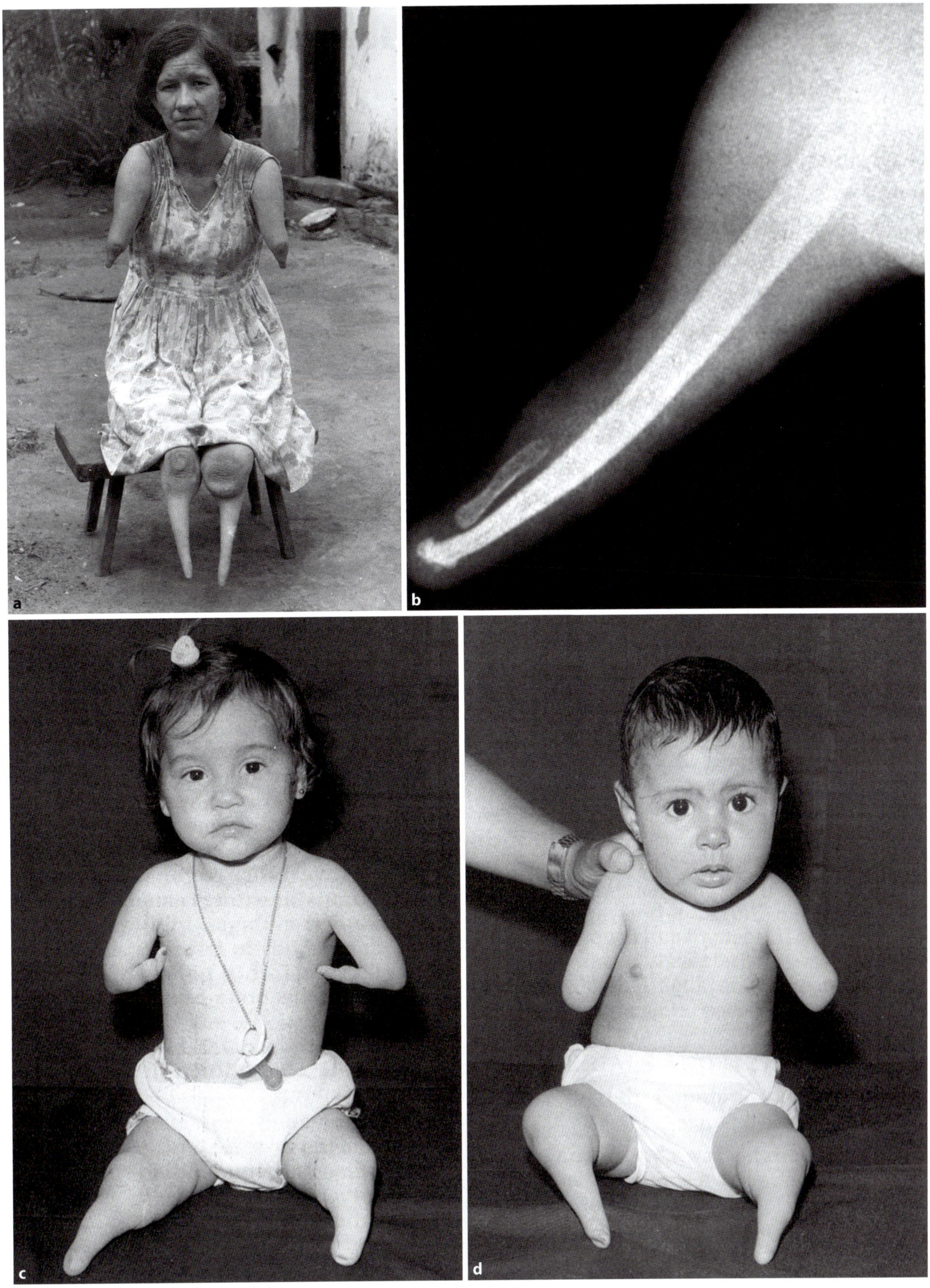

63 Al-Awadi/Raas–Rothschild/Schinzel Phocomelia Syndrome

MIM 228930

Includes
Fuhrmann Syndrome
MIM 276820

Synonyms
Limb/pelvis-hypoplasia/aplasia syndrome
Schinzel phocomelia syndrome

Major Clinical Findings
Al-Awadi/Raas–Rothschild/Schinzel phocomelia syndrome (AARRS) and Fuhrmann syndrome are two conditions of a phenotypic spectrum caused by mutations in the same gene. Individuals with AARRS exhibit gross lower-limb and severe upper-limb anomalies. These include ectrodactyly with nail dysplasia, oligodactyly, contractures, hypoplasia or aplasia of the elbow joint, reduction of the radius/ulna to a single bone, and monodactyly, as well as dysplastic nails in the upper limb. Also seen are dysplasia of the pelvis and absence of the distal lower limb with only a residual femur left.

In Fuhrmann syndrome, the upper limbs show hypoplasia/aplasia of the ulnar rays, shortening and bowing of the radius, hypoplastic 5th digits, and hypoplasia/aplasia of the nails with a radial-ulnar gradient. The dorsal side of the hands shows an abnormal texture, with hypoplastic flexion creases. Radiographic examination of the skeleton shows abnormalities of the pelvis, consisting of hypoplastic iliac wings and/or absent os ischia; dislocation and medial bending of the proximal ends of the femurs; absence of the patellae and other abnormalities of the knee joints (fusion); absence of the toenails; and loss of individual toes. The degree of severity varies within families, but per-person limb involvement is symmetrical. Because of limb shortening, the legs are more affected by major functional deficits than the arms are.

Genetic Transmission
Autosomal recessive.

Molecular Pathology
AARRS and Fuhrmann syndrome are both caused by mutations in *WNT7A*. Functional tests suggest that a partial loss of WNT7A function causes Fuhrmann syndrome, whereas the more severe limb truncation phenotypes observed in AARRS result from null mutations. Wnt7a belongs to a large family of secreted signaling proteins that signal through Frizzled, Lrp, and/or other receptors and the ß-catenin pathway. Wnt7a is involved in specifying cell fate in the developing limb. Together with Lmx1, Wnt7a has been shown to specify the dorsoventral axis. Accordingly, loss of Wnt7a leads to the acquisition of ventral characteristics in the distal dorsal limb regions (the loss of nails and formation of a palm on the dorsal side). The hypoplasia of the nails and patella as well as palmlike structures on the dorsum of the hands, as observed in Fuhrmann syndrome, are consistent with a loss of dorsal characteristics. The more severe phenotypes observed in AARRS are likely due to a collapse of the limb's entire signaling system (the feedback loop between dorsal ectoderm [Wnt7a], the apical ectodermal ridge [fibroblast growth factors], and the zone of polarizing activity [Shh]). Accordingly, the phenotype resembles the loss of Shh in the limb, as observed in Shh knockout mice.

References

Garavelli L, Wischmeijer A, Rosato S, Gelmini C, Reverberi S, Sassi S, et al. Al-Awadi–Raas-Rothschild (limb/pelvis/uterus-hypoplasia/aplasia) syndrome and WNT7A mutations: genetic homogeneity and nosological delineation. Am J Med Genet A. 2011 Feb;155A:332–6

Kantaputra PN, Mundlos S, Sripathomsawat W. A novel homozygous Arg222Trp missense mutation in WNT7A in two sisters with severe Al-Awadi/Raas–Rothschild/Schinzel phocomelia syndrome. Am J Med Genet A. 2010 Nov;152A(11):2832–7.

Riddle RD, Ensini M, Nelson C, Tsuchida T, Jessell TM, Tabin C. Induction of the LIM homeobox gene Lmx1 by WNT7a establishes dorsoventral pattern in the vertebrate limb. Cell. 1995 Nov 17;83(4):631–40.

Woods CG, Stricker S, Seemann P, Stern R, Cox J, Sherridan E, et al. Mutations in WNT7A cause a range of limb malformations, including Fuhrmann syndrome and Al-Awadi/Raas–Rothschild/Schinzel phocomelia syndrome. Am J Hum Genet. 2006 Aug;79(2):402–8.

S. Mundlos, D. Horn, *Limb Malformations*,
DOI 10.1007/978-3-540-95928-1_63, © Springer-Verlag Berlin Heidelberg 2014

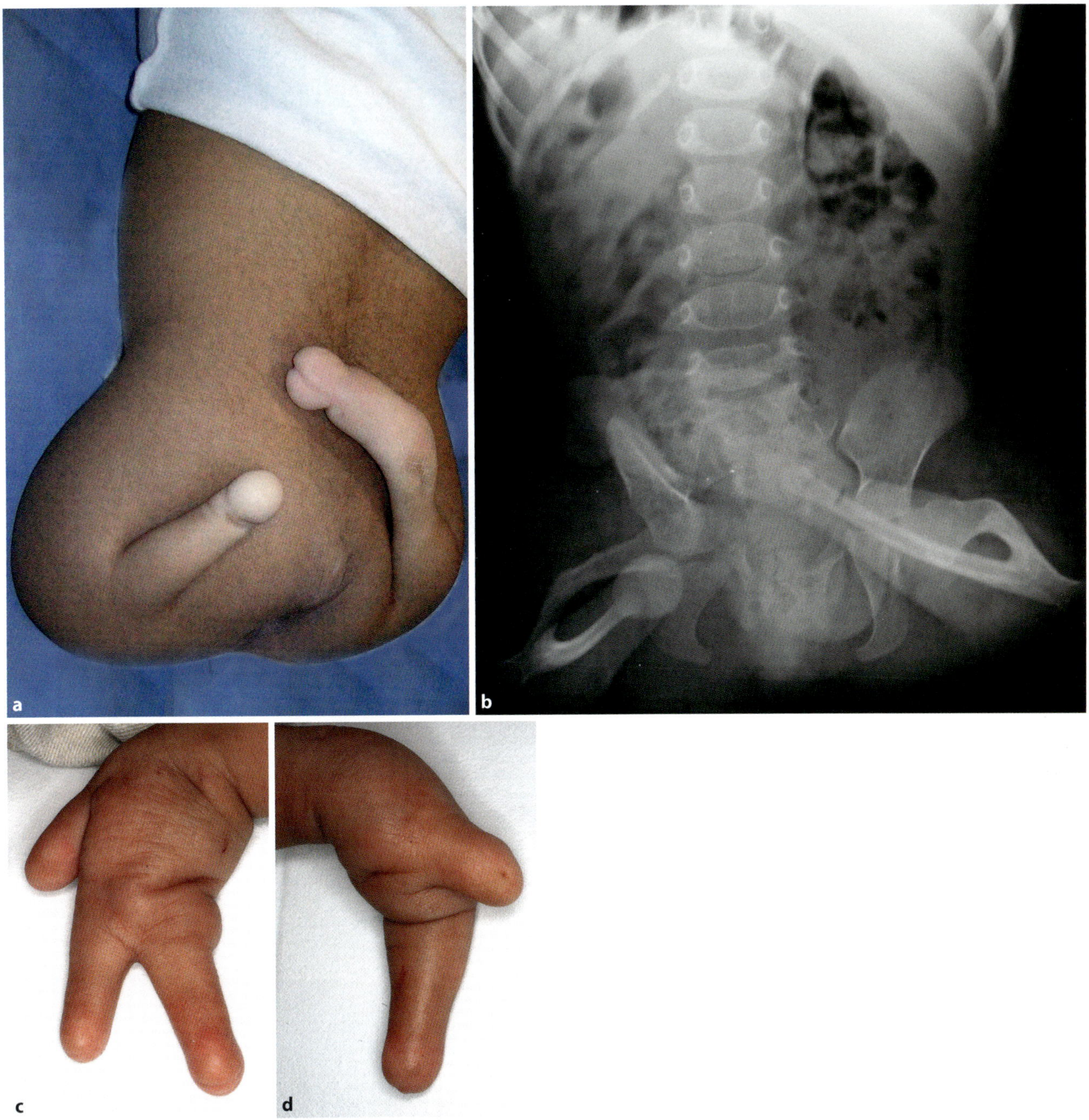

Fig. 63.1 **a** Lower limb malformation in severe case. Note truncation of the limb with total absence of distal structures. **b** Corresponding radiograph shows dysplastic ilia, hypoplastic ischia and sacrum, and Y-shaped femur, without distal structures. **c** Left hand with only three fingers and no nails. **d** Right hand with only two fingerlike structures. Note similarity of the palmar and dorsal skin.

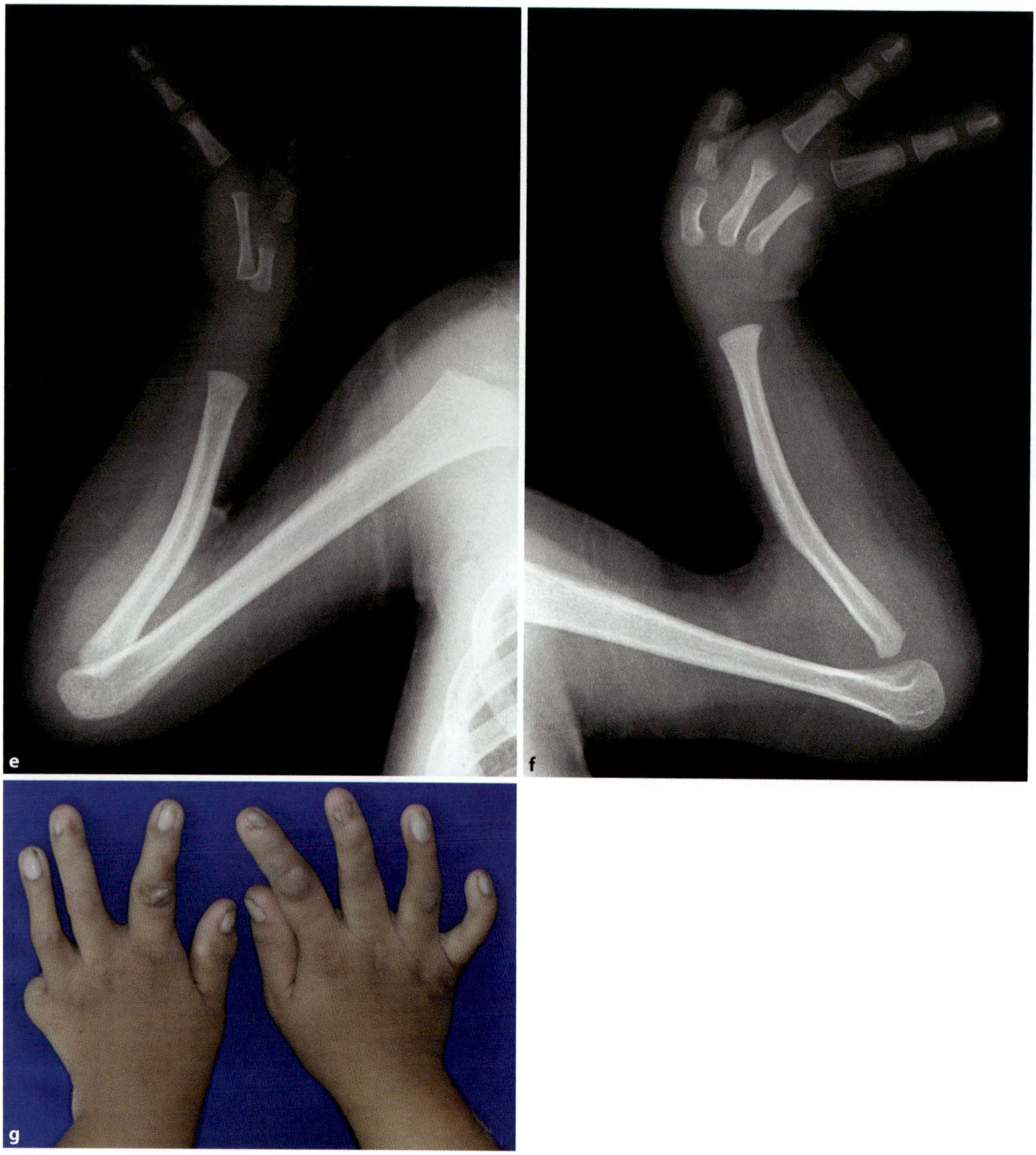

Fig. 63.1 (*continued*) **e, f** Corresponding radiographs show absence of the ulna and oligodactyly with absent fingers III–V on the left (**e**) and IV–V on the right (**f**). **g** Less severely affected hand with nail dysplasia and hypoplasia of left finger V. (**a–f** from Garavelli et al. 2011; **g** from Kantaputra et al. 2010)

64 Tetra-Amelia, Peromelia

MIM 273395

Major Clinical Findings

Variable degrees of limb reduction defects involving the loss of distal structures can be described using the term *peromelia*. They are usually symmetrical and involve amputation-like phenotypes at the level of the hands/feet or the forearm/calf with only stumps remaining. The complete absence of limbs is referred to as tetra-amelia. The latter may be associated with various other features, including cleft lip/palate, hypoplasia of the pelvis, pulmonary hypoplasia, and hydrocephalus.

Genetic Transmission

Sporadic, unknown. Recessive in some cases of tetra-amelia.

Molecular Pathology

Mutations in *WNT3* have been described in one family with tetra-amelia.

References

Niemann S, Zhao C, Pascu F, Stahl U, Aulepp U, Niswander L et al (2004) Homozygous WNT3 mutation causes tetra-amelia in a large consanguineous family. Am J Hum Genet 74:558–563

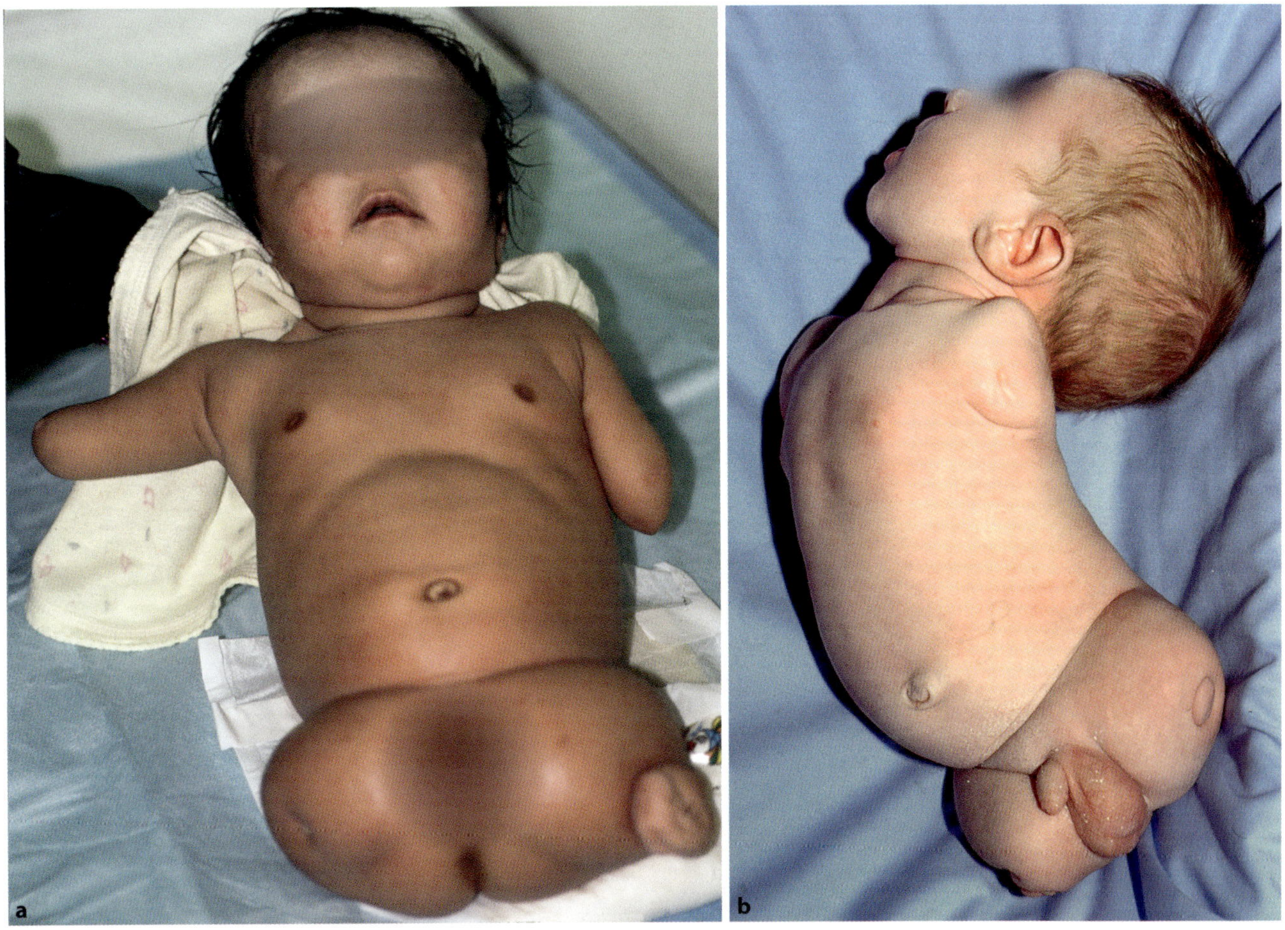

Fig. 64.1 **a** Peromelia with loss of structures at the level of the distal humerus. The lower limbs show complete loss of limb structures. Some remnants remain on the left. **b** Tetra-amelia

S. Mundlos, D. Horn, *Limb Malformations*,
DOI 10.1007/978-3-540-95928-1_64,

65 Hanhart Syndrome

MIM 103300

Synonyms

Hypoglossia–hypodactyly
Peromelia with micrognathism
Oromandibular limb hypoplasia
Aglossia–adactyly

Major Clinical Findings

Hanhart syndrome refers to a condition characterized by variable degrees of peromelia mainly affecting the more distal parts of the limbs (hands and feet) in combination with retrognathia, hypoplastic mandible, microstomia, hypoglossia, and other features affecting the oral cavity, such as glossopalatine ankylosis, ankylosis of the mandibular joint, and intraoral bands. The original family described by Hanhart featured peromelia and micrognathia. Other described cases showed variable degrees of limb truncations, oligodactyly, or ectrodactyly together with retrognathia and hypoglossia.

Genetic Transmission

Sporadic, unknown.

References

De Smet L, Schollen W (2001) Hypoglossia-hypodactyly syndrome: report of 2 patients. Genet Counsel 12:347–352

Hall BD (1971) Aglossia-adactylia. Birth Defects Orig Art Ser VII(7):233–236

Hanhart E (1950) Ueber die Kombination von Peromelie mit Mikrognathie, ein neues Syndrom beim Menschen, entsprechend der Akroteriasis congenita von Wriedt und Mohr beim Rind. Arch Klaus Stift Vererbungsforsch 25:531–543

S. Mundlos, D. Horn, *Limb Malformations*,
DOI 10.1007/978-3-540-95928-1_65, © Springer-Verlag Berlin Heidelberg 2014

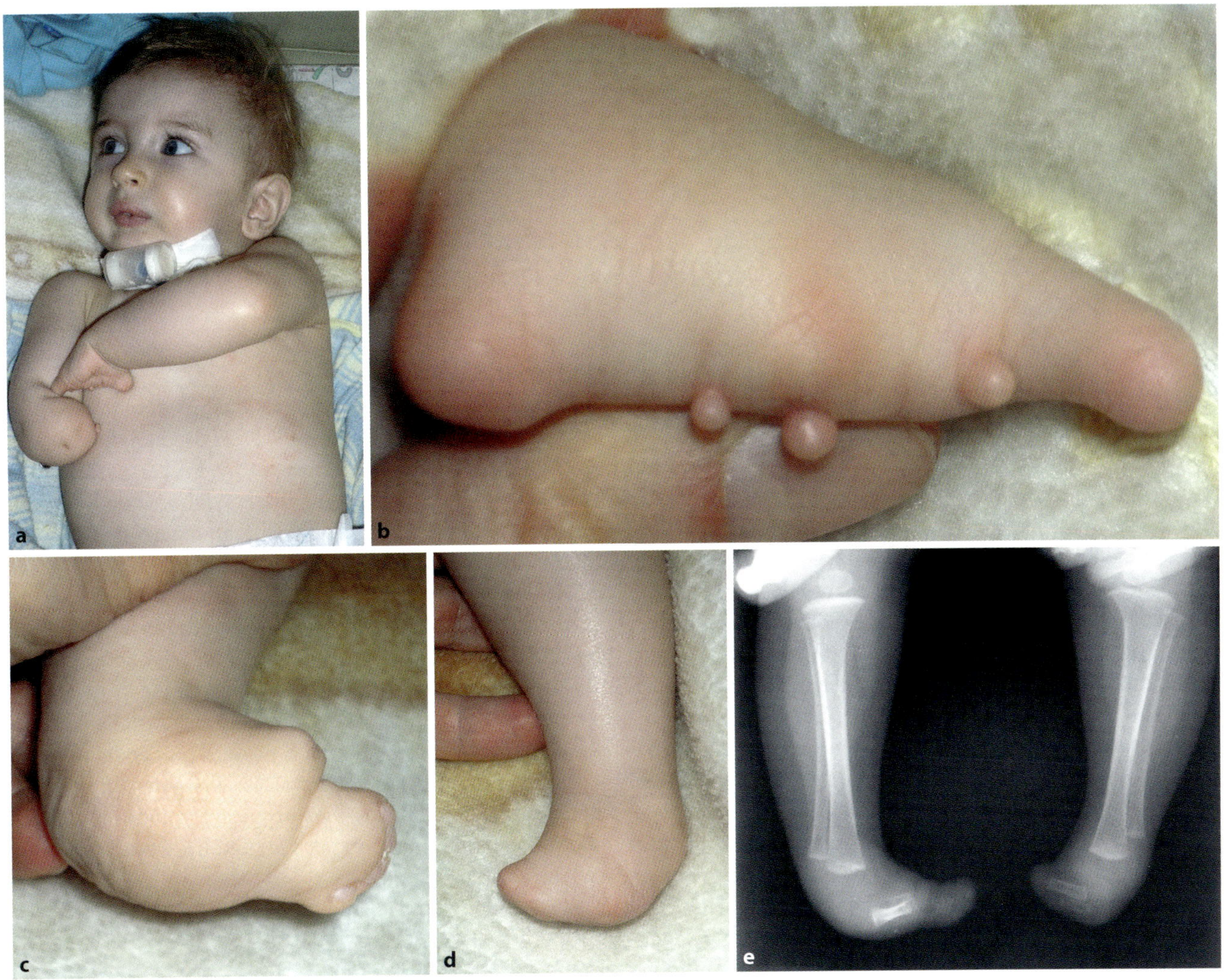

Fig. 65.1 **a** A 10-month-old boy with cleft palate, ankylosis of the temporomandibular joints, small mandible, hypoglossia, and laryngeal hypotonia requiring tracheostomy. There is distal peromelia affecting all limbs to variable degrees. **b** Left hand showing an ectrodactyly-like loss of digits with knoblike remnants of the middle digits remaining. **c, d** Right and left foot, respectively, with loss of distal elements. **e** Corresponding radiograph shows normal tibia/fibula, lack of tarsals, reduction in size and number of the metatarsals, no distal structures/toes on the left, and some remaining structures on the right (Courtesy of A. Jamsheer, Poznan University of Medical Sciences, Poland)

66 Roberts Syndrome

MIM 268300

Includes
SC Phocomelia Syndrome
MIM 269000

Synonyms
SC pseudothalidomide syndrome

Major Clinical Findings
Roberts syndrome is a variable condition mainly characterized by mesomelic limb shortening that is more severe in the upper limbs, severe prenatal and mild to severe postnatal growth deficiency, cleft lip/palate, and various abnormalities in other organ systems. The reduction anomalies of the long bones can be asymmetric and of variable degree, ranging from phocomelia of the arms and legs to oligodactyly and mild shortening. Flexion contractures occur in most of the large joints. The radius, ulna, tibia, and fibula as well as the thumb and the 1st and 5th metacarpals can be hypoplastic or absent. Cleft lip/palate, often bilateral, is present in 80%. Other craniofacial abnormalities include microcephaly, shallow orbits, hypertelorism, and sparse and silvery-blond scalp hair. Approximately 20% are stillborn. Among survivors, 50% show delayed psychomotor development. Premature centromere separation is found in the lymphocytes and/or fibroblasts of affected individuals.

SC phocomelia syndrome is an allelic, milder version of Roberts syndrome. The clinical phenotype consists of symmetrical limb malformations with hypoplasia of the humerus, hypoplasia/aplasia of the radius and ulna, and absence or hypoplasia of the thumbs in the upper limbs and similar changes in the lower limbs. Flexion contractures of various joints are a common finding. Other anomalies include intellectual disability; microcephaly; capillary hemangioma of the face, forehead, and ears; hypoplastic cartilage of the ears and nose; micrognathia; scanty, silvery-blond hair; and cloudy corneas.

Occasional Findings
Humeroradial and humeroulnar synostoses, femorotibial synostosis, hydrocephalus, encephalocele, seizures, enlarged penis or clitoris, cardiac and kidney anomalies.

Genetic Transmission
Autosomal recessive.

Differential Diagnosis
Roberts syndrome should be distinguished from other disorders with phocomelia, such as TAR syndrome. There is also overlap with thalidomide embryopathy. In cases with mainly radial ray involvement, Holt–Oram syndrome and Fanconi anemia should be considered as differential diagnoses.

Molecular Pathology
Roberts syndrome and SC phocomelia syndrome are caused by mutations in *ESCO2*. Both conditions can be caused by the same mutation in different members of the same family. The ESCO2 protein is required for the establishment of sister chromatid cohesion during S phase. This results in rather specific chromosomal abnormalities involving the heterochromatic C-banding regions of most chromosomes (puffing of heterochromatic regions around the centromeres and nucleolar organizers).

References

Parry DM, Mulvihill JJ, Tsai S, Kaiser-Kupfer MI, Cowan JM (1986) SC phocomelia syndrome, premature centromere separation and congenital cranial nerve paralysis in two sisters, one with malignant melanoma. Am J Med Genet 24:653–672

Schüle B, Oviedo A, Johnston K, Pai S, Francke U (2005) Inactivating mutations in ESCO2 cause SC phocomelia and Roberts syndrome: no phenotype-genotype correlation. Am J Hum Genet 77:1117–1128

Vega H, Waisfisz Q, Gordillo M, Sakai N, Yanagihara I, Yamada M et al (2005) Roberts syndrome is caused by mutations in ESCO2, a human homolog of yeast ECO1 that is essential for the establishment of sister chromatid cohesion. Nature Genet 37:468–470

Vega H, Trainer AH, Gordillo M, Crosier M, Kayserili H, Skovby F et al (2010) Phenotypic variability in 49 cases of ESCO2 mutations, including novel missense and codon deletion in the acetyltransferase domain, correlates with ESCO2 expression and establishes the clinical criteria for Roberts syndrome. J Med Genet 47:30–37

 S. Mundlos, D. Horn, *Limb Malformations*,
DOI 10.1007/978-3-540-95928-1_66, © Springer-Verlag Berlin Heidelberg 2014

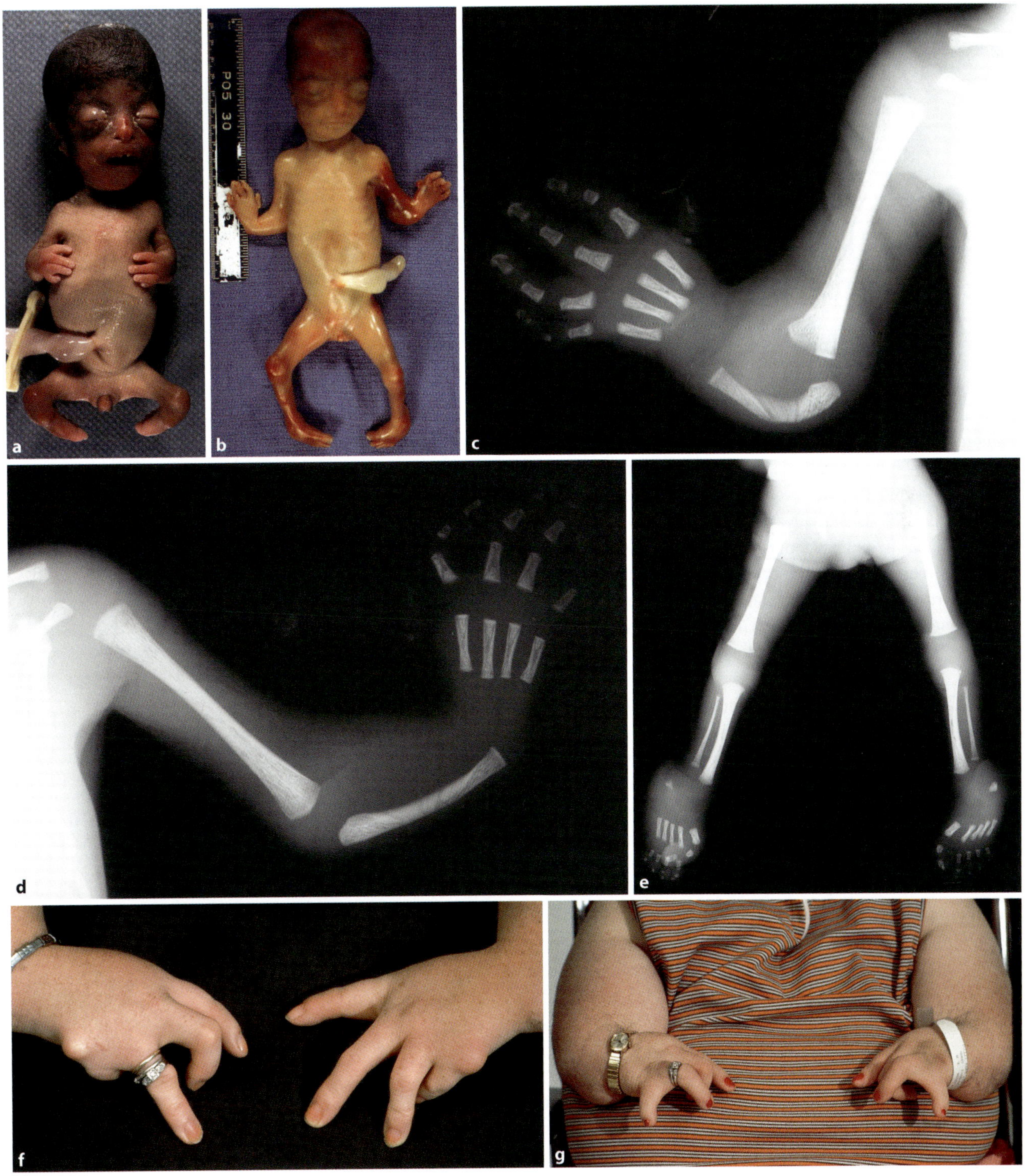

Fig. 66.1 **a** Fetus with Roberts syndrome. Note bulging eyes, beaked nose, hypoplasia of the nasal alae, micrognathia, severe shortening of the limbs, absence of thumbs bilaterally, and syndactyly of digits IV and V. **b** Less severely affected fetus with radial clubbed hands, hypoplastic thumbs, short lower legs, and clubfeet. **c–e** Corresponding radiographs. Bilateral 1st ray abnormality: absent radius bilaterally, rudimentary ossification of hypoplastic thumb, small middle phalanx of digit V with clinodactyly on the right, hypoplastic middle and distal phalanges of digits II and V on the left. Hypoplasia of fibulae. **f, g** Hands of sisters with SC phocomelia syndrome. (From Schüle et al. 2005)

67 Focal Dermal Hypoplasia

MIM 305600

Synonyms
Goltz syndrome
Goltz–Gorlin syndrome

Major Clinical Findings
Focal dermal hypoplasia (FDH) consists of various skin anomalies and abnormalities of the skeleton, especially the limbs. The skin features include focal absence of skin and linear or reticular hyperpigmentation or hypopigmentation of the skin, herniation of fat through the dermal defects, and multiple papillomas of the mucous membranes or skin, such as in the axilla and around the anus and vulva. Oral anomalies, in addition to lip papillomas, include hypoplastic teeth. Spotty hypotrichosis of the scalp or pubic hair has been described. Digital anomalies comprise syndactyly, postaxial polydactyly, brachydactyly, camptodactyly, and absence deformities such as oligodactyly. The combination of split-hand/foot with syndactyly is common. Limb anomalies are often asymmetric. Short stature occurs. Right-sided clavicular pseudoarthrosis is frequently found. Ocular anomalies, including strabismus, microphthalmia, and coloboma of the iris, choroid, and retina, may be present in some cases. Delayed psychomotor development occurs in many patients. Striated bones are a frequent feature. Hypodontia is a frequent teeth anomaly, but supernumerary teeth, enamel dysplasia, and malocclusion are also seen.

Occasional Findings
Rib anomalies, scoliosis, multiple giant cell tumor of long bones, anomalies of the genitourinary system, umbilical hernia, omphalocele, cleft lip/palate, ectopia lentis, aniridia, mixed hearing loss, spina bifida.

Genetic Transmission
Focal dermal hypoplasia is inherited as an X-linked dominant disorder with in utero lethality in males. Somatic mosaicism has been documented. The majority of cases have been sporadic.

Differential Diagnosis
FDH should be distinguished from microphthalmia with linear skin defects (MIDAS syndrome, involving microphthalmia, dermal aplasia, and sclerocornea) by the presence of limb defects and skin involvement over the entire body. Other syndromic and nonsyndromic forms of split-hand/foot malformation should also be considered.

Molecular Pathology
Focal dermal hypoplasia is caused by heterozygous mutations or deletions of the *PORCN* gene. PORCN encodes a putative O-acyltransferase and is potentially crucial for the cellular export of Wnt signaling proteins.

References

Bornholdt D, Oeffner F, Konig A, Happle R, Alanay Y, Ascherman J et al (2009) PORCN mutations in focal dermal hypoplasia: coping with lethality. Hum Mutat 30:E618–E628

Goltz RW (1992) Focal dermal hypoplasia syndrome: an update. (Editorial). Arch Derm 128:1108–1111

Grzeschik K-H, Bornholdt D, Oeffner F, Konig A, del Boente MC, Fritz B et al (2007) Deficiency of PORCN, a regulator of Wnt signaling, is associated with focal dermal hypoplasia. Nature Genet 39:833–835

Maas SM, Lombardi MP, van Essen AJ, Wakeling EL, Castle B, Temple IK et al (2009) Phenotype and genotype in 17 patients with Goltz–Gorlin syndrome. J Med Genet 46:716–720

Fig. 67.1 **a** Typical skin lesions in focal dermal hypoplasia. Note atrophy and linear pigmentation of the skin and herniation of fat through the dermal defects. **b, c** Foot of affected individual. Note ectrodactyly type malformation with fusion of the middle toes. **d** Other foot of individual in **b** and **c**, having only minor abnormalities and syndactyly of toes IV and V. **e** Syndactyly of toes II–V, distal hypoplasia of toe II. **f, g** Syndactyly III/IV, dorsal and palmar views. **h** Left hand of same individual. Note ectrodactyly-like malformation. **i** Central cleft and postaxial polydactyly

S. Mundlos, D. Horn, *Limb Malformations*,
DOI 10.1007/978-3-540-95928-1_67, © Springer-Verlag Berlin Heidelberg 2014

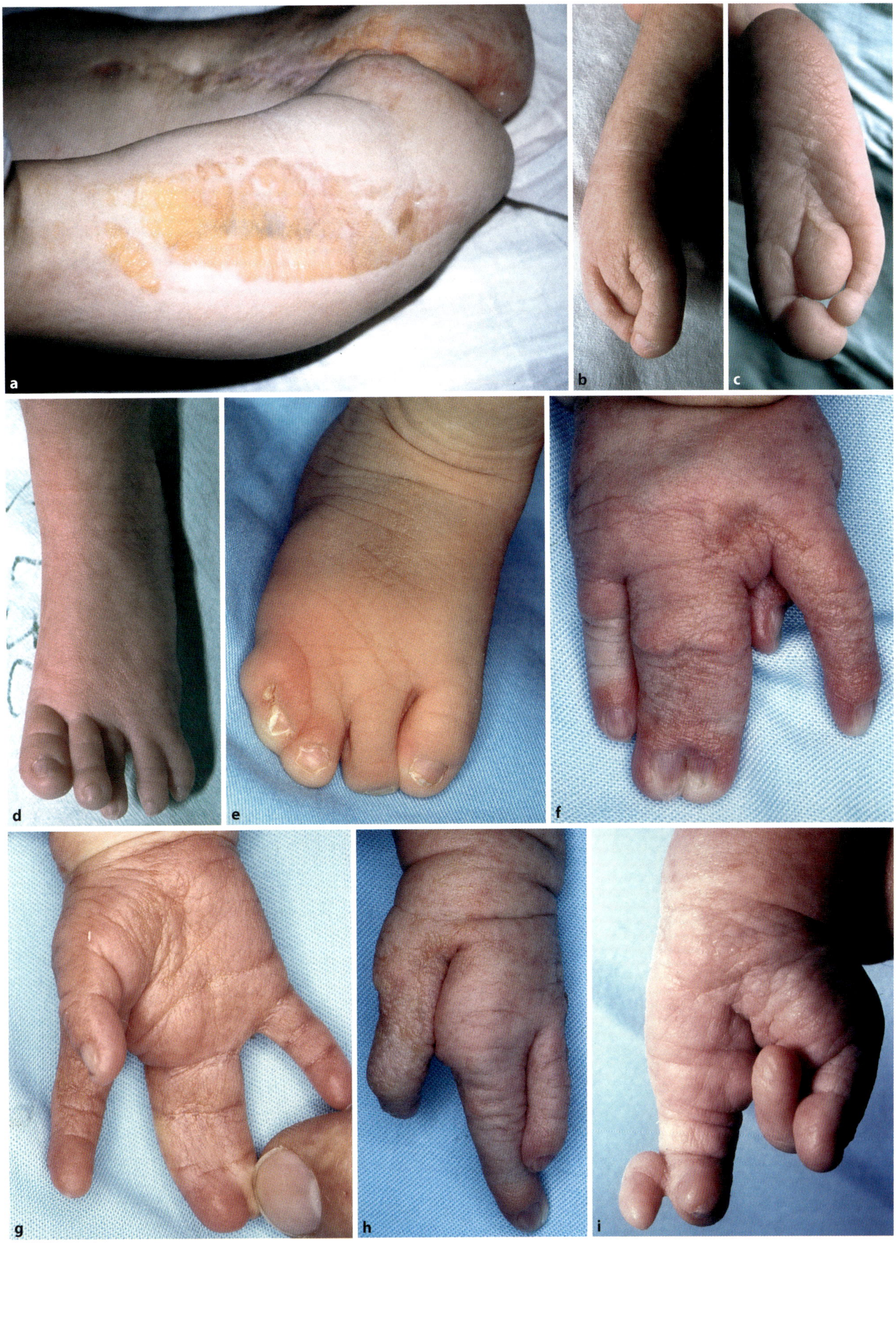
a
b
c
d
e
f
g
h
i

Part XI

Reduction Anomalies: Lower Limbs

68 Deficiency of Long Bones with Clubfoot and Mirror-Image Polydactyly

MIM 119800

Includes
Clubfoot, congenital

Major Clinical Findings

This condition is characterized by abnormalities of the lower limb only, consisting of deficiency of the long bones (tibial hemimelia with a preference for the right side, hypoplasia of the tibia), clubfoot, and mirror-image polydactyly. Further radiographic anomalies include patellar hypoplasia, oblique talus manifesting as pes planus, and hip dysplasia. A reduction in the overall size of the affected limb with reduced muscle and bone volumes, especially in the distal parts, has been observed in magnetic resonance imaging studies of an affected individual. Dysmorphic facial features may be present, including downward slanting palpebral fissures, mild hypertelorism, flat nasal bridge, and low-set ears. Further anomalies reported include hypoplasia of the corpus callosum, enlargement of the cisterna magna, a median cleft palate, cardiomegaly, and bilateral popliteal pterygia. The upper limbs are normal.

Congenital talipes equinovarus, also known as clubfoot, is a lower limb deformity defined as fixation of the foot in cavus, adductus, varus, and equinus positions. It is a relatively frequent malformation with an incidence of approximately 10 per 10,000 live births for the isolated form. However, clubfoot frequently occurs as part of a skeletal dysplasia or syndrome.

Genetic Transmission

Long bone deficiency with clubfoot and polydactyly follows an autosomal dominant trait.

Isolated clubfoot appears to be a multifactorial trait. In a few families, clubfoot segregates as an autosomal dominant condition with incomplete penetrance and variable expressivity.

Differential Diagnosis

Tibial hemimelia with polydactyly is also a feature of Mesomelic dysplasia Werner type. However, in this condition the upper limbs are affected as well.

Concordant with isolated clubfoot following a multifactorial trait, there can be multiple affected individuals within one family. Clubfoot can be part of skeletal dysplasias. In multiple epiphyseal dysplasia, recessive type, as well as diastrophic dysplasias that are caused by mutations of the *DTDST* gene, congenital clubfoot is a prominent clinical sign at birth. The mode of inheritance as well as additional clinical and radiographic features differentiate these entities.

Molecular Pathology

Long bone deficiency with clubfoot and mirror-image polydactyly can be caused by mutations or deletions in *PITX1*. Pitx1 is a master transcription factor expressed throughout the developing hindlimb but not the forelimb. The function of Pitx1 has been elucidated in knockout mice and by overexpression of Pitx1 in the forelimb. Pitx1 inactivation resulted in structural changes in the tibia and fibula as well as patterning alterations in the patella and proximal tarsus, causing the hindlimb to resemble the corresponding forelimb structures. Accordingly, misexpression of Pitx1 in the forelimb resulted in the acquisition of morphologic characteristics of hindlimbs. Thus, Pitx1 is a master regulator for hindlimb identity (see also Liebenberg syndrome Chap. 54).

Clubfoot is a heterogeneous disorder. A polygenetic threshold model has been used to explain its inheritance patterns. A key developmental pathway in its pathogenesis appears to involve the PITX1–TBX4 pathway. Isolated clubfoot has also been associated with deletions or duplications involving the *TBX4* gene, which is a transcriptional target of PITX1, and with mutations and deletions involving PITX1. Interestingly, clubfoot-like anomalies occur in Pitx1+/- mice with a penetrance of 9%, and skeletal muscle gene expression was significantly reduced in the hind limb buds, suggesting early disturbed muscle development.

References

Alvarado DM, Aferol H, McCall K, Huang JB, Techy M, Buchan J, Cady J, Gonzales PR, Dobbs MB, Gurnett CA (2010) Familial isolated clubfoot is associated with recurrent chromosome 17q23.1q23.2 microduplications containing TBX4. Am J Hum Genet 87(1):154–160

Alvarado DM, McCall K, Aferol H, Silva MJ, Garbow JR, Spees WM et al (2011) Pitx1 haploinsufficiency causes clubfoot in humans and a clubfoot-like phenotype in mice. Hum Molec Genet 20:3943–3952

Dobbs MB, Gurnett CA (2012) Genetics of clubfoot. J Pediatr Orthop B 21(1):7–9

Gurnett CA, Alaee F, Kruse LM, Desruisseau DM, Hecht JT, Wise CA et al (2008) Asymmetric lower-limb malformations in individuals with homeobox PITX1 gene mutation. Am J Hum Genet 83:616–622

Klopocki E, Kahler C, Foulds N, Shah H, Joseph B, Vogel H et al (2012) Deletions in PITX1 cause a spectrum of lower-limb malformations including mirror-image polydactyly. Europ J Hum Genet 20:705–708

S. Mundlos, D. Horn, *Limb Malformations*,
DOI 10.1007/978-3-540-95928-1_68, © Springer-Verlag Berlin Heidelberg 2014

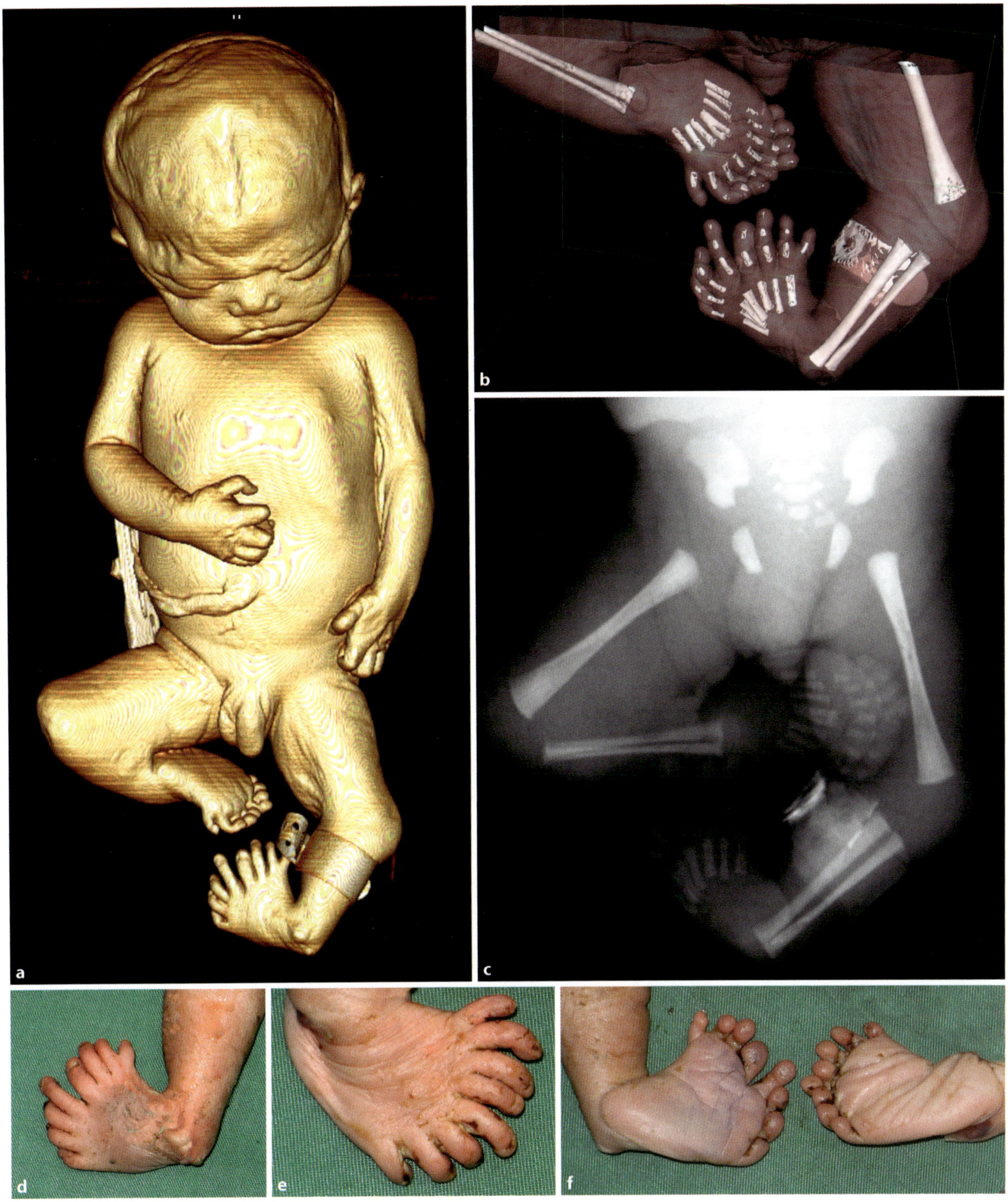

Fig. 68.1 **a** Three-dimensional (3D) scan of fetus showing clubfeet and foot polydactyly. **b** 3D image of the lower limb bones. Note thin tibia/fibula on the right side and polydactyly with eight toes bilaterally. **c** Corresponding plain film showing clubfoot on the left and polydactyly. Note also the unilateral absence of pubic ossification, high/narrow iliac wings, and very straight, thin long bones. **d, e** Polydactyly of feet, mirror-image-like. **f** Plantar view

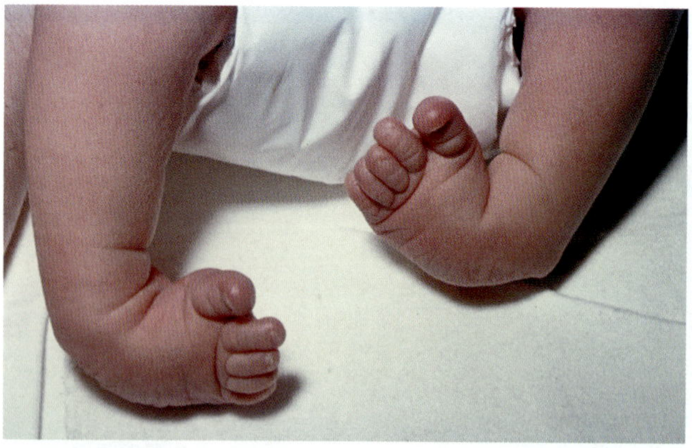

Fig. 68.2 Clubfeet

69 Femoral-Facial Syndrome

MIM 134780

Synonyms

Femoral hypoplasia unusual facies syndrome

Major Clinical Findings

Femoral-facial syndrome (FFS) is a multiple congenital anomaly syndrome with bilateral femoral hypoplasia. Shortening is often asymmetric and associated with bowing. The condition is probably heterogeneous, with some individuals having characteristic facial features, including short nose with broad tip, hypoplastic alae nasi, long philtrum, thin upper lip, and micrognathia with or without cleft palate. The ears may be dysplastic or low set. Other features may include renal hypoplasia; genital anomalies including cryptorchidism, microphallus, hypoplastic labia, absent uterus and vagina with normal ovaries; bilobed lungs; and hydrocephalus. Other rare skeletal associations include short proximal arms with absent elbow flexion and extension, humeroradial synostosis, and clubfeet.

Genetic Transmission

Sporadic. Some familial cases with dominant inheritance have been described.

Differential Diagnosis

Caudal regression syndrome should be considered.

Molecular Pathology

FFS-like phenotypes have been observed in severe fetal constraint secondary to oligohydramnios and have been associated with maternal diabetes.

References

Burn J, Winter RM, Baraitser M, Hall CM, Fixsen J (1984) The femoral hypoplasia-unusual facies syndrome. J Med Genet 21(5):331–340

Johnson JP, Carey JC, Gooch WM 3rd, Petersen J, Beattie JF (1983) Femoral hypoplasia-unusual facies syndrome in infants of diabetic mothers. J Pediatr 102(6):866–872

Robinow M, Sonek J, Buttino L, Veghte A (1995) Femoral-facial syndrome—prenatal diagnosis—autosomal dominant inheritance. Am J Med Genet 57(3):397–399

S. Mundlos, D. Horn, *Limb Malformations*,
DOI 10.1007/978-3-540-95928-1_69,

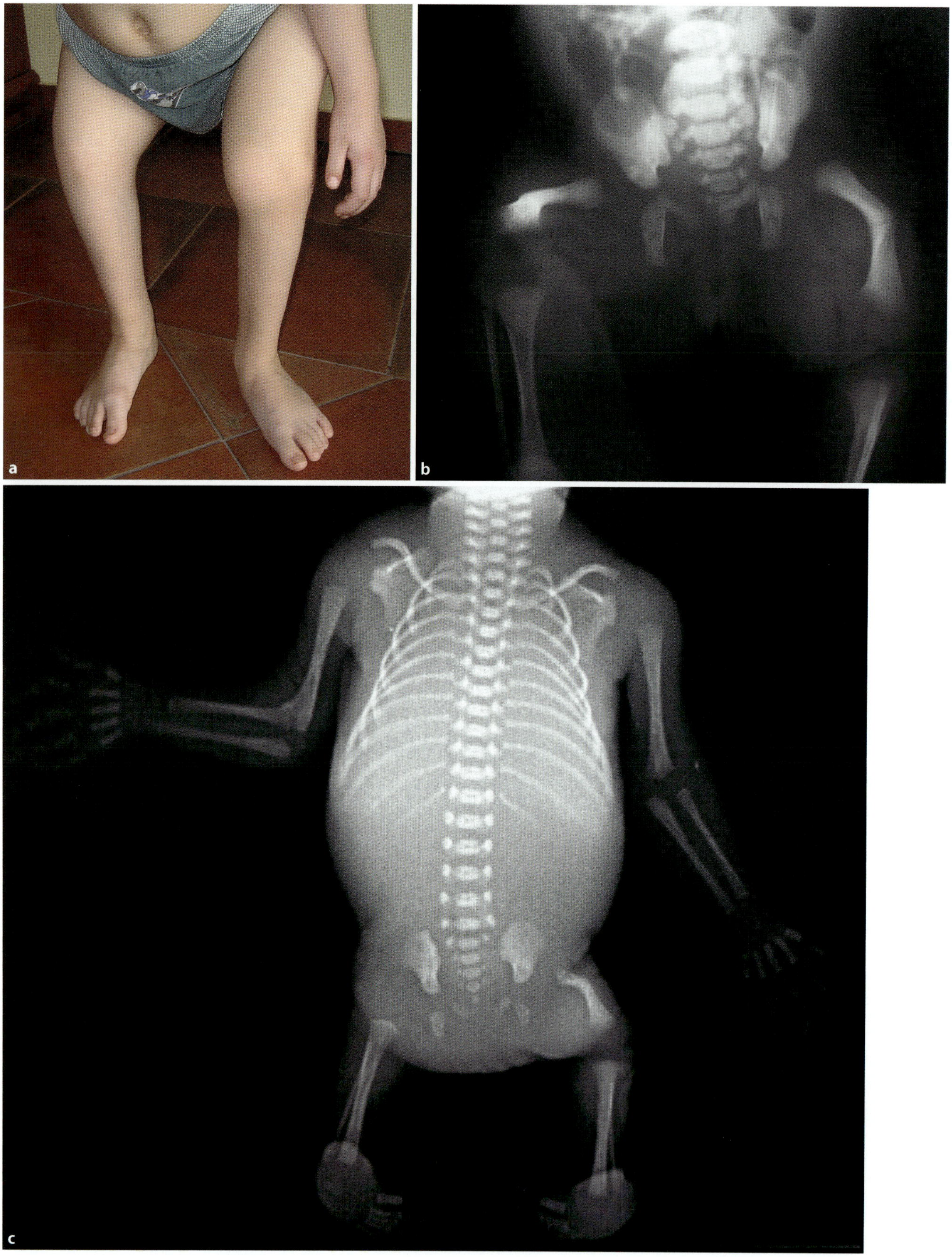

Fig. 69.1 **a** Asymmetric shortening of both femurs. **b** Radiograph of pelvis and upper part of the lower limbs. Hypoplasia of dislocated and bowed femurs, more severe on the right. **c** Radiograph of newborn with femoral-facial syndrome. Absent right femur; hypoplastic left, bowed femur; clubfeet; unilateral elbow fusion

Gollop–Wolfgang Complex

MIM 228250

70

Synonyms
Femur, unilateral bifid, with monodactylous ectrodactyly

Major Clinical Findings
Gollop–Wolfgang complex refers to the rare finding of unilateral bifurcation of the femur. In addition, absence of the tibia, monodactyly of the feet, and ectrodactyly of the hands have been described. Congenital heart defects may be additional features.

Genetic Transmission
Reported recurrence in siblings is suggestive of autosomal recessive inheritance.

Differential Diagnosis
Other forms of ectrodactyly. However, bifid femur is a specific sign.

References

Fiogbe MA, Hounnou GM, Gbenou AS, Biaou O, Sossou R, Laleye A et al (2010) Femoral bifurcation associated with tibial aplasia: about 3 cases. Genet Counsel 21:1–7

Gollop TR, Lucchesi E, Martins RMM, Nione AS (1980) Familial occurrence of bifid femur and monodactylous ectrodactyly. Am J Med Genet 7:319–322

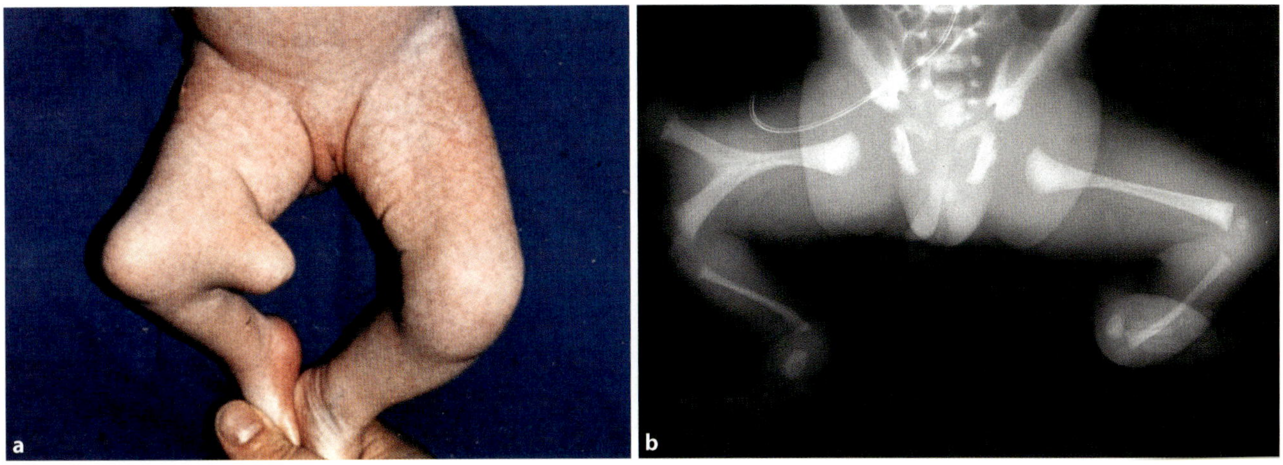

Fig. 70.1 **a** Newborn with bifurcation of femur on the right. **b** Radiograph of another individual showing Y-shaped femur on the right and bilaterally absent tibias

S. Mundlos, D. Horn, *Limb Malformations*,
DOI 10.1007/978-3-540-95928-1_70, © Springer-Verlag Berlin Heidelberg 2014

71 Sirenomelia

Major Clinical Findings

Sirenomelia describes an anomaly in which the lower limbs are replaced by a single midline limb. Several types and degrees of severity have been described: fusion of limbs with thigh and leg bones present, absent or fused fibulae, partial or complete fusion of the femurs and/or tibias, or, as the most severe manifestation, replacement of the limbs by a single femur. About a third of cases show upper limb anomalies, most commonly radial ray defects. Half of the cases with sirenomelia also present with genital, large bowel, and urinary defects. Approximately 60 % show sacral or sacrococcygeal absence. Anal atresia is the most common abnormality, present in approximately 90 % of cases. Less frequent anomalies include cardiac defects, abnormalities of the central nervous system, esophageal atresia/fistula, single or anomalous umbilical artery, and abdominal wall defects. There is a greater than expected association of sirenomelia with other very rare defects such as bladder exstrophy, cyclopia/holoprosencephaly, and acardia–acephaly. Except for very rare instances, sirenomelia is a lethal condition.

Genetic Transmission

Sporadic. There is an increase in the incidence of sirenomelia in monozygotic twins over that in singletons and dizygotic twins. Recurrence in siblings has been reported.

Molecular Pathology

It is debated whether sirenomelia is a severe form of caudal regression syndrome. But in contrast to caudal regression syndrome, sirenomelia appears not to be associated with maternal diabetes. Known teratogenic substances such as cadmium and retinoic acid (in mice), as well as the vasoconstrictive effect of cocaine, have been implicated as possible environmental agents. A "vascular steal" effect has been postulated via abnormal vitelline arteries that might cause reduced blood flow to the caudal end of the embryo, resulting in an aberrant formation of the lower extremities.

References

Gabriele T, Gianpaolo G (2013) Sirenomelia: a review on embryonic and environmental theories, novel three-dimensional ultrasound imaging and first trimester diagnosis in a case of mosaic 69,XXX/46XX fetus. Arch Gynecol Obest 288:3–11

Orioli IM, Amar E, Arteaga-Vazquez J, Bakker MK, Bianca S, Botto LD et al (2011) Sirenomelia: an epidemiologic study in a large dataset from the International Clearinghouse of Birth Defects Surveillance and Research, and literature review. Am J Med Genet C Semin Med Genet 157C(4):358–373

Stevenson RE, Jones KL, Phelan MC, Jones MC, Barr M Jr, Clericuzio C et al (1986) Vascular steal: the pathogenetic mechanism producing sirenomelia and associated defects of the viscera and soft tissues. Pediatrics 78(3):451–457

S. Mundlos, D. Horn, *Limb Malformations*,
DOI 10.1007/978-3-540-95928-1_71, © Springer-Verlag Berlin Heidelberg 2014

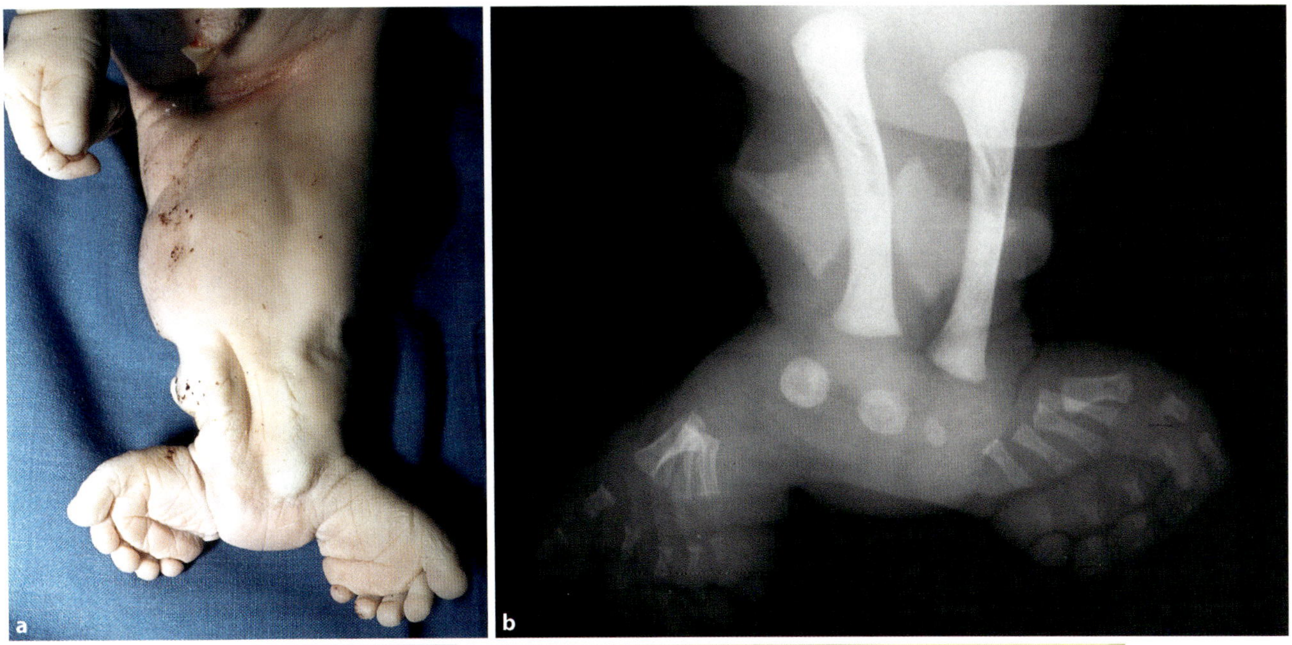
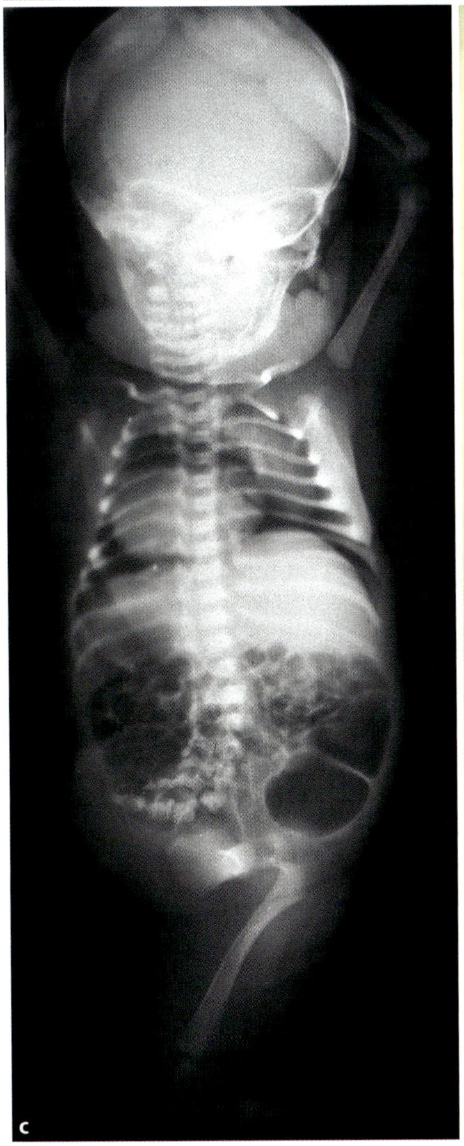
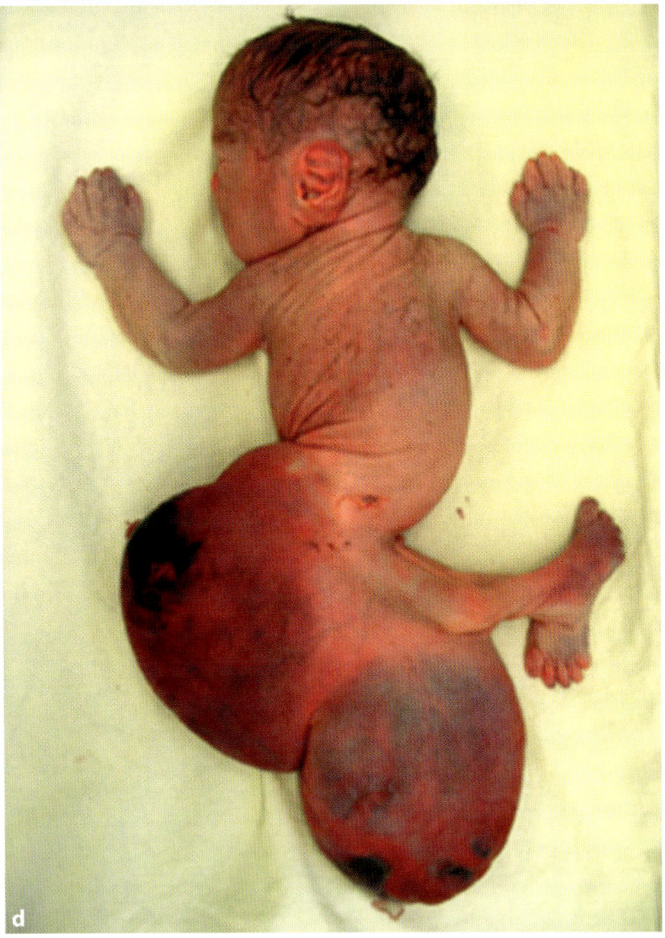

Fig. 71.1 **a** Newborn with sirenomelia. Fusion of the lower limb with separate feet. **b** Corresponding radiograph shows two tubular bones and two triangular bones. There is fusion of dorsal elements of the feet. **c** Sirenomelia with complete fusion of the lower limb to one bone and highly abnormal spine/pelvis. **d** Sirenomelia associated with/due to large teratocarcinoma

Part XII

Reduction Anomalies: Unilateral

72 Poland Syndrome

MIM 173800

Synonyms
Poland syndactyly
Poland anomaly
Poland sequence

Major Clinical Findings
Poland syndrome is defined as unilateral hand anomalies together with the ipsilateral absence or hypoplasia of the pectoralis muscle and breast. The digit phenotype includes various degrees of symbrachydactyly. The middle phalanges can be hypoplastic or absent, resulting in only one interphalangeal joint. Syndactyly is usually incomplete but may involve all fingers and frequently includes the thumb. Digits II–IV are the most severely affected, and in some cases this may include the metacarpals, resulting in an ectrodactyly-like phenotype. In those cases that extend more proximally, absence, fusion, or size reduction of the carpal bones can be observed. Most frequently the sternocostal portion of the pectoralis major muscle is involved, but the serratus anterior and latissimus dorsi as well as other muscles of the shoulder girdle may be affected. Other abnormalities of the chest include hypoplasia of subcutaneous tissue, absence of costal cartilages or ribs II–V, and deformed sternum. The nipple of the affected side may be small, displaced, or absent. In females, the breasts can be small or even absent. The chest wall defect is often associated with a lung hernia. Other skeletal anomalies include hemivertebrae, fused ribs, hypoplasia of the clavicle, and Sprengel anomaly. All features are unilateral and occur on the right side more often (75 % of cases). The condition is three times more common in males.

Occasional Findings
Poland syndrome can be associated with Moebius syndrome. In left-sided Poland syndrome, dextrocardia may occur. Triphalangeal thumb may be present.

Genetic Transmission
Commonly sporadic, but pedigrees with autosomal dominant inheritance pattern have been described.

Differential Diagnosis
Unilaterality and a Poland-like phenotype may occur in split-hand/foot malformation. Terminal transverse defects have overlapping features and may be part of Poland spectrum. Other genetic distal limb reduction defects are bilateral.

References

Fuhrmann W, Mosseler U, Neuss H (1971) Zur Klinik und Genetik des Poland-Syndroms. Dtsch Med Wschr 96:1076–1078

Ireland DCR, Takayama N, Flatt AE (1976) Poland's syndrome: a review of forty-three cases. J Bone Joint Surg Am 58:52–58

Konig R, Lenz W (1983) Pektoralis-Handdefekte (Poland-Syndaktylia). Z Orthop 121:244–253

Urschel HC Jr. (2009) Poland syndrome. Semin Thorac Cardiovasc Surg 21(1):89–94

S. Mundlos, D. Horn, *Limb Malformations*,
DOI 10.1007/978-3-540-95928-1_72,

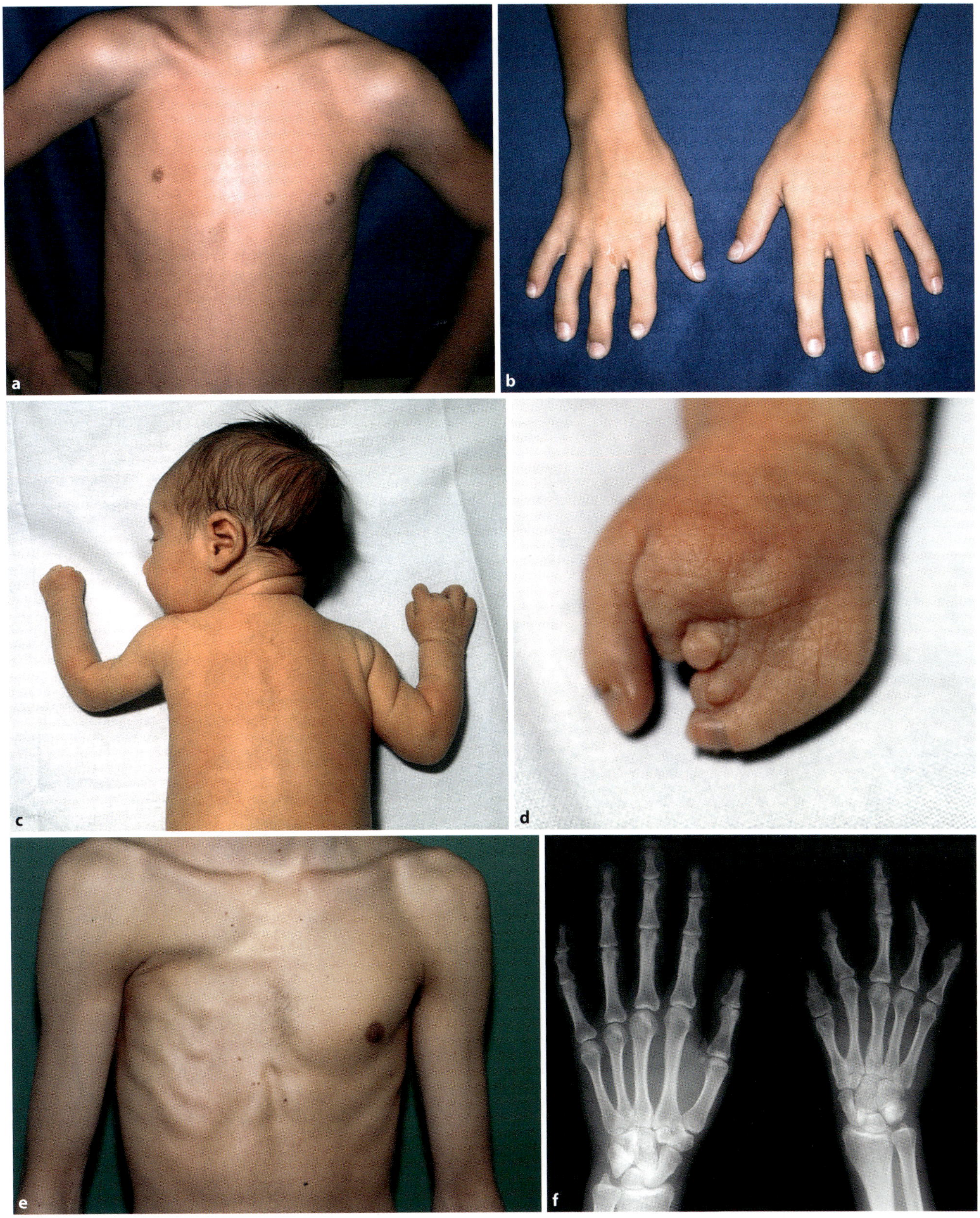

Fig. 72.1 **a** Hypoplastic pectoral musculature on the right. **b** The right hand is smaller; symbrachydactyly after surgical correction on the right. **c** Newborn with left sided Poland anomaly and symbrachydactyly. **d** Note rudimentary digits II–V and normal thumb. **e** Aplasia of the right pectoralis musculature and nipple. **f** Anteroposterior radiograph of both hands showing generalized smaller bones of the right hand; unilateral absent middle phalanges II, IV, and V; broad middle and distal phalanx of the thumb; and thin, elongated 1st metacarpal

73 Terminal Transverse Defect

MIM 102650

Synonyms
Adactylia, unilateral

Major Clinical Findings
Terminal transverse defects are characterized by the unilateral absence of the terminal portions of the digits or the entire hand, with tiny digit/nail remnants on the stump. The other hand and both feet are clinically and radiologically normal.

Genetic Transmission
The condition is considered sporadic, but pedigrees with autosomal dominant inheritance pattern have been described.

Differential Diagnosis
Poland syndrome must be considered. However, the severity of the reduction defects, the occurrence of digit remnants, and the absence of pectoral abnormalities distinguishes the two conditions.

References

Graham JM Jr, Brown FE, Struckmeyer CL, Hallowell C (1986) Dominantly inherited unilateral terminal transverse defects of the hand (adactylia) in twin sisters and one daughter. Pediatrics 78(1):103–106

Neumann L, Pelz J, Kunze J (1998) Unilateral terminal aphalangia in father and daughter—exogenous or genetic cause? Am J Med Genet 78(4):366–370

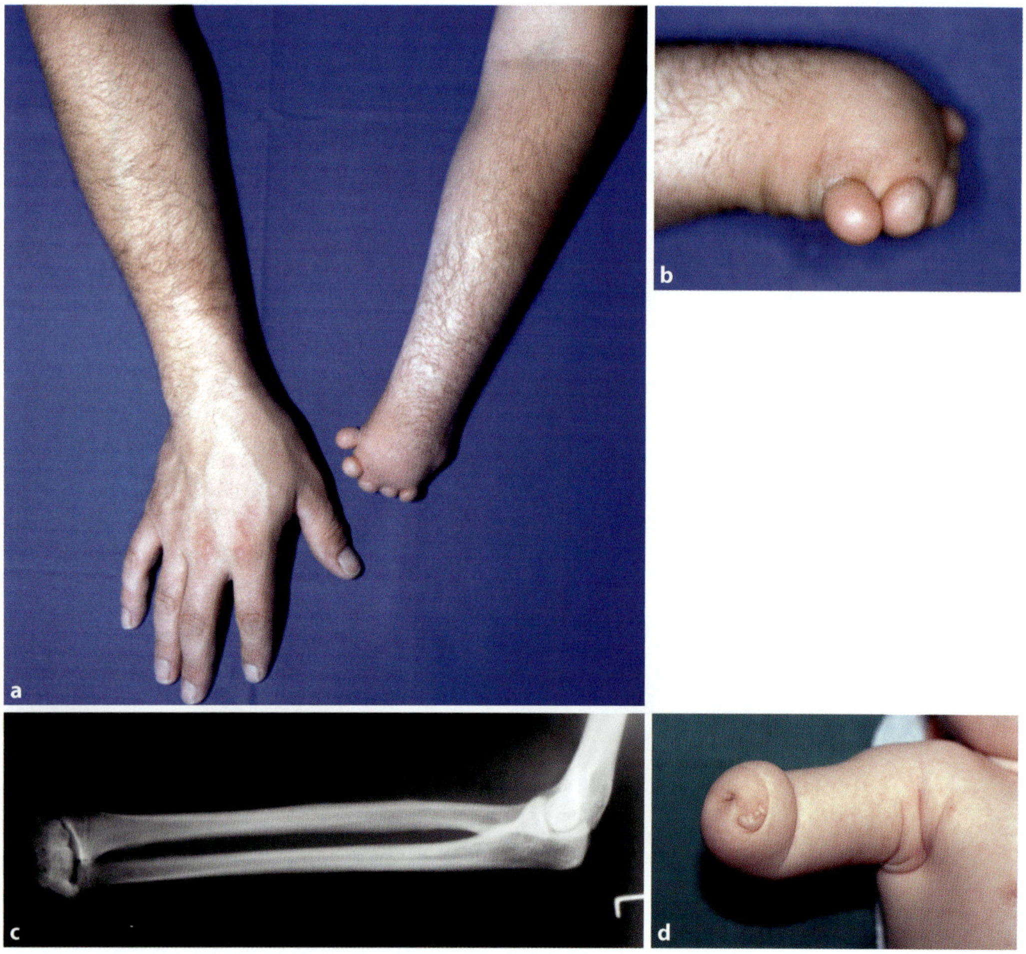

Fig. 73.1 **a** Unilateral loss of distal structures at the level of the wrist. **b** Rudimentary knoblike digits. **c** Corresponding anteroposterior elbow-to-wrist radiograph reveals relatively normal structures to the carpal region, ending in a conglomerate of bones. **d** Terminal transverse defect with knoblike digits

S. Mundlos, D. Horn, *Limb Malformations*,
DOI 10.1007/978-3-540-95928-1_73, © Springer-Verlag Berlin Heidelberg 2014

Part XIII

Reduction Anomalies: Radial Ray

74 Thrombocytopenia-Absent Radius Syndrome

MIM 274000

Synonyms

TAR syndrome

Major Clinical Findings

Typical clinical features of thrombocytopenia-absent radius (TAR) syndrome are bilateral absence or hypoplasia of the radius in the presence of both thumbs and a reduction in the number of platelets (thrombocytopenia; <50 platelets/nl). Additional skeletal features include shortening and, less commonly, aplasia of the ulna and/or humerus. In the latter situation, the five-fingered hand arises from the shoulder. The hands may show limited extension of the fingers and radial deviation. There may be hypoplasia of the carpal and phalangeal bones. The musculature of the hands, arms, and shoulders can be hypoplastic. The lower limbs are frequently involved (~50 %) but to a lesser extent than the upper limbs. Dislocation of the hips and subluxation of the knees resulting in coxa vara are common. Extraskeletal manifestations comprise cardiac abnormalities, such as tetralogy of Fallot and atrial and ventricular septal defects (15–25 %), and abnormalities of the genitourinary tract (renal anomalies and agenesis of the uterus, cervix, and upper part of the vagina). Craniofacial features include brachycephaly, micrognathia, strabismus, ptosis, and a small, upturned nose. Cow's milk allergy or intolerance appears to be relatively common among patients with TAR syndrome and may provoke eosinophilia.

Patients with TAR syndrome typically present with petechiae and severe bleeding during the first years of life. Platelet counts are often <50/nl (normal range 150–400/nl) due to impaired presence or maturation of megakaryocytic progenitors in the bone marrow. Although platelet counts ameliorate over time, patients remain thrombocytopenic with continued risk of bleeding. In addition, young patients with TAR syndrome have been reported to have leukemoid reactions with white blood counts exceeding 35,000 cells/mm^3. Similar to the thrombocytopenia, these reactions are transient in nature and are not associated with true leukemia.

Treatment

Treatment consists of platelet transfusion for thrombocytopenia as needed. Other measures are generally not indicated, given the transient nature of the thrombocytopenia. Orthopedic intervention is provided as needed to maximize limb function. Affected individuals may avoid cow's milk.

Genetic Transmission and Recurrence Risk

Autosomal recessive. TAR syndrome follows an unusual inheritance pattern as the recurrence risk has been shown to be less than 25 %. This is because TAR syndrome is caused by compound heterozygosity for a null allele (a common microdeletion) and a hypomorphic allele (a single nucleotide polymorphism [SNP] in the *RBM8A* gene), and because the 200-kb minimally deleted region occurs as a de novo event in a substantial proportion (25 %) of cases. The presence of compound heterozygosity explains why consanguinity of the parents is rare in TAR syndrome. Furthermore, the relatively high frequency of the pathogenic SNP (approximately 3.5 %) accounts for the observed parent-to-child transmission that is otherwise rare in recessive conditions. Likewise, affected 2nd-degree and 3rd-degree relatives with no manifestation in between account for the same mechanism.

Differential Diagnosis

Other conditions with radial ray hypoplasia should be considered. Holt–Oram syndrome, Roberts syndrome, Okihiro syndrome, VACTERL association (vertebral defects, anal atresia, cardiac defects, tracheoesophageal fistula, renal anomalies, and limb abnormalities), and Fanconi anemia also feature hypoplasia of the radial ray, but in these conditions the thumb is usually absent or severely hypoplastic, and thrombocytopenia is not a feature. However, Fanconi disease pancytopenia may be present, and because of the dramatic consequences the diagnosis must be considered in all unclear cases. Thalidomide embryopathy may show overlapping features, particularly in severe cases. No other phenotypes are known to be associated with the 200-kb minimally deleted region at 1q21.1. However, recurrent deletion or duplication of nearby DNA segments at 1q21.1 gives rise to the variable phenotypes associated with 1q21.1 deletion/duplication, and occasionally these rearrangements may extend into the 200-kb minimally deleted TAR region.

Molecular Pathology

TAR syndrome is associated with a common microdeletion (chr1:144.1–144.3 Mb) that encompasses 200 kb and 11 genes on chromosome 1q21.1. The deletion is present in the great majority of patients. It is inherited from one of the unaffected parents in most cases but occurs de novo in approximately 25 %. This finding led to the hypothesis that other factors are needed to generate TAR syndrome. Two SNPs located on

S. Mundlos, D. Horn, *Limb Malformations*,
DOI 10.1007/978-3-540-95928-1_74, © Springer-Verlag Berlin Heidelberg 2014

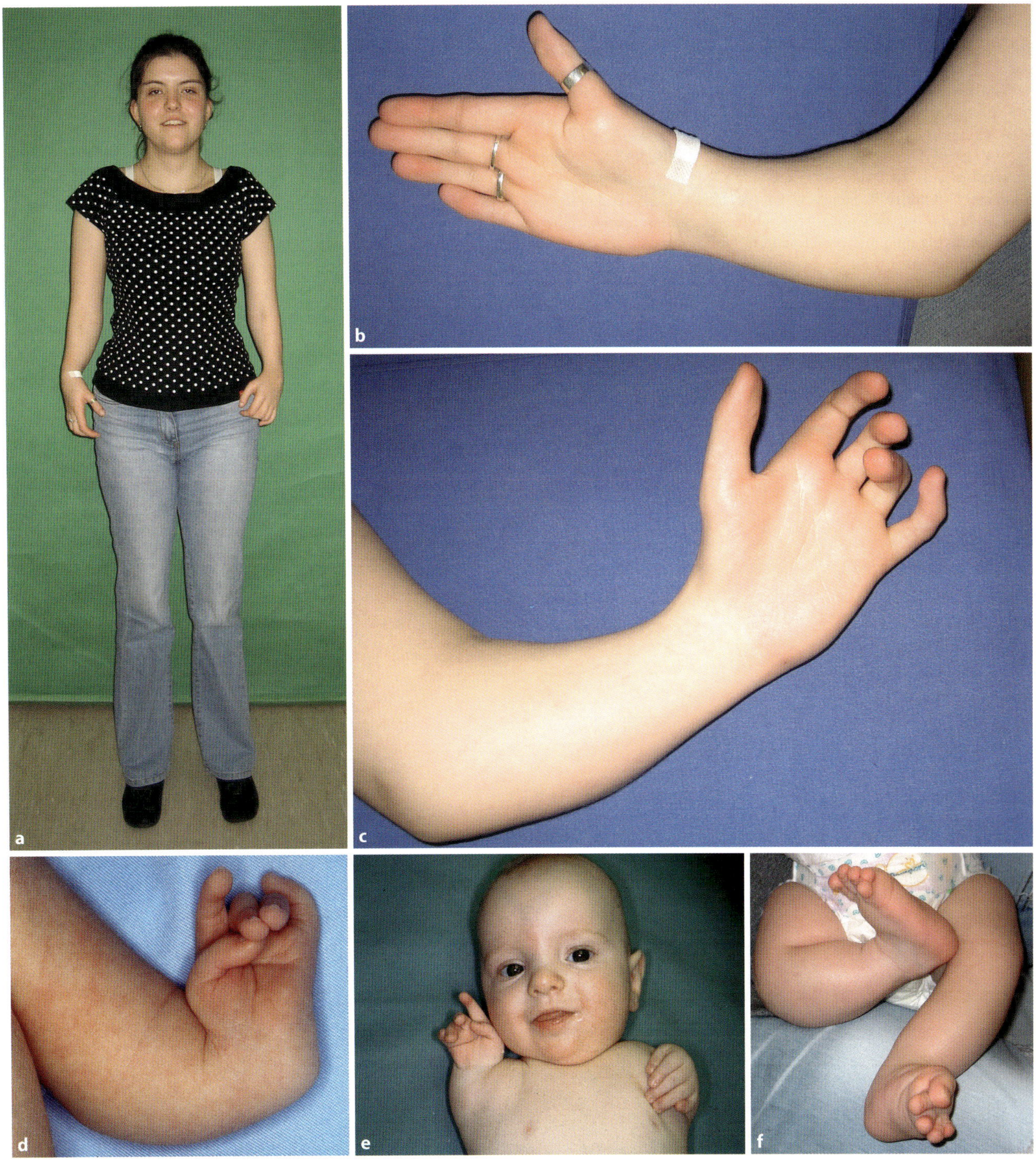

Fig. 74.1 **a** Individual with TAR syndrome and radial hypoplasia. **b** Palmar view of the right arm. Note radial deviation of the hand, normal thumb, and short forearm. **c** Left arm. Note contracture of the digits and hypoplastic musculature of the arm/palm. **d** TAR syndrome in a newborn. Very short forearm, radial deviation of the hand, normal thumb. **e** Severe TAR phenotype with phocomelia of the upper limbs. **f** TAR phenotype in the lower limbs. Tibial torsion on the right and subluxation of the knee joint. (**a, e** from Klopocki et al. 2007)

the other allele in the regulatory regions of the RBM8A gene have been identified as causative. Thus, in the vast majority of cases, compound inheritance of a rare null allele (the deletion) and one of two low-frequency noncoding SNPs with a frequency of 3.05% and 0.42%, respectively, cause TAR syndrome. In rare cases without deletion, coding mutation in RBM8A can be detected instead. Together, the mutations result in diminished RBM8A transcription. RBM8A encodes for Y14, a subunit of the exon junction complex with a conserved RNA-binding motif. The protein is preferentially associated with mRNAs produced by splicing, including both nuclear mRNAs and newly exported cytoplasmic mRNAs.

References

Albers CA, Paul DS, Schulze H, Freson K, Stephens JC, Smethurst PA et al (2012) Compound inheritance of a low-frequency regulatory SNP and a rare null mutation in exon-junction complex subunit RBM8A causes TAR syndrome. Nat Genet 44(4):435–439 (1–2)

Hall JG, Levin J, Kuhn JP, Ottenheimer EJ, van Berkum KA, McKusick VA (1969) Thrombocytopenia with absent radius (TAR). Medicine (Baltimore) 48(6):411–439

Klopocki E, Schulze H, Strauss G, Ott CE, Hall J, Trotier F et al (2007) Complex inheritance pattern resembling autosomal recessive inheritance involving a microdeletion in thrombocytopenia-absent radius syndrome. Am J Hum Genet 80(2):232–240

Fanconi Anemia

MIM 227650

75

Synonyms
Fanconi pancytopenia syndrome

Major Clinical Findings
Fanconi anemia is a clinically heterogeneous disorder mainly characterized by progressive bone marrow failure, predisposition to cancer, and a broad range of congenital anomalies. In about 50% of patients, upper limb anomalies are present that typically present as defects of the radial ray, ranging from bilateral aplasia of the thumbs and radii to a unilateral hypoplastic or bifid thumb. Prenatal and postnatal growth retardation, abnormalities of the kidneys, and congenital malformations of the heart are other findings. In addition, patients show cutaneous abnormalities (brownish pigmentation) and a typical facial appearance with microphthalmia or small eyes, ptosis, and microcephaly. About a third of patients exhibit only hematologic manifestations without congenital malformations.

Occasional Findings
A wide range of other abnormalities may be present, including cryptorchidism, abnormalities of the central nervous system, gastrointestinal anomalies, and diverse skeletal manifestations (congenital hip dislocation, scoliosis, rib anomalies).

Genetic Transmission
Autosomal recessive mode of inheritance in most cases. One type has X-linked recessive inheritance (*FANCB* gene).

Differential Diagnosis
Some cases show an overlapping phenotype with VACTERL association (vertebral defects, anal atresia, cardiac defects, tracheoesophageal fistula, renal anomalies, and limb abnormalities). Other syndromes with radial ray involvement, such as Holt–Oram syndrome, should be considered.

Molecular Pathology
Fanconi anemia results from a defect in DNA repair and consecutive genomic instability. This is reflected by the cellular phenotype showing a high frequency of chromosomal aberrations. Extensive genetic heterogeneity has been documented. More than 10 different Fanconi anemia complementation groups and corresponding genes (*FANCA-O*, for example) have been identified.

Clinical Management
Bone marrow failure and the risk of leukemic transformation are the major, life-threatening problems in Fanconi anemia. Allogeneic hematopoietic stem cell transplantation with a human leukocyte antigen (HLA)-identical sibling can successfully cure the disease. To minimize the adverse effects of blood transfusions, the possible toxicity of long-term, high-dose androgen therapy, and the risk of leukemic transformation, it has been suggested to transplant all patients as soon as pancytopenia develops.

References

Deakyne JS, Mazin AV (2011) Fanconi anemia: at the crossroads of DNA repair. Biochemistry 76:36–48

Grompe M, D'Andrea A (2001) Fanconi anemia and DNA repair. Hum Molec Genet 10:2253–2259

Joenje H, Levitus M, Waisfisz Q, D'Andrea A, Garcia-Higuera I, Pearson T et al (2000) Complementation analysis in Fanconi anemia: assignment of the reference FA-H patient to group A. Am J Hum Genet 67:759–762

S. Mundlos, D. Horn, *Limb Malformations*,
DOI 10.1007/978-3-540-95928-1_75, © Springer-Verlag Berlin Heidelberg 2014

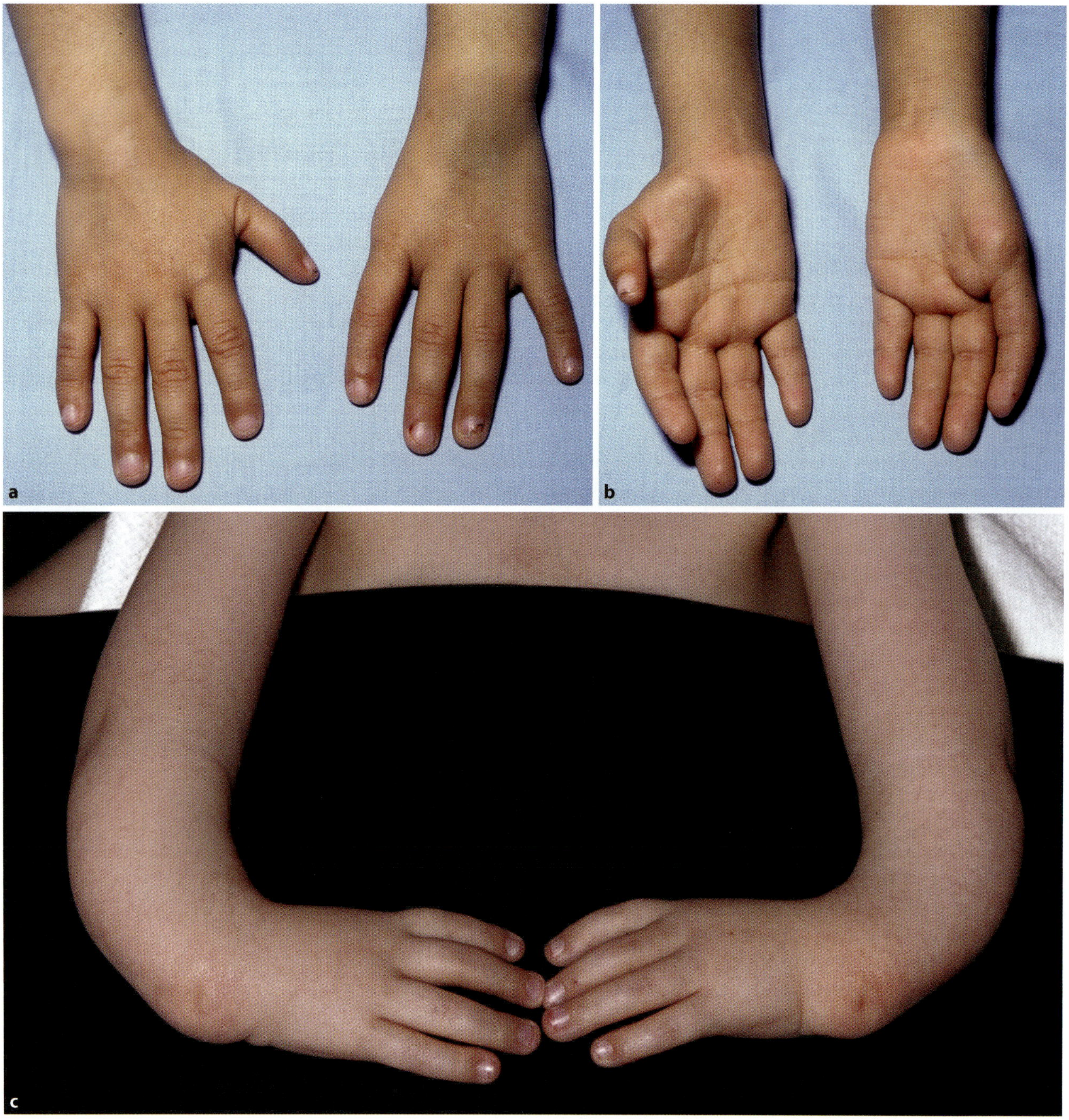

Fig. 75.1 **a, b** Dorsal and palmar views of hands, respectively. Absence of thumb on the left, inability to bend the thumb at the interphalangeal joint on the right. **c** Hypoplasia of radius with absent thumbs bilaterally

76 Holt–Oram Syndrome

MIM 142900

Synonyms
Heart–hand syndrome
Atriodigital dysplasia
Cardiomelic syndrome

Major Clinical Findings
Holt–Oram syndrome (HOS) is characterized by the combination of upper limb anomalies, in particular of the radial ray, and congenital heart defects. Abnormalities of the thumbs – aplasia, hypoplasia, or triphalangeal thumb – are the most common finding, often associated with hypoplastic thenar, limited supination of the forearm, or both. Other common findings are reduced digit length, clinodactyly of the 5th finger, and hypoplasia of individual fingers, most commonly involving the index and middle fingers. Hypoplasia of the radius occurs in approximately 50 %, and aplasia of the radius is present in approximately 25 %. Ulnar hypoplasia occurs only in individuals with radial defects. In the most severe cases, the defect extends up to the humerus, resulting in upper extremity phocomelia. Carpal bones may be abnormal, including bipartite scaphoid. Narrow, sloping shoulders are common, accompanied by mildly hypoplastic clavicles, hypoplasia/aplasia of the pectoralis major muscle, and pectus excavatum or carinatum. Limb defects are always bilateral and often asymmetrical, with the left side being more severely affected. Vertebral anomalies and thoracic scoliosis are further skeletal abnormalities.

Cardiac involvement is present in more than 90 % of cases, with secundum atrial septal defect and ventricular septal defect being the most common defects, but more complex cardiac defects such as hypoplastic left heart, total anomalous pulmonary venous return, and truncus arteriosus also occur in a substantial number of affected individuals. Cardiac conduction defects are often observed, resulting in atrioventricular block and/or atrial fibrillation. In some cases, only electrocardiographic abnormalities can be found. Antiarrhythmic medications and surgery may be necessary. Individuals with severe heart block may require pacemaker implantation.

Occasional Findings
Postaxial/central polydactyly, absence of fingers, agenesis of the lung.

Genetic Transmission
Autosomal dominant.

Differential Diagnosis
Other conditions with defects of the radial ray must be considered, including Okihiro syndrome, Fanconi anemia, Townes–Brooks syndrome, and TAR syndrome. None of these conditions shows consistent heart involvement, and in TAR syndrome the thumbs are always present. VACTERL syndrome may show overlapping features. Individuals with the mildest cases or with no upper limb malformations or congenital heart malformations may escape diagnosis. Late-onset cardiac abnormalities such as pulmonary hypertension, high-grade atrioventricular block, and atrial fibrillation should be considered.

Molecular Pathology
HOS is caused by loss of function mutations in *TBX5*, which encodes a transcription factor of the T-box family. Tbx5 is one of the few genes that is expressed in the upper limb only, hence the restriction of malformations. A closely related T-box gene, Tbx4, and a paired-like homeodomain factor, Pitx1, are both expressed in a reciprocal pattern in the developing hindlimb mesenchyme. Misexpression experiments in the chick have demonstrated that ectopic expression of Tbx5 in the leg bud is capable of transforming the hindlimb to a more forelimb character, indicating that Tbx5 plays a role in forelimb versus hindlimb specification. In the mouse, Tbx5 is required at early limb bud stages for forelimb bud development, as inactivation results in completely absent forelimbs but unaffected hindlimbs. Tbx5 specifically affects muscle and tendon patterning. Tbx5 associates with Nkx2–5 and synergistically promotes cardiomyocyte differentiation. Alpha-myosin heavy chain (MYH6), a structural protein expressed at high levels in the developing atria, is regulated by Tbx5. Mutations in MYH6 result in atrial septal defects.

There appears to be a phenotype–genotype correlation in that defects predicted to create null alleles are associated with abnormalities both in the heart and limb, whereas certain missense mutations produce significant cardiac malformations with only minor skeletal abnormalities, and vice versa. Structural data of Tbx5 suggest that organ-specific effects correlate with altered interactions with different target DNA sequences.

S. Mundlos, D. Horn, *Limb Malformations*,
DOI 10.1007/978-3-540-95928-1_76, © Springer-Verlag Berlin Heidelberg 2014

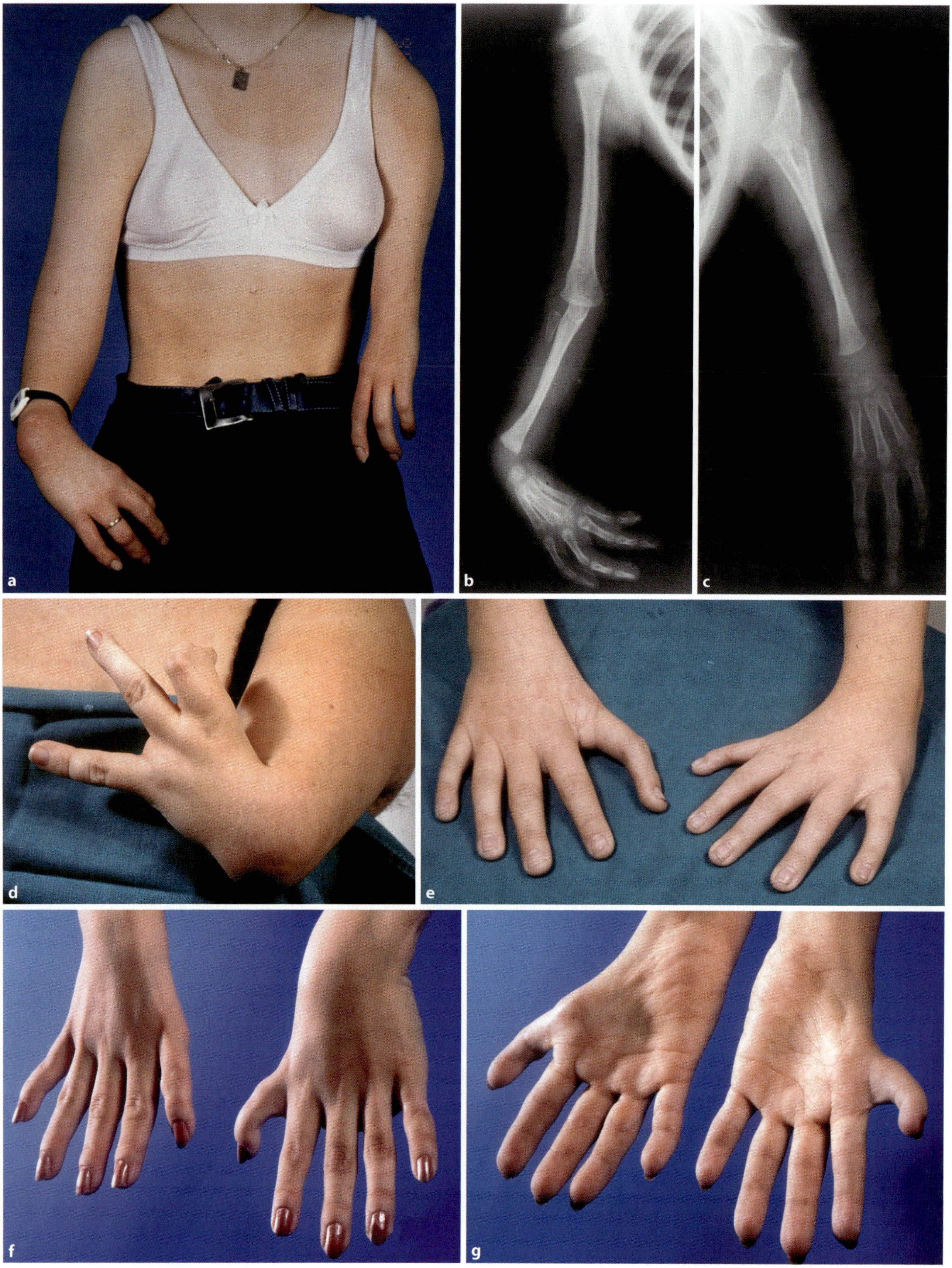
a
b
c
d
e
f
g

References

Basson CT, Huang T, Lin RC, Bachinsky DR, Weremowicz S, Vaglio A et al (1999) Different TBX5 interactions in heart and limb defined by Holt–Oram syndrome mutations. Proc Natl Acad Sci U S A 96(6):2919–2924

Bruneau BG, Nemer G, Schmitt JP, Charron F, Robitaille L, Caron S et al (2001) A murine model of Holt–Oram syndrome defines roles of the T-box transcription factor Tbx5 in cardiogenesis and disease. Cell 106(6):709–721

Kohlhase J, Schubert L, Liebers M, Rauch A, Becker K, Mohammed SN et al (2003) Mutations at the SALL4 locus on chromosome 20 result in a range of clinically overlapping phenotypes, including Okihiro syndrome, Holt–Oram syndrome, acro-renal-ocular syndrome, and patients previously reported to represent thalidomide embryopathy. J Med Genet 40(7):473–478

Li QY, Newbury-Ecob RA, Terrett JA, Wilson DI, Curtis AR, Yi CH et al (1997) Holt–Oram syndrome is caused by mutations in TBX5, a member of the Brachyury (T) gene family. Nat Genet 15(1):21–29

Newbury-Ecob RA, Leanage R, Raeburn JA, Young ID (1996) Holt–Oram syndrome: a clinical genetic study. J Med Genet 33(4):300–307

Rallis C, Bruneau BG, Del Buono J, Seidman CE, Seidman JG, Nissim S et al (2003) Tbx5 is required for forelimb bud formation and continued outgrowth. Development 130(12):2741–2751

Smith J (1997) Brachyury and the T-box genes. Curr Opin Genet Dev 7(4):474–480

Fig. 76.1 **a** Asymmetry with severe reduction on the left side. There are four fingers on the right but only three on the left side. **b, c** Corresponding radiographs. The right side (**b**) shows radial deviation of the hand with aplasia of thumb and a single large carpal bone (os centralis). The radius is virtually absent; only a very small portion is visible near the elbow. The left side (**c**) shows only three digits, proximal humeral deficiency, and relatively normal distal. The ulna is thin but proximally intact; the radius is either very hypoplastic or fused proximally to the ulna. **d** Severely affected individual with very short arm, radial deviation of the hand, and only three digits, one with contracture deformity. **e** Triphalangeal thumb on the right and a small, rudimentary thumb on the left. **f, g** Dorsal and palmar views, respectively, showing small, digit-like thumbs with contractures on the left side. Note hypoplasia of the thenar eminence

77 Okihiro Syndrome

MIM 607323

Synonyms
Duane radial ray syndrome
Duane anomaly with radial ray abnormalities and deafness
Acrorenoocular syndrome

Major Clinical Findings
Okihiro syndrome is characterized by upper limb anomalies, in particular radial ray deficiencies, ocular anomalies, and, in some cases, renal anomalies. Radial malformations are present in the great majority of affected individuals, are highly variable, and may include hypoplasia of the thenar musculature, triphalangeal thumb, absence of the thumb and 1st metacarpal, and, in more severe cases, hypoplastic/absent radius, hypoplastic humerus, and hypoplastic ulna. Preaxial polydactyly, syndactyly, and radial deviation of the hands may be present. The musculature of the shoulder girdle may be involved, including pectoralis hypoplasia and other upper limb muscle hypoplasia. The ocular phenotype includes a wide range of anomalies including optic disc hypoplasia/dysplasia, retinal coloboma, iris coloboma, and Duane anomaly (unilateral or bilateral limitation of abduction of the eye associated with retraction of the globe and narrowing of the palpebral fissure on adduction, caused by aberrant innervation of the extraocular muscles by axons of brainstem motor neurons; undiagnosed in children, it can lead to amblyopia). External ear malformations, sensorineural deafness, and slitlike openings of the exterior auditory meatus are further features. Renal anomalies are less common but may feature a wide range of anomalies including renal hypoplasia, agenesis, dystopic kidney, horseshoe kidney, hydronephrosis, and vesicoureteric reflux.

Occasional Findings
Gastrointestinal anomalies such as imperforate anus. Choanal stenosis/atresia, fused cervical vertebrae, scoliosis. Congenital defects of the heart.

Genetic Transmission
Autosomal dominant.

Differential Diagnosis
Holt–Oram syndrome, caused by mutation in the *TBX5* gene, shows similar anomalies of the upper limb but can be differentiated from Okihiro syndrome by the absence of ocular and renal anomalies and the presence of severe congenital heart defects. Other conditions with radial ray defect have to be considered, including Fanconi anemia, TAR syndrome, and Townes–Brooks syndrome. Overlap with thalidomide embryopathy has been reported. Other forms of Duane retraction syndrome should be considered.

Molecular Pathology
Okihiro syndrome is caused by mutation in SALL4, a zinc finger transcription factor. Sall4 has been shown to act together with Tbx5 in a positive and negative feed-forward circuit during embryonic development of the limb and heart. Their close functional relationship correlates well with the similarities in associated phenotypes.

References

Al-Baradie R, Yamada K, St Hilaire C, Chan W-M, Andrews C, McIntosh N et al (2002) Duane radial ray syndrome (Okihiro syndrome) maps to 20q13 and results from mutations in SALL4, a new member of the SAL family. Am J Hum Genet 71:1195–1199

Kohlhase J, Heinrich M, Schubert L, Liebers M, Kispert A, Laccone F et al (2002) Okihiro syndrome is caused by SALL4 mutations. Hum Mol Genet 11(23):2979–2987

Kohlhase J, Schubert L, Liebers M, Rauch A, Becker K, Mohammed SN et al (2003) Mutations at the SALL4 locus on chromosome 20 result in a range of clinically overlapping phenotypes, including Okihiro syndrome, Holt–Oram syndrome, acro-renal-ocular syndrome, and patients previously reported to represent thalidomide embryopathy. J Med Genet 40(7):473–478

Koshiba-Takeuchi K, Takeuchi JK, Arruda EP, Kathiriya IS, Mo R, Hui CC et al (2006) Cooperative and antagonistic interactions between Sall4 and Tbx5 pattern the mouse limb and heart. Nat Genet 38(2):175–183

Fig. 77.1 **a–c** Radial ray deficiency bilaterally. **d–j** Mild Okihiro syndrome spectrum in family with SALL4 mutation. **d, e** Hypoplastic thumb with contracture bilaterally. **f** Corresponding radiograph shows hypoplastic, triphalangeal thumbs; long, thin metacarpals; navicular absence; and carpal fusions with contracture deformities bilaterally. **g, h** Finger-like triphalangeal thumb; note two flexion creases in thumb. **i** Feet of same individual showing duplication of the right hallux and small, laterally deviated toe on the left (hallux valgus). **j** Corresponding radiograph showing broad proximal phalanx and duplication of the distal phalanx of the hallux on the right, short and broad metatarsal I, and narrow proximal phalanx of the hallux on the left. (**d–j** Courtesy of Aleksander Jamsheer, Poznan University of Medical Sciences, Poland)

S. Mundlos, D. Horn, *Limb Malformations*,
DOI 10.1007/978-3-540-95928-1_77, © Springer-Verlag Berlin Heidelberg 2014

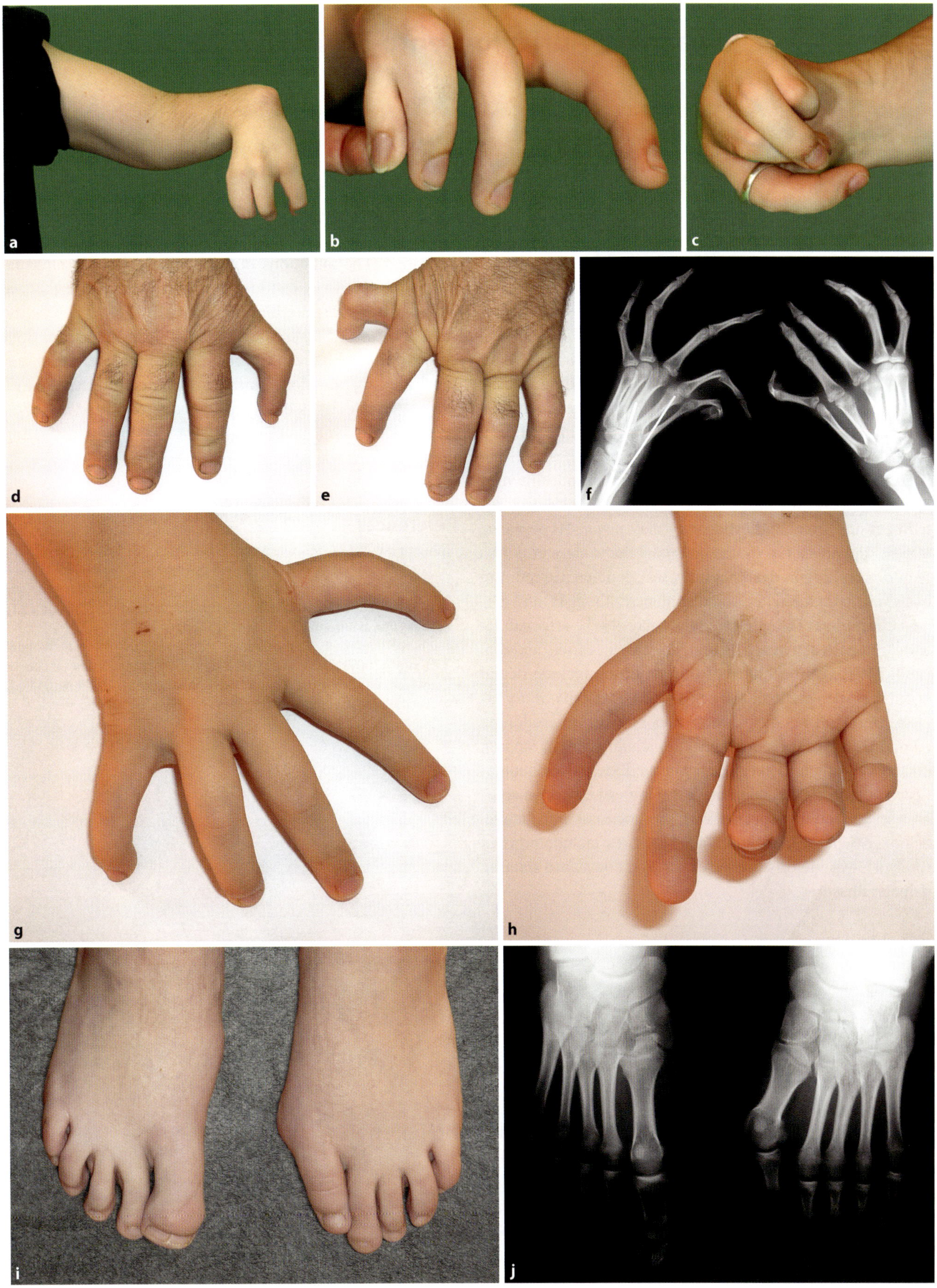
a
b
c
d
e
f
g
h
i
j

78 Lacrimo-Auriculo-Dento-Digital (LADD) Syndrome

MIM 149730

Synonyms

Levy–Hollister syndrome

Major Clinical Findings

Lacrimo-auriculo-dento-digital (LADD) syndrome is characterized by limb anomalies, abnormalities of the lacrimal ducts, malformed ears and deafness, and tooth abnormalities. Most frequent are malformed thumbs, including aplasia, hypoplasia, bifid, and triphalangeal thumb. Thenar muscle hypoplasia and synostosis of interphalangeal joints can be a minor manifestation. Syndactyly of fingers II/III and clinodactyly of fingers III–V are seen. The radius and ulna may be short. The lower limbs are less commonly affected, but halluces are broad and syndactyly may occur. Hypoplasia, atresia, and aplasia of the nasolacrimal ducts are a common feature, resulting in dacryocystitis, tear deficiency, recurrent or chronic conjunctivitis, keratoconjunctivitis sicca, and corneal ulcerations. The salivary glands may also be affected, resulting in poor saliva production, dry mouth, caries, and oral candidiasis. Other features of this condition include dental anomalies such as small and peg-shaped lateral maxillary incisors, mild enamel dysplasia, hypodontia, and microdontia. Abnormalities of the parotid glands, including absent Stensen duct or parotid gland aplasia, may occur. External ear anomalies including cup-shaped, small, and low-set ears are a common feature, often associated with sensorineural, conductive, or mixed-type hearing loss. Facial features include a broad forehead, hypertelorism, telecanthus, and downward slanting palpebral fissures.

Rare Findings

Radial-ulnar synostosis, renal agenesis, nephrosclerosis, hypospadias.

Genetic Transmission

Autosomal dominant.

Differential Diagnosis

Other conditions with hypoplastic, triphalangeal thumbs. LADD syndrome shows similarities to other ectodermal syndromes, including p63-associated conditions.

Molecular Pathology

LADD syndrome is caused by mutations in the fibroblast growth factor receptors (FGFRs) 1 or 2. The mutations are localized within the tyrosine kinase domain of the receptors. In addition, mutations in the FGFR ligand FGF10 have been identified. The mutations in the FGFRs appear to alter the configuration of key residues in the catalytic pocket that are essential for substrate binding and activation, whereas the mutations in FGF10 lead to impaired ligand function. Both types of mutations result in reduced functional activity and thus a loss of function. This is in contrast to other FGFR-associated mutations observed in chondrodysplasias or craniosynostosis syndromes that are associated with activating mutations.

References

Hollister DW, Klein SH, Dejager HJ, Lachman RS, Rimoin DL (1973) The lacrimo-auriculo-dento-digital syndrome. J Pediat 83:438–444

Rohmann E, Brunner HG, Kayserili H, Uyguner O, Nürnberg G, Lew ED et al (2006) Mutations in different components of FGF signaling in LADD syndrome. Nat Genet 38(4):414–417

Shams I, Rohmann E, Eswarakumar VP, Lew ED, Yuzawa S, Wollnik B et al (2007) Lacrimo-auriculo-dento-digital syndrome is caused by reduced activity of the fibroblast growth factor 10 (FGF10)-FGF receptor 2 signaling pathway. Mol Cell Biol 27(19):6903–6912

S. Mundlos, D. Horn, *Limb Malformations*,
DOI 10.1007/978-3-540-95928-1_78, © Springer-Verlag Berlin Heidelberg 2014

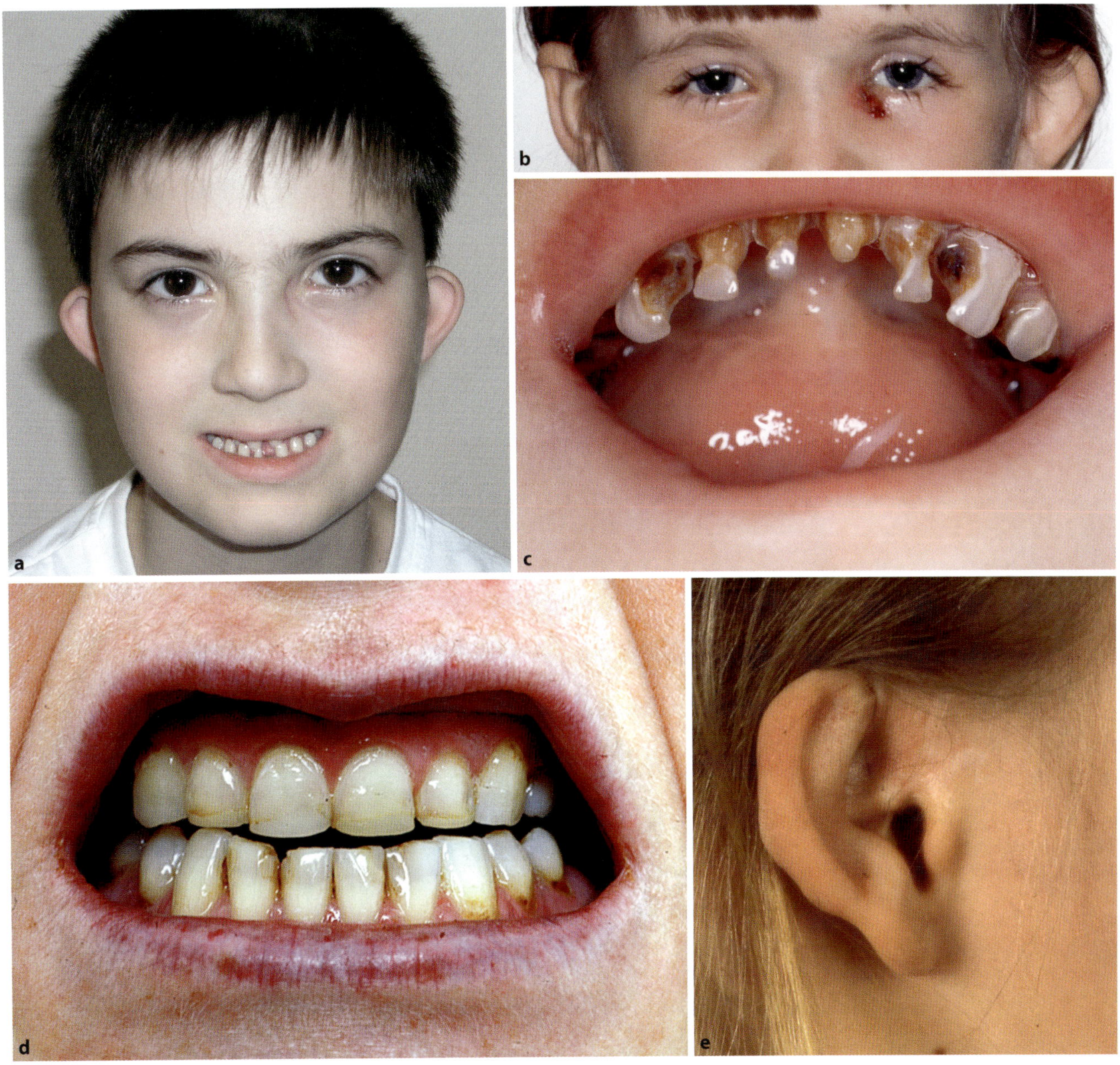

Fig. 78.1 **a** Facial features in LADD syndrome. Surgical correction of lacrimal duct aplasia, cup-shaped ears, microdontia. **b** Occlusion of lacrimal duct on the left by infection. **c** Dental caries. **d** Enamel abnormalities. **e** Abnormally shaped ear. (**a, c–e** Courtesy of Bernd Wollnik, University of Cologne, Germany)

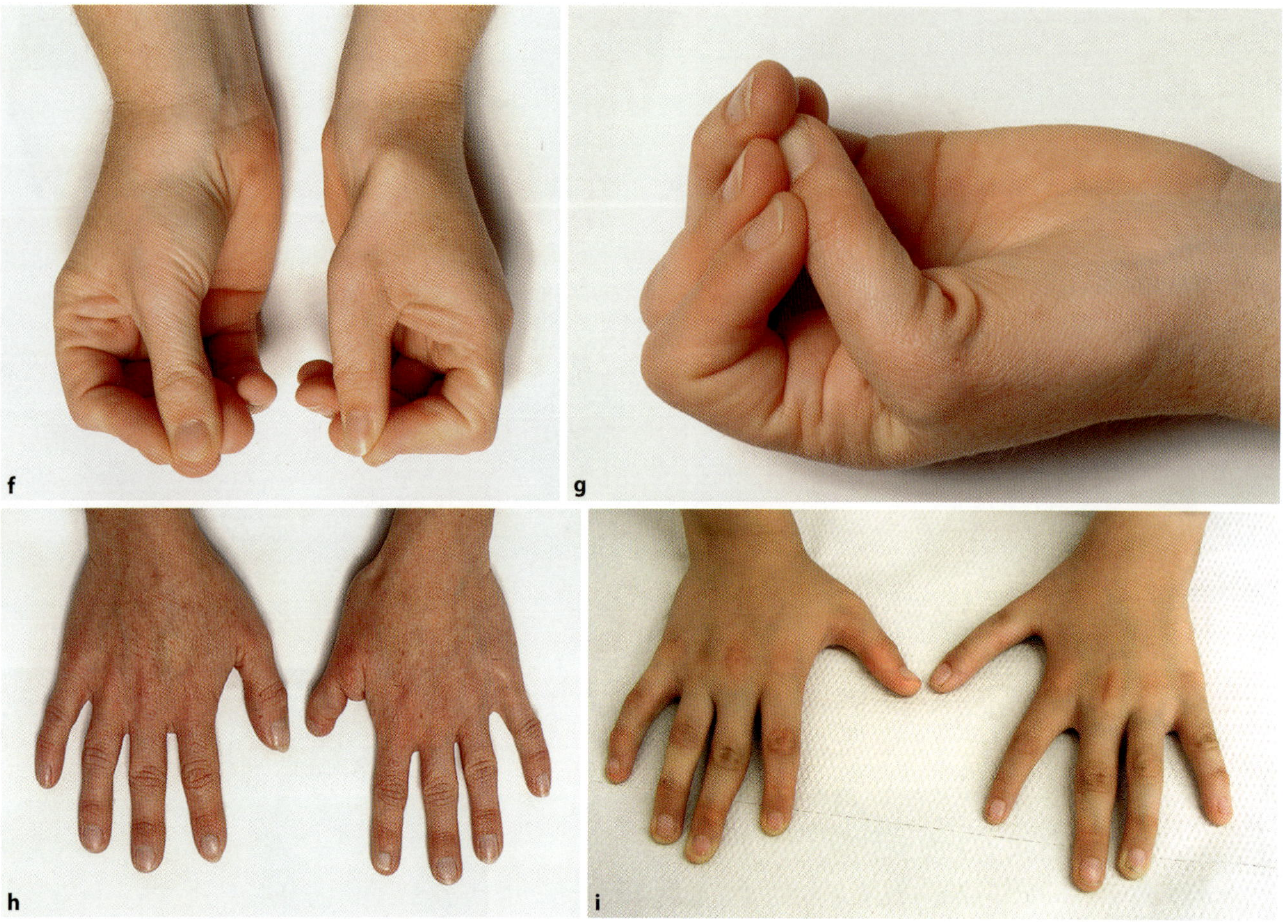

Fig. 78.1 (*continued*) **f** Thenar hypoplasia on the left. **g** Inability to bend thumb in interphalangeal joint. **h** Hypoplastic left thumb. **i** Triphalangeal, finger-like thumb and thin, hypoplastic digit II on the left. Abnormal ulnar deviation in proximal interphalangeal joint of digit III on the right. (**f–i** courtesy of A. Jamsheer, Poznan University of Medical Sciences, Poland)

79 Nager Syndrome

MIM 154400

Synonyms

Nager acrofacial dysostosis
Acrofacial dysostosis 1, Nager type

Major Clinical Findings

Nager syndrome is characterized by anomalies of the craniofacial skeleton and the distal upper limbs. The major facial signs are zygomatic and mandibular hypoplasia with downward slanting palpebral fissures, micrognathia, reduced number of eyelashes, lower eyelid coloboma, and ear malformations. Limb anomalies include radial ray defects, such as thumb hypoplasia and aplasia, triphalangeal thumbs, duplication of distal parts of the thumbs, hypoplasia of the radius, and radioulnar synostosis. The thumb anomalies are usually asymmetric.

Occasional Findings

Short stature, hip dislocation, laryngeal and epiglottal hypoplasia, genitourinary abnormalities.

Genetic Transmission

Most cases are autosomal dominant. Affected siblings have been reported, suggesting the possibility of autosomal recessive inheritance.

Differential Diagnosis

The presence of radial defects and the lack of lower limb involvement distinguishes Nager syndrome from Miller syndrome, another type of acrofacial dysostosis. The craniofacial aspect of Nager syndrome is similar to that of Treacher–Collins syndrome.

Molecular Pathology

Nager syndrome is caused by different heterozygous *SF3B4* mutations. The SF3B4 protein is a component of the pre-mRNA spliceosomal complex. Further genetic heterogeneity seems to be likely because SF3B4 mutations were only identified in two-thirds of a large cohort of patients with Nager syndrome.

References

Aylsworth AS, Lin AE, Friedman PA (1991) Nager acrofacial dysostosis: male-to-male transmission in 2 families. Am J Med Genet 41:83–88

Bernier FP, Caluseriu O, Ng S, Schwartzentruber J, Buckingham KJ, Innes AM et al (2012) Haploinsufficiency of SF3B4, a component of the pre-mRNA spliceosomal complex, causes Nager syndrome. Am J Hum Genet 90(5):925–933

Czeschik JC, Voigt C, Alanay Y, Albrecht B, Avci S, Fitzpatrick D et al (2013) Clinical and mutation data in 12 patients with the clinical diagnosis of Nager syndrome. Hum Genet 132(8):885–898

Wieczorek D (2013) Human facial dysostoses. Clin Genet 83(6):499–510

S. Mundlos, D. Horn, *Limb Malformations*,
DOI 10.1007/978-3-540-95928-1_79, © Springer-Verlag Berlin Heidelberg 2014

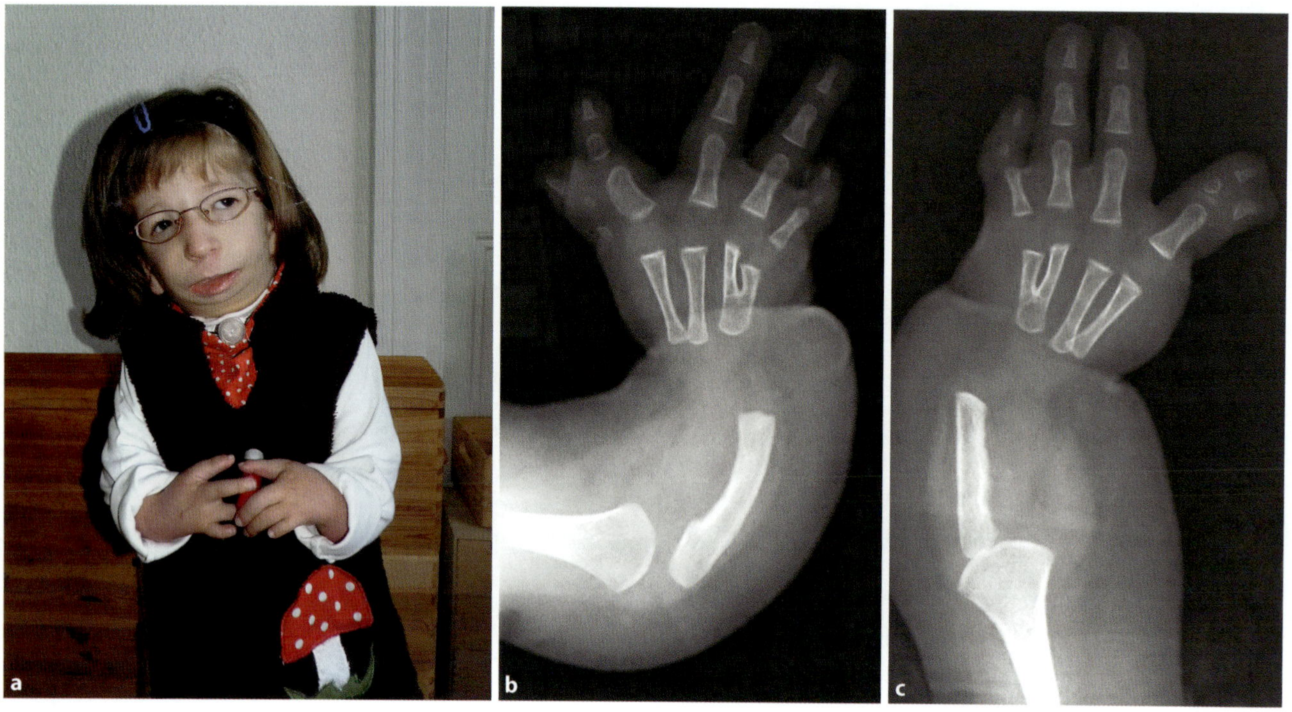

Fig. 79.1 **a** Nager syndrome. Note facial dysmorphism with downward slanting palpebral fissures, partial absence of the lower eyelashes, micrognathia, high nasal bridge, and abnormal ears. **b** Radiograph of right arm showing aplasia of the radius, distally truncated ulna, aplasia of metacarpal I, hypoplastic phalanges I, soft tissue syndactyly of fingers I/II, short and radially bowed metacarpal II, delta phalanx of 2nd proximal phalanx II, proximal fusion of metacarpals IV and V, and hypoplastic middle/distal phalanges V. **c** Radiograph of left arm showing aplasia of the radius, absence of metacarpal I and middle phalanx of thumb, duplication of the distal phalanx of digit II (likely to be associated rudimentary thumb), proximal fusion of metacarpals IV and V, and delta phalanx of middle phalanx II. (**a** from Wieczorek 2013; **b, c** courtesy of R. Habenicht, Wilhelmsstift, Hamburg)

Baller–Gerold Syndrome

MIM 218600

80

Synonyms

Craniosynostosis with radial defects
Craniosynostosis-radial aplasia syndrome

Major Clinical Findings

The main features of Baller–Gerold syndrome are craniosynostosis and radial ray deficiency. In addition to radial deficiency, absent/malformed thumbs, fused/absent carpal bones, absent metacarpals and phalanges, oligodactyly of the feet, and short, curved ulna can be present. A peculiar facial appearance with micrognathia, downward slanting palpebral fissures, and malformed, low-set, and posteriorly rotated ears is recognized. Craniosynostosis of the coronal, metopic, and lambdoid sutures results in turribrachycephaly. Skeletal anomalies of the spine and pelvis as well as general growth retardation are frequent. Anteriorly placed anus and imperforate anus with either perineal fistula or rectovaginal fistula are further features. Anomalies of the heart and urogenital system and mental and/or motor retardation have been noted in some patients.

Genetic Transmission

Autosomal recessive.

Differential Diagnosis

There is considerable clinical overlap with other conditions, including RAPADILINO syndrome, an autosomal recessive disorder characterized by short stature, radial ray defects, and infantile diarrhea, but no significant cancer risk. Other conditions with craniosynostosis and/or radial ray defects have to be considered.

Molecular Pathology

Baller–Gerold syndrome is caused by mutations in *RECQL4*. RECQL4 protein has a DNA strand-annealing activity, but in contrast to other RecQ helicases, RECQL4 does not possess DNA helicase activity. It is crucial for the initiation of DNA replication. Mutations in *RECQL4* also cause RAPADILINO syndrome and Rothmund–Thomson syndrome, a progeria condition with skin atrophy, telangiectasia, hyperpigmentation and hypopigmentation, congenital skeletal abnormalities, short stature, and increased risk of malignant disease.

References

Dietschy T, Shevelev I, Stagljar I (2007) The molecular role of the Rothmund–Thomson-, RAPADILINO- and Baller–Gerold-gene product, RECQL4: recent progress. Cell Mol Life Sci 64(7–8):796–802

Gripp KW, Stolle CA, Celle L, McDonald-McGinn DM, Whitaker LA, Zackai EH (1999) TWIST gene mutation in a patient with radial aplasia and craniosynostosis: further evidence for heterogeneity of Baller–Gerold syndrome. Am J Med Genet 82(2):170–176

Siitonen HA, Sotkasiira J, Biervliet M, Benmansour A, Capri Y, Cormier-Daire V et al (2009) The mutation spectrum in RECQL4 diseases. Eur J Hum Genet 17(2):151–158

Van Maldergem L, Siitonen HA, Jalkh N, Chouery E, De Roy M, Delague V et al (2006) Revisiting the craniosynostosis-radial ray hypoplasia association: Baller–Gerold syndrome caused by mutations in the RECQL4 gene. J Med Genet 43(2):148–152

Van Maldergem L, Verloes A, Lejeune L, Gillerot Y (1992) The Baller–Gerold syndrome. J Med Genet 29(4):266–268

S. Mundlos, D. Horn, *Limb Malformations*,
DOI 10.1007/978-3-540-95928-1_80, © Springer-Verlag Berlin Heidelberg 2014

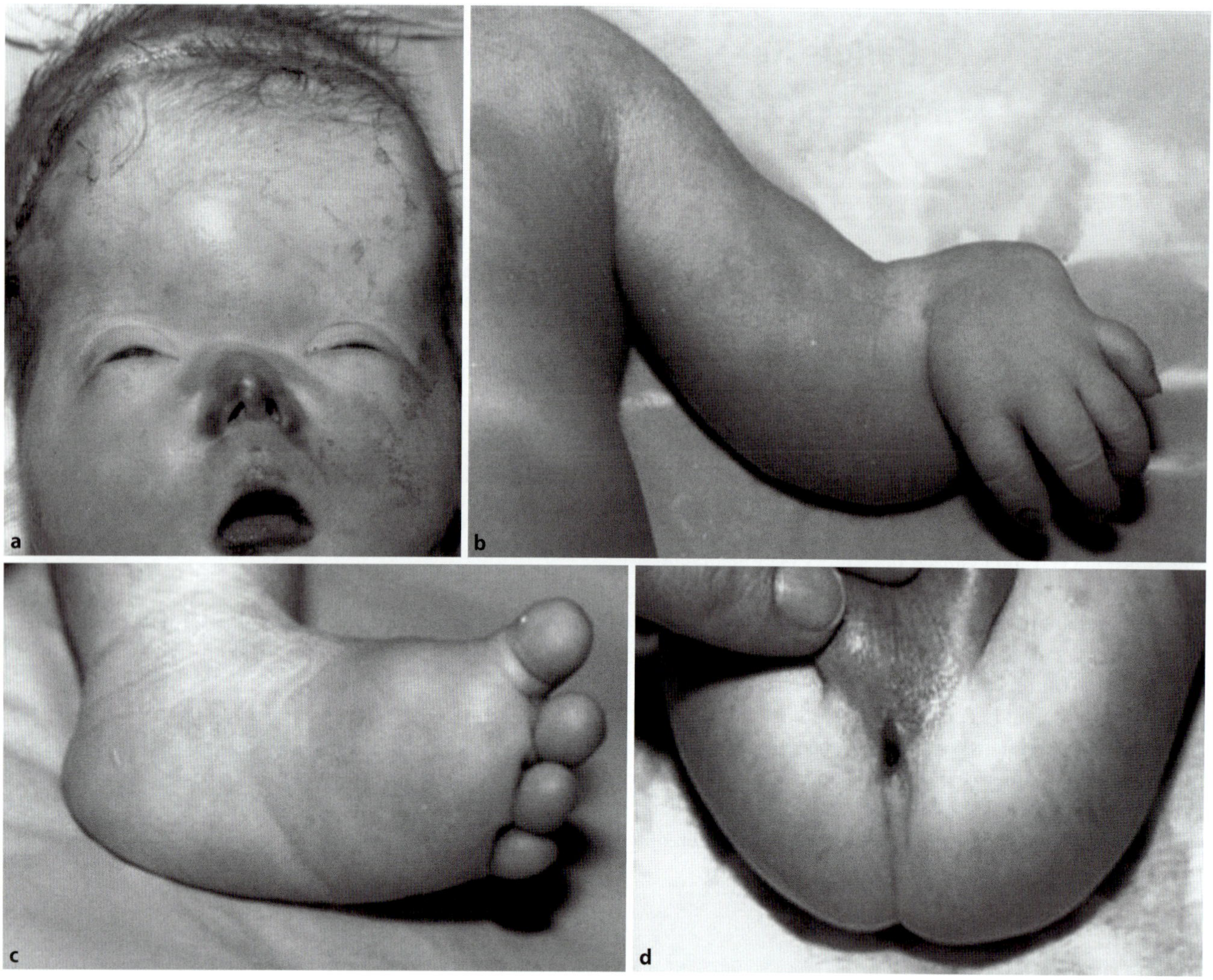

Fig. 80.1 **a** Fetus with Baller–Gerold syndrome. Note turricephalus with bulging forehead; wide-set eyes with small, downward slanting palpebral fissures; small, upturned nose; and micrognathia. **b** Upper limb with radial ray defect, absent thumb. **c** Foot with absence of the 5th ray. **d** Anteriorly placed anus. (Courtesy of Lionel van Maldergem, University de Franche-Comté, Besançon, France)

81 Richieri-Costa–Pereira Syndrome

MIM 268305

Synonyms
Robin sequence with cleft mandible and limb anomalies

Major Clinical Findings
Richieri-Costa–Pereira syndrome belongs to the group of acrofacial dysostoses syndromes. The facial phenotype is characterized by a midline cleft of the mandible, microstomia, micrognathia, cleft palate (Robin sequence), absence of the central lower incisors, and prominent, low-set ears. Radiographically, there is considerable variability in the mandibular involvement, ranging from abnormal fusion of the midline with a well-developed jaw to a wide gap at the mandibular symphysis with very little mandibular bone. The larynx may also be affected, resulting in airway obstruction due to an absent or abnormal epiglottis or aryepiglottic folds. Learning and language difficulties appear to be a common problem but are not present in all affected individuals. The most common abnormality of the limbs is hypoplastic and/or proximally placed thumbs, as well as hypoplasia of the radius. In contrast to other conditions with radial ray defects, the ulnar side is also affected, ranging from 5th-finger clinodactyly to hypoplasia of the 5th finger, metacarpal IV/V fusion, and hypoplasia of the ulna. Fusion of carpal bones is also seen. The lower limbs are commonly affected, including clubfeet, tibial deviation of the halluces, and small halluces. The tibia and fibula may be short, resulting in mesomelic limb shortening.

Genetic Transmission
Autosomal recessive.

Differential Diagnosis
The condition shows overlap with Nager syndrome.

Molecular Pathology
Richieri-Costa–Pereira syndrome is caused by a noncoding repeat expansion in the 5' untranslated region of *EIF4A3*. This region contains a polymorphic repeat that ranges from 3–12 repeats per allele in unaffected individuals to a repeat length of 15–16 in affected individuals. There appears to be a founder effect because all mutations detected so far have originated from a similar region in Brazil. *EIF4A3* encodes a DEAD box helicase that is involved in coordinating the downstream processes of mRNA splicing and nonsense-mediated decay.

References

Favaro FP, Alvizi L, Zechi-Ceide RM, Bertola D, Felix TM, de Souza J et al (2014) A noncoding expansion in EIF4A3 causes Richieri-Costa–Pereira syndrome, a craniofacial disorder associated with limb defects. Am J Hum Genet 94:120–128

Favaro FP, Zechi-Ceide RM, Alvarez CW, Maximino LP, Antunes LFBB, Richieri-Costa A et al (2011) Richieri-Costa–Pereira syndrome: a unique acrofacial dysostosis type: an overview of the Brazilian cases. Am J Med Genet 155A:322–331

S. Mundlos, D. Horn, *Limb Malformations*,
DOI 10.1007/978-3-540-95928-1_81, © Springer-Verlag Berlin Heidelberg 2014

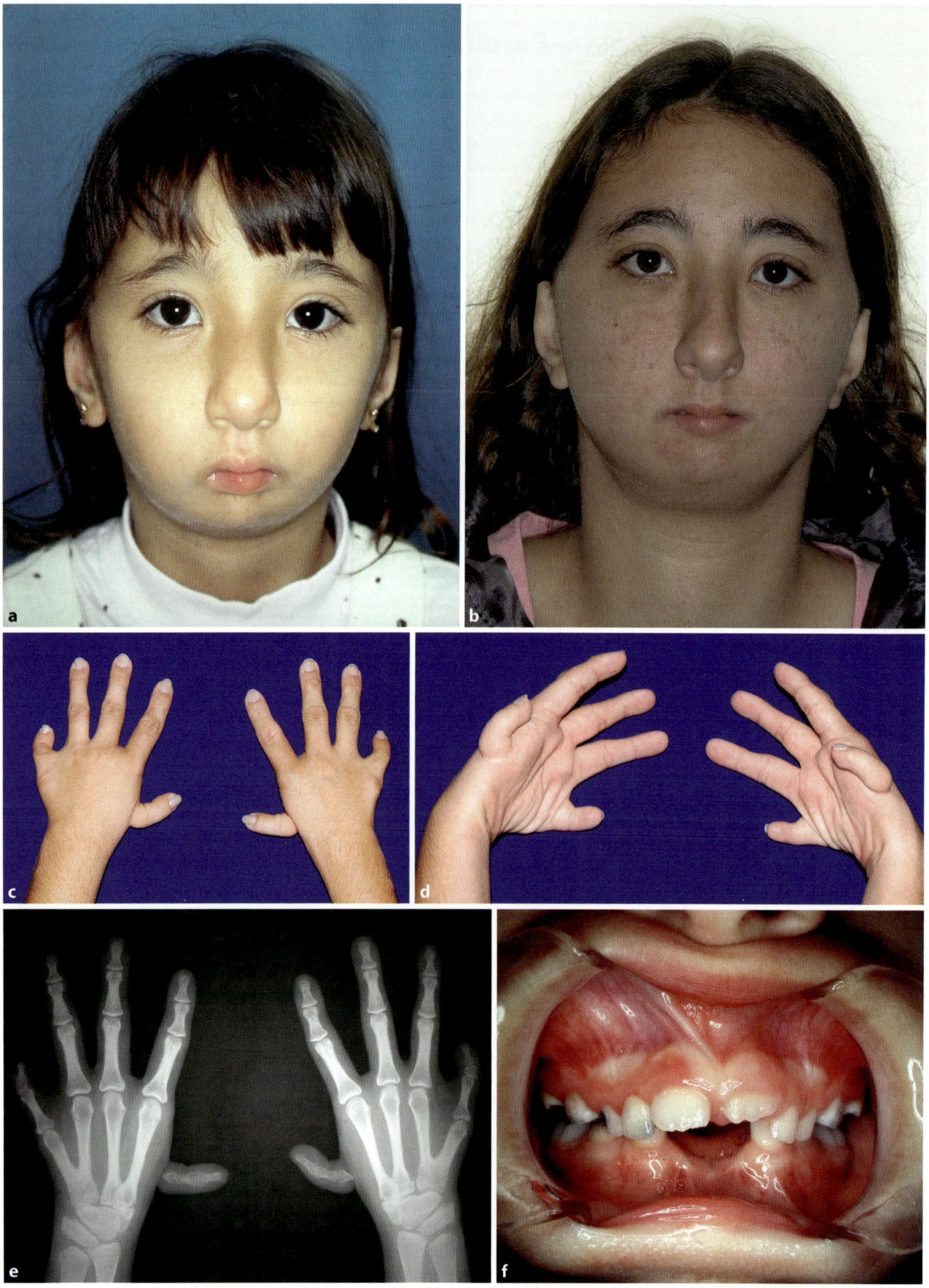

Fig. 81.1 **a, b** Facial expression in Richieri-Costa–Pereira syndrome. Note microstomia, micrognathia, and long and narrow nose. **c, d** Dorsal and lateral views, respectively, of hands showing hypoplastic, proximally set thumbs and short 5th fingers. **e** Corresponding radiograph shows an extremely hypoplastic metacarpal I without connection to the carpals, very small 1st phalanges, a short metacarpal V that is proximally fused with metacarpal IV, small middle phalanges of fingers V, and fusion of carpals. **f** Midline mandibular cleft with missing central lower incisors. (**a–f** courtesy of Antonio Richieri-Costa and Maria Leine Guion-Almeida, HRAC-USP, Bauru, Sao Paulo, Brazil)

Part XV

Reduction Anomalies: Ulnar Ray

82 Femur–Fibula–Ulna Syndrome

MIM 228200

Synonyms
FFU complex

Major Clinical Findings
Femur–fibula–ulna (FFU) syndrome describes the association of asymmetric reduction defects of the femur, fibula, and/or ulna. Some rare anomalies of the upper limbs such as amelia, peromelia of the humerus, humeroradial synostosis, and defects of the ulna fall into this category. One, two, three, and four limbs can be affected, with a striking asymmetry in presence and degree. The malformations are more often unilateral than bilateral, and the upper limbs are affected more often than the lower limbs. Despite the nonspecificity of the clinical phenotype, the limb malformations in FFU syndrome appear to be different from those seen in most other types of limb defects.

Genetic Transmission
Sporadic.

Differential Diagnosis
Other conditions with reduction defects of the long bones.

References

Lenz W, Zygulska M, Horst J (1993) FFU complex: an analysis of 491 cases. Hum Genet 91(4):347–56

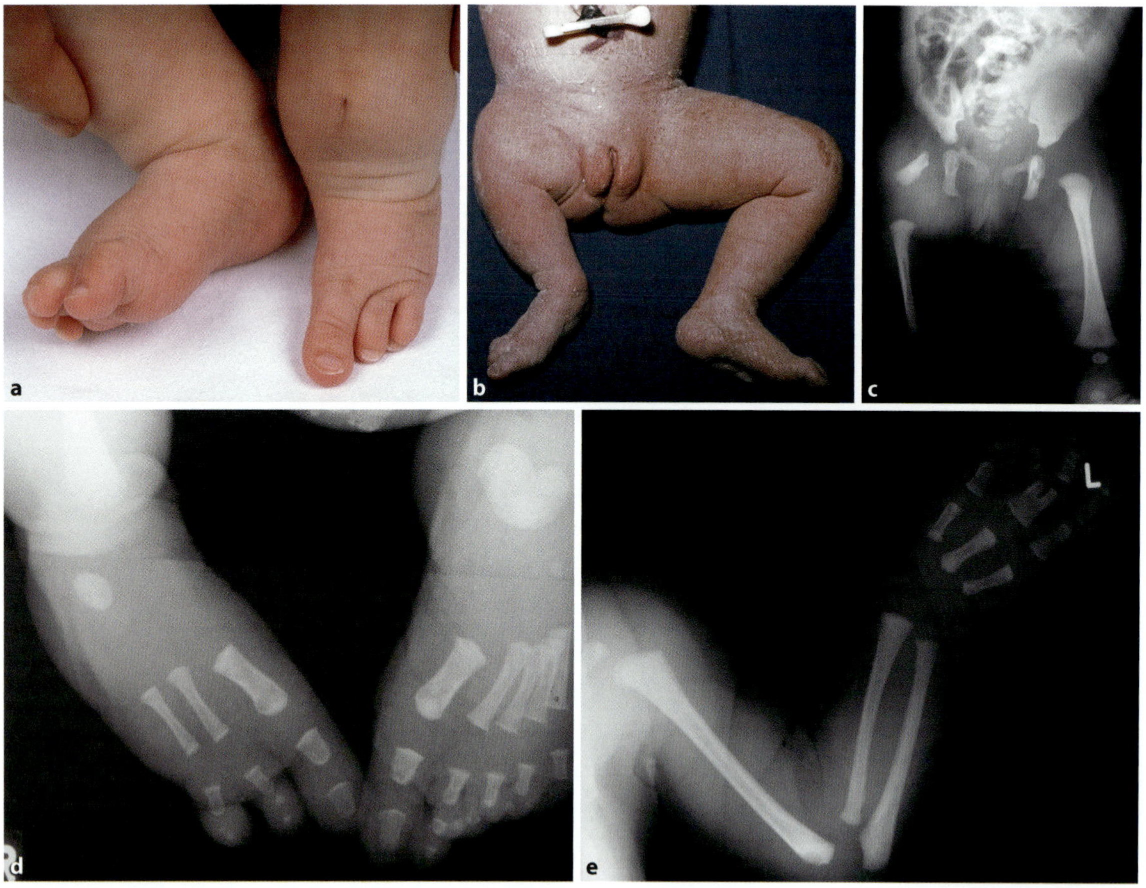

Fig. 82.1 **a** Aplasia of the fibula with short tibia, anterior dimple, and loss of toes IV and V on the left. **b** Lower limb phenotype in femur–fibula–ulna syndrome with short/hypoplastic right leg. **c** Corresponding radiograph shows hypoplastic femur and aplasia of the fibula on the right side. **d** Feet of the same individual with unilateral (right foot) loss of lateral toes IV and V, hypoplasia of distal phalanges bilaterally, and right-sided marked tarsal ossification delay. **e** Complex hand malformation in the same individual with fusions and loss of ulnar digits

S. Mundlos, D. Horn, *Limb Malformations*,
DOI 10.1007/978-3-540-95928-1_82, © Springer-Verlag Berlin Heidelberg 2014

Ulnar-Mammary Syndrome

MIM 181450

83

Synonyms

Pallister ulnar-mammary syndrome
Schinzel syndrome

Major Clinical Findings

Ulnar-mammary syndrome (UMS) is characterized by ulnar ray defects, delayed growth and onset of puberty, and hypoplasia of the breasts/nipples and apocrine glands. Postaxial limb defects range from shortening of digit V to absence of digits III–V and ulna with radial shortening. The most severe cases show complete absence of the radius/ulna and hand. Further features include fusion of the interphalangeal joints with hypoplastic/absent flexion creases, ventral duplication of the nail of digit V, clinodactyly of digit V, postaxial polydactyly, and wide space between digits IV and V. Generally, the feet are not affected, but toes IV and V can be short. Apocrine abnormalities in UMS include diminished or absent axillary hair, reduced or absent perspiration, hypoplasia/aplasia of the breasts, supernumerary nipples as well as hypoplasia of the nipples, and hypopigmentation and/or hypoplasia of the areola. Hypogonadism and delayed puberty are seen in males. Dental abnormalities include ectopic, hypoplastic, and absent canine teeth. Genital anomalies, such as micropenis, shawl scrotum, and imperforate hymen are further features. A wide range of phenotypic expression exists in UMS. Up to a third of mutation carriers have nearly normal limbs and show only a few minor anomalies. Affected individuals may have a similar facial appearance with a broad nasal tip, broad jaw, prominent chin, and tongue frenulum.

Occasional Findings

Ventricular septal defect, Wolff–Parkinson–White arrhythmia, subglottic stenosis, anal atresia, anal stenosis, pyloric stenosis. Abnormalities of the pituitary including anterior pituitary hypoplasia, thin pituitary stalk, and ectopic posterior pituitary.

Genetic Transmission

Autosomal dominant.

Differential Diagnosis

Acro-dermato-ungual-lacrimal-tooth (ADULT) syndrome, featuring sparse hair, lacrimal duct stenosis, oligodontia, dystrophic nails, reduced sweating, ectrodactyly, and nail dysplasia, may phenotypically overlap with UMS.

Molecular Pathology

UMS is caused by heterozygous mutation in *TBX3*, a member of the T-box family of transcription factors. The T-box is characterized by a highly conserved sequence encoding a DNA-binding domain, called the T-domain, that binds specific sequences in the promoters of target genes. During organogenesis, TBX3 is expressed in the primordia of many tissues and organs, notably in the apical ectodermal ridge, the anterior and posterior margins of the developing limbs, and the epithelium of the mammary buds. *TBX3* is located in close vicinity to *TBX5*, the gene that causes Holt–Oram syndrome. Deletions encompassing both genes that result in overlapping phenotypes have been described. Mild gonadotropin deficiency may be the primary cause for abnormal external genitalia in UMS.

References

Bamshad M, Le T, Watkins WS, Dixon ME, Kramer BE, Roeder AD et al (1999) The spectrum of mutations in TBX3: genotype/phenotype relationship in ulnar-mammary syndrome. Am J Hum Genet 64(6):1550–1562

Bamshad M, Lin RC, Law DJ, Watkins WC, Krakowiak PA, Moore ME et al (1997) Mutations in human TBX3 alter limb, apocrine and genital development in ulnar-mammary syndrome. Nat Gene 16(3):311–315

Davenport TG, Jerome-Majewska LA, Papaioannou VE (2003) Mammary gland, limb and yolk sac defects in mice lacking Tbx3, the gene mutated in human ulnar mammary syndrome. Development 130(10):2263–2273

Schinzel A (1987) Ulnar-mammary syndrome. J Med Genet 24(12):778–781

Wollnik B, Kayserili H, Uyguner O, Tukel T, Yuksel-Apak M (2002) Haploinsufficiency of TBX3 causes ulnar-mammary syndrome in a large Turkish family. Ann Genet 45(4):213–217

S. Mundlos, D. Horn, *Limb Malformations*,
DOI 10.1007/978-3-540-95928-1_83, © Springer-Verlag Berlin Heidelberg 2014

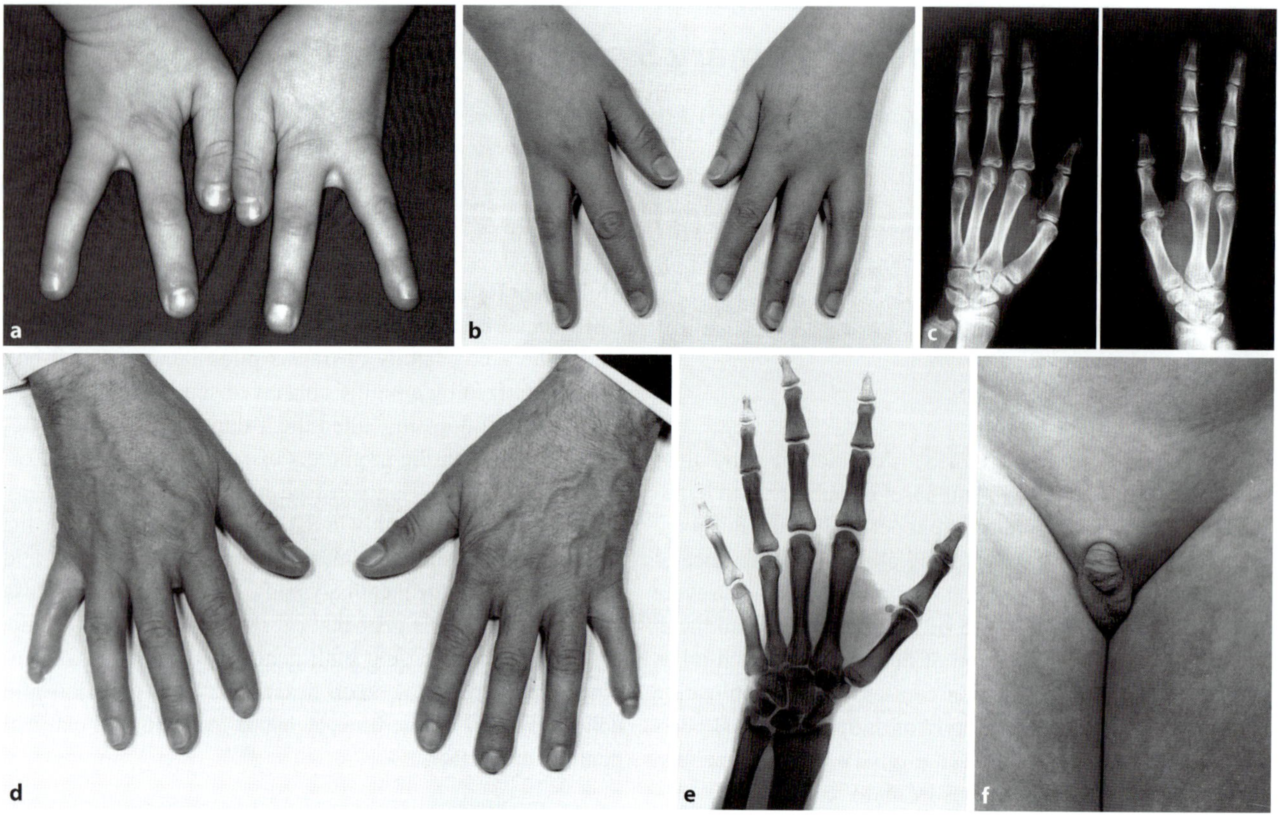

Fig. 83.1 **a** Absence of digits IV and V bilaterally. **b** Similar case, but digit IV is also missing on the right hand. **c** Corresponding radiographs. Note the normal formation of residual digits but bilateral short ulnas. **d** A more mildly affected individual from the same family. Note distally hypoplastic digits V with missing creases and distal hypoplasia of digit III on the left. **e** Corresponding radiograph of the left hand showing distal hypoplasia of digit V and hypoplasia of distal tufts of digits II and IV. **f** Affected male with micropenis. (Courtesy of Albert Schinzel, University of Zurich, Switzerland)

Genée–Wiedemann Syndrome

84

MIM 263750

Synonyms
Miller syndrome
Postaxial acrofacial dysostosis

Major Clinical Findings
Genée–Wiedemann syndrome is characterized by hypoplasia or aplasia of the ulnar ray, manifesting as small or missing digits and toes V and occasionally II and IV. In addition, the thumb may be small and proximally placed. The ulna and radius can be hypoplastic and the olecranon small or missing, and there may be radioulnar synostosis. Facial abnormalities include micrognathia, cleft lip and/or palate, coloboma of the eyelids, ectropion, downward slanting palpebral fissures, cup-shaped ears, low-set ears, hearing loss, choanal atresia, and tooth abnormalities. Further anomalies include rib abnormalities, pectus excavatum, supernumerary nipples, postnatal growth, pyloric stenosis, and midgut malrotation.

Genetic Transmission
Autosomal recessive, but possibly dominant pedigrees have been described.

Differential Diagnosis
The pattern of malformations observed in individuals with Genée–Wiedemann syndrome is similar to those in individuals with fetal exposure to methotrexate. Other types of hypoplasia of the ulnar ray should also be considered.

Molecular Pathology
Genée–Wiedemann syndrome is caused by mutations in *DHODH*, which encodes a key enzyme in the pyrimidine de novo biosynthesis pathway. Interestingly, methotrexate is an inhibitor of de novo purine biosynthesis. The drug has antiproliferative actions that are thought to be due to its inhibition of dihydrofolate reductase and folate-dependent transmethylations. This may explain the overlap in phenotypes between Genée–Wiedemann syndrome and methotrexate-associated malformations. One of the classical phenotypes in Drosophila melanogaster reported by T.H. Morgan is "rudimentary," characterized by wing anomalies, defective oogenesis, and malformed posterior legs. For this mutant, a nutritional requirement for pyrimidines was reported, suggesting that the rudimentary mutation causes a block in one of the first two steps of pyrimidine biosynthesis. Mutations in the pyrimidine pathway were subsequently confirmed. This is the same pathway affected by mutations in *DHODH*, which result in Genée–Wiedemann syndrome.

References

Ng SB, Buckingham KJ, Lee C, Bigham AW, Tabor HK, Dent KM et al (2010) Exome sequencing identifies the cause of a mendelian disorder. Nature Genet 42:30–35

Ogilvy-Stuart AL, Parsons AC (1991) Miller syndrome (postaxial acrofacial dysostosis): further evidence for autosomal recessive inheritance and expansion of the phenotype. J Med Genet 28:695–700

Wiedemann HR (1973) Missbildungs-Retardierungs-Syndrom mit Fehlen des 5: Strahls an Haenden and Fuessen, Gaumenspalte, dysplastischen Ohren und Augenlidern und radioulnarer Synostose. Klin Paediat 185:181–186

S. Mundlos, D. Horn, *Limb Malformations*,
DOI 10.1007/978-3-540-95928-1_84, © Springer-Verlag Berlin Heidelberg 2014

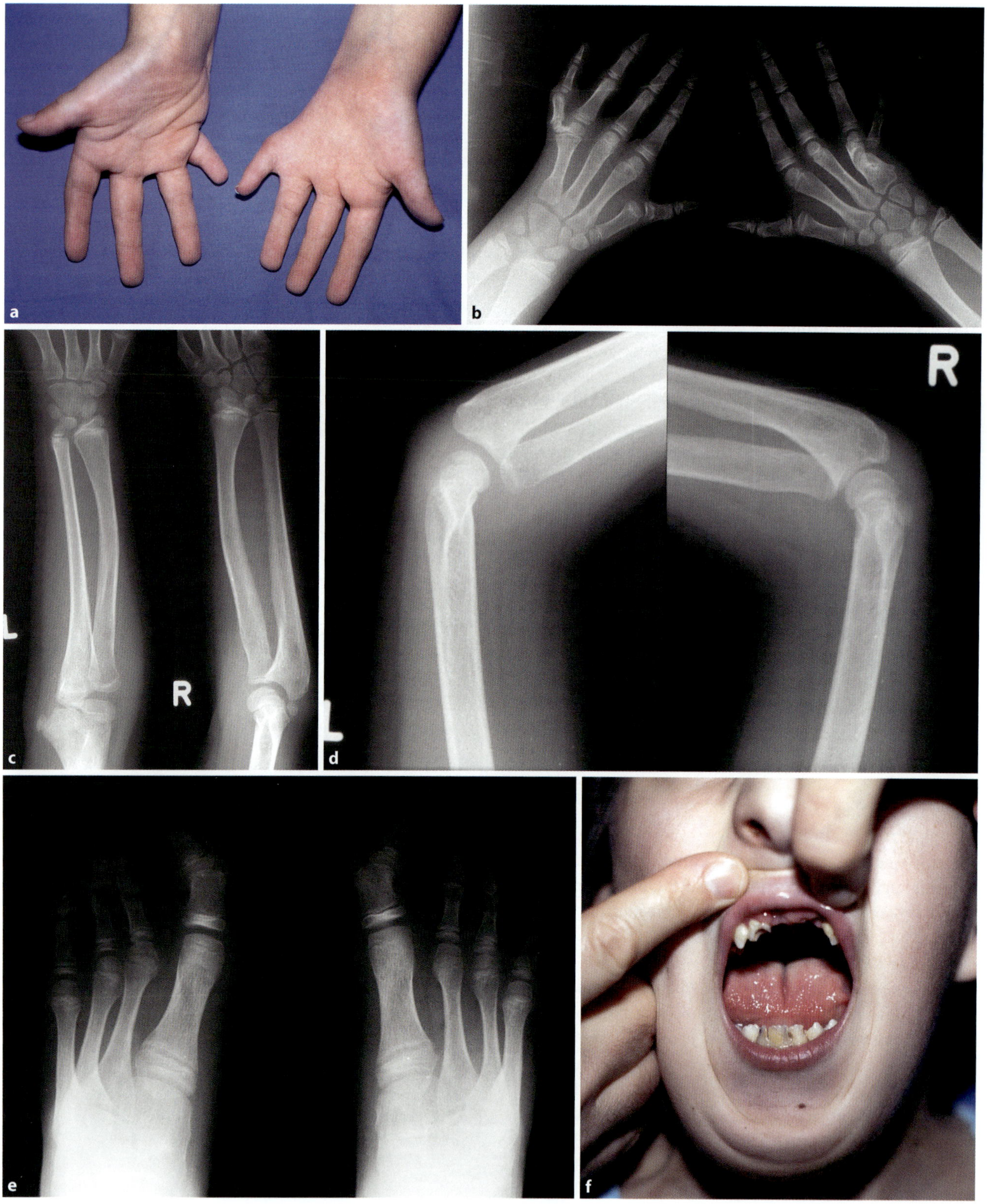

Fig. 84.1 **a** Palmar view of hands showing proximally placed, hypoplastic digits V. **b** Corresponding radiograph shows hypoplasia and fusion of metacarpals IV/V on the right and similar but more complete metacarpal fusion on the left. Note fusion of hamate and capitate on the left, bilateral hypoplastic 5th digits, abnormal 1st metacarpophalangeal joints with subluxation of thumb, and proximal phalangeal cone epiphyses. **c** Forearms of the same individual. Note bowing of the radius, wedged (Madelung-like) distal epiphysis of the radius, and distally thin/hypoplastic ulna on the left. **d** Elbow region: hypoplasia/aplasia of the olecranon. **e** Radiographs of feet. Note missing 5th rays and relatively long proximal phalanges of the great toes. **f** Abnormally shaped and discolored teeth

Cornelia de Lange Syndrome

85

MIM 122470

Synonyms

Brachmann de Lange syndrome

Major Clinical Findings

Cornelia de Lange syndrome (CDLS) is a malformation syndrome characterized by typical facial dysmorphism, prenatal and postnatal growth retardation, microcephaly, intellectual disability, and upper limb anomalies. Facial features include "penciled" and arched eyebrows; synophrys; high-set, short anteverted nose; a long, flat, and poorly structured philtrum; thin upper lip; downturned corners of the mouth; and micrognathia. The teeth are often widely spaced. Cleft palate occurs in 20 %. Body hair is increased, and cutis marmorata is often present. The hands and feet are small, with short and curved fingers V and proximally placed thumbs. The upper limb involvement is often asymmetric and ranges from thumb hypoplasia to severe general hypoplasia with monodactyly. About 25 % of affected individuals exhibit severely malformed upper limbs. Radiographically, the radius and ulna, and in some cases also the humerus, are shortened. The metacarpophalangeal profile is characteristic, with the 1st metacarpal being shorter than the others. The middle phalanges of the index fingers are hypoplastic. Bone age is delayed. Dislocations of the radial head are observed in 80 %. Coxa valga is a constant feature.

Gastroesophageal reflux is a frequent complication, and structural anomalies of the kidney and urinary tract have been documented in many patients. Conductive or sensorineural hearing loss and frequent otitis media with effusion have been documented in the majority of patients. Cardiac anomalies are present in about a third. A wide variety of behavioral problems frequently occur, especially hyperactivity, self-injury, aggressive behavior, and sleep disturbance. These correlate closely with the degree of intellectual disability; 80 % of patients show severe or profound developmental delay/intellectual disability.

Occasional Findings

Seizures, muscular hypertonia, vermian hypoplasia, ophthalmologic abnormalities, cutaneous syndactyly of the 2nd and 3rd toes, single palmar crease.

Genetic Transmission

Autosomal dominant. Most cases are sporadic. Rarely, affected siblings have been reported.

Differential Diagnosis

There is clinical overlap with the phenotype seen in patients with duplication 3q syndrome. Facial features of Coffin–Siris syndrome may occasionally be confused with those of CDLS.

Patients with Gorlin–Chaudhry–Moss syndrome may show some facial resemblance to individuals with CDLS.

Molecular Pathology

CDLS can be caused by heterozygous mutations in the *NIPBL* gene, which encodes a component of the cohesion complex. About 50–60 % of CDLS cases are due to a mutation in *NIPBL*, and about 5 % show deletions. A high frequency of somatic mosaicism mutations has been detected, such as in buccal cells from patients with CDLS in whom no mutations were detectable in lymphocytes. Two milder variants of CDLS have been identified: CDLS3, caused by mutation in the *SMC3* gene, and CDLS4, caused by mutation in the *RAD21* gene. One X-linked form of the disorder can be caused by mutation in the *SMC1A* gene. Another X-linked form, CDLS5, is caused by mutation in the *HDAC8* gene, the vertebrate histone deacetylase of SMC3.

NIPBL and the other genes involved in CDLS are part of the cohesin complex, a family of proteins involved in formation of the spindle apparatus during mitosis and meiosis. Cohesin counteracts the force of spindle microtubules on sister kinetochores and allows chromosomes to align at the mitotic spindle. Furthermore, the cohesin complex has been shown to physically and functionally connect enhancers and core promoters of active genes, thereby enabling loop formation, a process that is important for long-range gene regulation via enhancers. Studies in Nipbl-deficient mice and cells have shown that DNA replication and repair and chromosome segregation are not affected; rather, Nipbl deficiency results in visible chromatin decompaction, which appears to affect gene expression by deregulating transcription.

References

Allanson JE, Hennekam RCM, Ireland M (1997) De Lange syndrome: subjective and objective comparison of the classical and mild phenotypes. J Med Genet 34:645–650

Berney TP, Ireland M, Burn J (1999) Behavioural phenotype of Cornelia de Lange syndrome. Arch Dis Child 81:333–336

Huisman SA, Redeker EJW, Maas SM, Mannens MM, Hennekam RCM (2013) High rate of mosaicism in individuals with Cornelia de Lange syndrome. J Med Genet 50:339–344

S. Mundlos, D. Horn, *Limb Malformations*,
DOI 10.1007/978-3-540-95928-1_85,

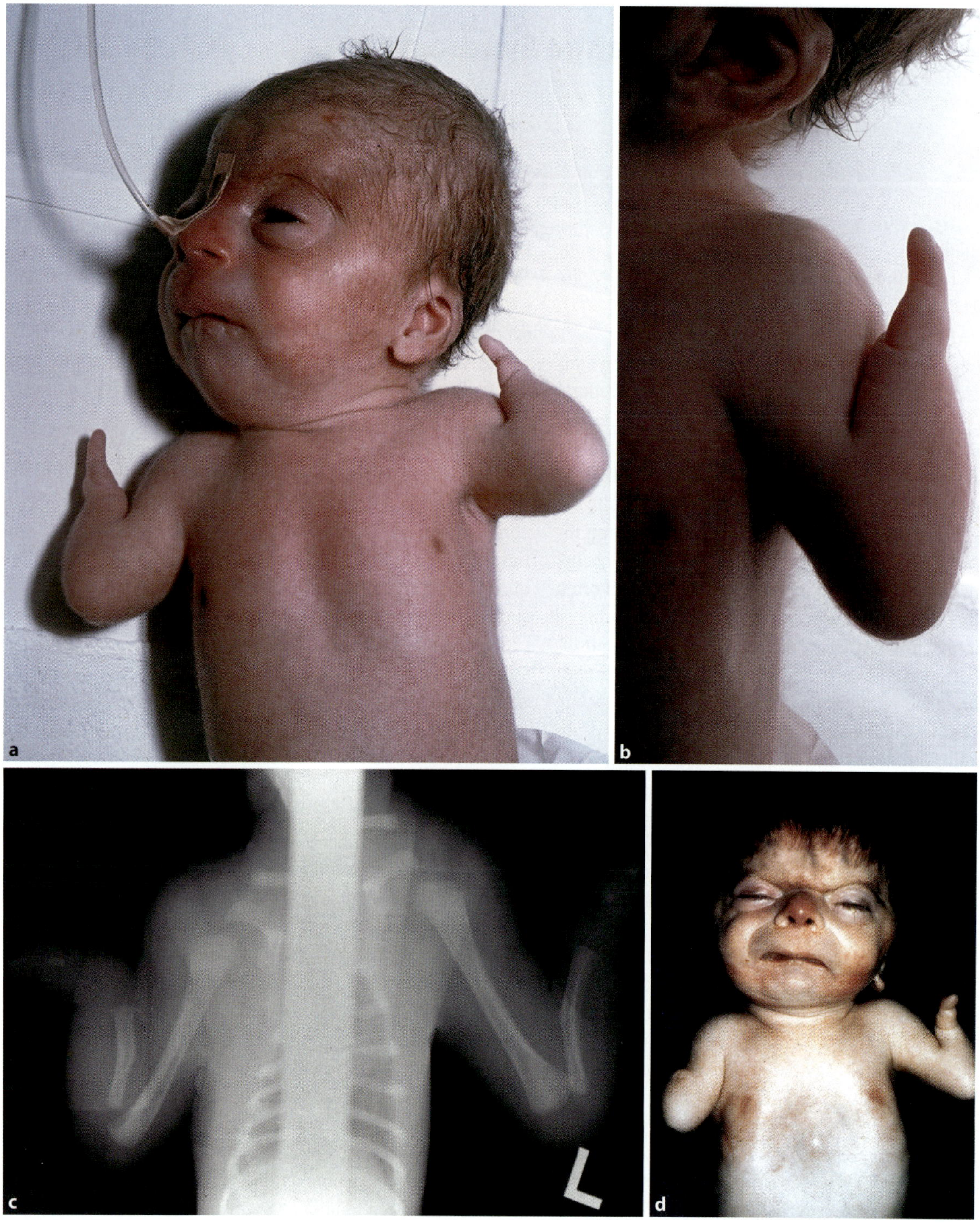

Fig. 85.1 **a** Severely affected child with typical features, including arched eyebrows that grow across the base of the nose (synophrys), low anterior hairline, anteverted nares, maxillary prognathism, long philtrum, thin lips, and crescent-shaped mouth. Prenatal and postnatal growth retardation. Severe reduction deformity of the arms with contracture deformity of the elbows and monodactyly. **b** Close-up of left arm. **c** Corresponding radiograph of both upper limbs shows ulnar hemimelia, asymmetric radial shortening, and monodactyly. **d** Note typical facial expression and severe reduction defects of the arms, with monodactyly on the left and truncation on the right side

Krantz ID, McCallum J, DeScipio C, Kaur M, Gillis LA, Yaeger D et al (2004) Cornelia de Lange syndrome is caused by mutations in *NIPBL*, the human homolog of Drosophila melanogaster Nipped-B. Nature Genet 36:631–635

Rohatgi S, Clark D, Kline AD, Jackson LG, Pie J, Siu V et al (2010) Facial diagnosis of mild and variant CdLS: insights from a dysmorphologist survey. Am J Med Genet 152A:1641–1653

Tonkin ET, Wang T-J, Lisgo S, Bamshad MJ, Strachan T (2004) NIPBL, encoding a homolog of fungal Scc2-type sister chromatid cohesion proteins and fly Nipped-B, is mutated in Cornelia de Lange syndrome. Nature Genet 36:636–641

Part XV

Reduction Anomalies: Nongenetic

86 Amnion Rupture Sequence

MIM 217100

Synonyms
Amniotic band syndrome
Amniotic band lesions
Streeter anomaly

Includes
ADAM complex

Major Clinical Findings
Amnion rupture sequence can result in limb reduction defects, amputations, ring constrictions, and distal syndactyly as well as various other anomalies such as craniofacial clefts and body wall deficiency. The severity of anomalies varies from a single ring constriction to severe abnormalities incompatible with life. Limb defects are most frequently observed. The lower limbs are more severely and more frequently affected, and distal structures are more often and more severely involved than are proximal structures. Limb abnormalities include congenital amputations of one or more limbs or digits, ring constrictions, lymphedema below the ring constriction, distal syndactyly, and talipes equinovarus. Less frequent limb abnormalities include a missing forearm bone or lower leg bone, radial and ulnar hypoplasia, ectrodactyly, and absence of an entire limb. The birth prevalence for the amnion rupture sequence is 1.17 per 10,000 live births.

ADAM complex (amniotic deformity, adhesions, mutilations) refers to the association of constriction bands with cleft lip and palate as well as other facial malformations. Limb and/or body wall defect refers to constriction bands that affect internal organs, most frequently the head, lungs, heart, diaphragm, kidneys, and gonads.

Occasional Findings
Neural tube defects, encephalocele, cleft palate, brain abnormalities, eye anomalies, different types of body wall deficiencies.

Genetic Transmission
The condition is generally considered nongenetic. However, familial instances of limb involvement have been reported.

Differential Diagnosis
Amniotic band defects affecting the digits may resemble brachydactyly type B and syndactyly type IV. Limb anomalies in Goltz–Gorlin syndrome (focal dermal hypoplasia) may look like amniotic band defects.

Molecular Pathology
Anomalies due to amnion band sequence have been found to be associated with amniocentesis. The cause of amnion band sequence is still unclear.

References

Christianson C, Huff D, McPherson E (1999) Limb deformations in oligohydramnios sequence: effects of gestational age and duration of oligohydramnios. Am J Med Genet 96:430–433

Garza A, Cordero JF, Mulinare J (1988) Epidemiology of the early amnion rupture spectrum of defects. Am J Dis Child 142:541–544

Jamsheer A, Materna-Kiryluk A, Badura-Stronka M, Wiśniewska K, Wieckowska B, Mejnartowicz J et al (2009) Comparative study of clinical characteristics of amniotic rupture sequence with and without body wall defect: further evidence for separation. Birth Defects Res A Clin Mol Teratol 85(3):211–215

S. Mundlos, D. Horn, *Limb Malformations*,
DOI 10.1007/978-3-540-95928-1_86,

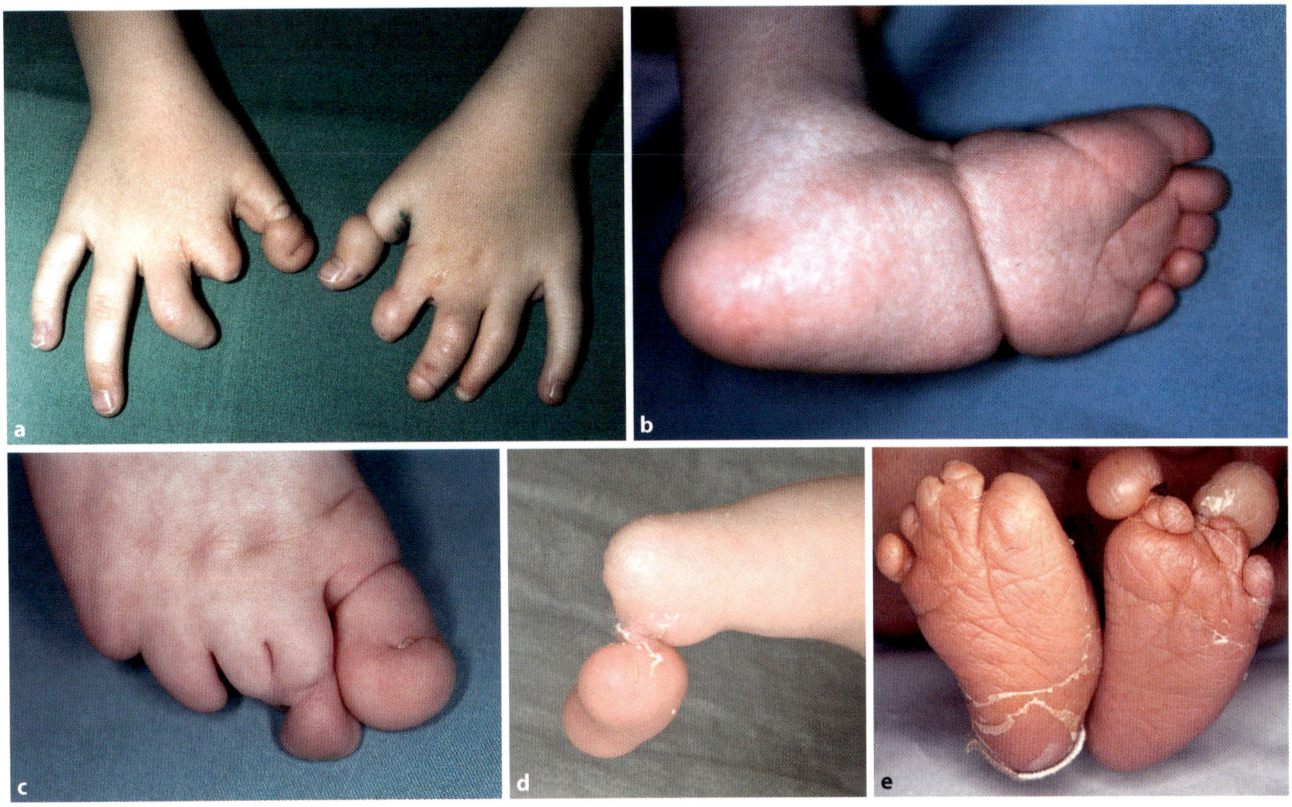

Fig. 86.1 **a** Visible constriction rings in both thumbs with nail hypoplasia on the right. Amputation of distal digits II–IV on the left and II and III on the right. **b** Constriction ring around foot. **c** Amputation of toes II and V, syndactyly of toes II and III, constriction ring at hallux. **d** Constriction ring below the knee with visible remnants. **e** Amputation of toes and swelling due to constriction

87 Thalidomide Embryopathy

Major Clinical Findings

Thalidomide causes a wide variety of birth defects that are highly correlated with the timing of thalidomide exposure in pregnancy. With exposure at embryonic days 41–44, severe reduction anomalies of the upper limbs occur; with exposure at days 44–48, the lower limbs are affected. The bones of the upper limb are affected in a recurrent recognizable pattern. The thumb is affected most frequently, followed by the radius, the humerus, the ulna, and finally the fingers on the ulnar side of the hand. Consequently, the most severe defects consist of one or more digits directly attached to the shoulder, or with a bone interposed between the shoulder and the digits. The least severe cases may show abnormalities of the thumbs only. They may include complete absence or hypoplasia of the thumb, thenar muscle, or both; partial fusion to the adjacent index finger; or a triphalangeal thumb. The other fingers may be thin, flexed, and weak. Reduction deformities of the radius tend to start at the distal end and extend toward the elbow. In addition to being short, the radius is often bowed, may be thicker than normal, and can be fused to some degree with the ulna. The humerus also tends to be affected from the distal to the proximal end. The muscles that would normally attach to the missing bones are hypoplastic, but the extent of this muscle hypoplasia does not always correspond exactly to the loss of bone.

Upper limbs are more commonly affected than lower limbs. A minority of affected individuals have defects of all limbs, and defects of the lower limbs with normal upper limbs are uncommon. Abnormalities of the lower limb include hypoplasia of the femur (extending from proximal to distal), tibia, or both. In the most severe cases, the feet arise from the hip areas. Polydactyly may occur. Talipes (clubfoot) is common. Hips may be dislocated or unstable at birth and may develop Perthes disease later. Arthritis appears to be a common problem of later life.

Thalidomide embryopathy affects the entire body. Apart from severe limb malformations, craniofacial, cardiac, bowel, and urogenital abnormalities have been observed. Craniofacial anomalies include anophthalmia/microphthalmia, colobomas, ear abnormalities such as microtia, and hemangiomas of the forehead, nose, and upper lip. Frequent visceral anomalies include esophageal and duodenal atresia and heart defects such as tetralogy of Fallot.

Occurrence

Thalidomide was a sedative used between 1957 and 1961 until it was recognized as a teratogenic agent. Approximately 10,000 individuals with thalidomide embryopathy were born during that time. The drug has been out of use but has had a recent revival for a variety of other indications, including leprosy and the dermatological complications of AIDS and other severe dermatoses, and as an antitumor agent (including multiple myeloma).

Differential Diagnosis

Thalidomide embryopathy should be differentiated by the complex phenotype caused by *SALL4* mutations such as Okihiro syndrome. A further differential diagnosis includes Roberts syndrome, which can be distinguished by the neurological involvement and mode of inheritance. In certain instances, VACTER(L) association (vertebral defects, anal atresia, cardiac defects, tracheoesophageal fistula, renal anomalies, and limb abnormalities) can be a differential. Thalidomide embryopathy is universally bilateral and does not include distal transverse type defects.

Molecular Pathology

Loss of immature blood vessels appears to be a cause of thalidomide-induced teratogenesis. In chick embryos it was shown that thalidomide temporarily blocks outgrowth and remodeling of more mature blood vessels, whereas newly formed, rapidly developing angiogenic vessels are lost. This loss of vessels occurs before changes in limb morphogenesis and gene expression and results in developmental defects. This effect is probably due to inhibition of cytokines, including tumor necrosis factor-α and vascular endothelial growth

Fig. 87.1 Clinical variability of thalidomide-associated malformations. **a** Complete absence of left arm. Single digit and a very short arm remnant on the right. **b** Hypoplasia of thumbs bilaterally with flexion contracture. **c** Corresponding radiograph of the right hand showing thin and elongated metacarpal I and a small additional phalanx between the proximal and distal phalanges, resulting in a triphalangeal thumb. **d** Radiograph showing bilateral aplasia of thumb. Note camptodactyly due to abnormal proximal interphalangeal joints of digits II and V bilaterally and aplasia of the radial carpal bones. **e** Aplasia of the radius and thumb on the right; hypoplasia on the left. Short ulna and club hand deformity.

S. Mundlos, D. Horn, *Limb Malformations*,
DOI 10.1007/978-3-540-95928-1_87, © Springer-Verlag Berlin Heidelberg 2014

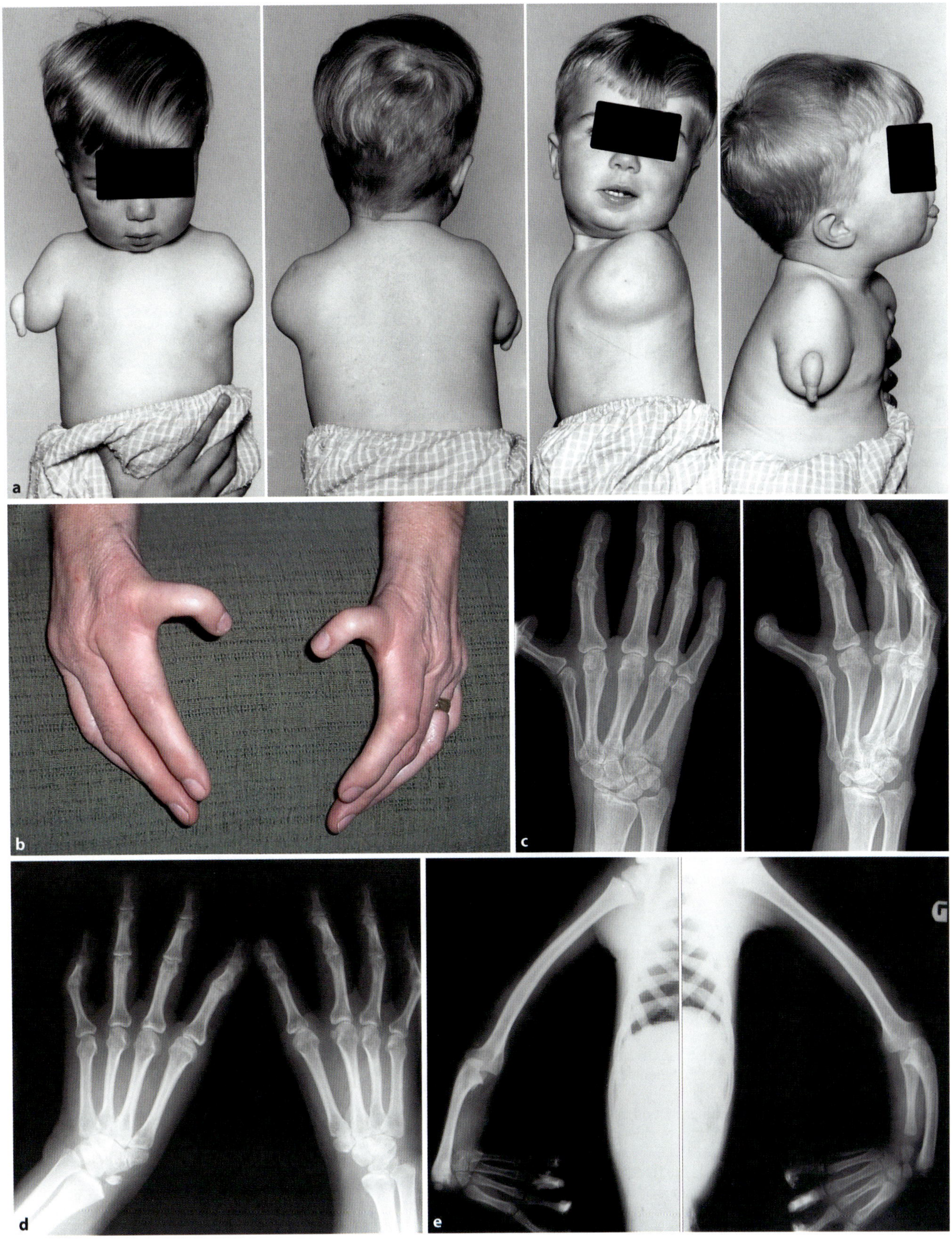
a
b
c
d
e
G

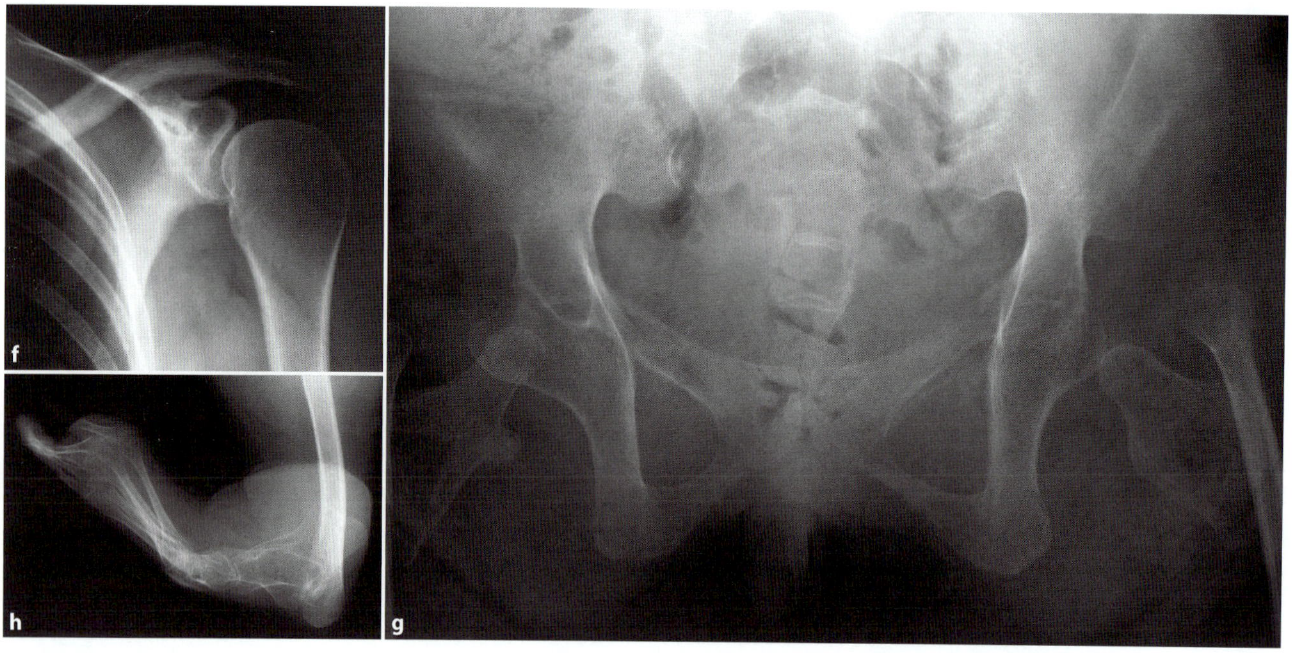

Fig. 87.1 (*continued*) Clinical variability of thalidomide-associated malformations. **f** Shoulder joint showing hypoplastic glenoid neck. **g** Pelvis and hips of a severely affected individual. The tibia projects over the left femur. The femurs are severely hypoplastic/dislocated, and there are sacral vertebral anomalies with sacral scoliosis. **h** Lower limb of the same person, with a single bone likely representing the tibia. The foot is abnormally rotated and projects laterally and superiorly. (**a** from Newman 1985; **d–h** courtesy of U. M. Peters, Nümbrecht, Germany)

factor. A further effect of thalidomide appears to be its ability to induce apoptosis. Furthermore, cereblon (CRBN), a protein encoded by a candidate gene for mild mental retardation, has been identified as a primary target of thalidomide teratogenicity. CRBN forms an E3 ubiquitin ligase complex with Cul4A that is important for limb outgrowth and expression of fibroblast growth factor 8 (FGF8). FGF8 is expressed in the apical ectodermal ridge (AER) and is important for limb outgrowth and AER function. Thus, thalidomide initiates its teratogenic effects by binding to CRBN and inhibiting the associated ubiquitin ligase activity, thereby inhibiting FGF8.

References

D'Amato RJ, Loughnan MS, Flynn E, Folkman J (1994) Thalidomide is an inhibitor of angiogenesis. Proc Natl Acad Sci U S A 91(9):4082–4085

Ito T, Ando H, Suzuki T, Ogura T, Hotta K, Imamura Y et al (2010) Identification of a primary target of thalidomide teratogenicity. Science 327(5971):1345–1350

Knobloch J, Rüther U (2008) Shedding light on an old mystery: thalidomide suppresses survival pathways to induce limb defects. Cell Cycle 7(9):1121–1127

Kohlhase J, Schubert L, Liebers M et al (2003) Mutations at the SALL4 locus on chromosome 20 result in a range of clinically overlapping phenotypes, including Okihiro syndrome, Holt–Oram syndrome, acro-renal-ocular syndrome, and patients previously reported to represent thalidomide embryopath. J Med Genet 40:473–478

Lenz W (1988) A short history of thalidomide embryopathy. Teratology 38(3):203–215

Lenz W (1961) Kindliche Missbildungen nach Medikamenten-Einnahme während der Gravidität. Dtsch Med Wochenschr 191:2555–2556

Newman CG (1985) Teratogen update: clinical aspects of thalidomide embryopathy—a continuing preoccupation. Teratology 32(1):133–144

Smithells RW, Newman CG (1992) Recognition of thalidomide defects. J Med Genet 29:716–723

Valproate Embryopathy

88

Synonyms
Fetal valproate syndrome

Major Clinical Findings
Valproic acid, or valproate, has been associated with the highest risk of malformations among all antiepileptic drugs. The relative risk is seven times greater for the offspring of women taking valproic acid compared to women in the general population as well as to women who use other antiepileptic drugs. A dose–response relationship has been documented. Limb anomalies include distal phalangeal hypoplasia, nail hypoplasia, radial ray defects, hypoplasia or digitalization of the thumb, contractures of the hands or fingers, overlapping fingers, and foot deformities. Facial dysmorphism includes midface hypoplasia, hypertelorism, short nose with a broad and depressed nasal root, long and flat philtrum, thin upper lip, and posteriorly rotated ears. Cardiac anomalies have been reported in about 25 % of individuals with valproate embryopathy, and neural tube defects have been documented in 1–5 %. Developmental delay and muscular hypotonia are present in a considerable proportion of affected children. The incidence of autistic disorders is increased in these children.

Occasional Findings
Genital abnormalities, absent radius, preaxial polydactyly, craniosynostosis.

Differential Diagnosis
Clinical features resemble those of other antiepileptic embryopathies, such as hydantoin and carbamazepine embryopathy. Syndromes with developmental delay and hypoplastic distal phalanges such as hyperphosphatasia with mental retardation syndrome should be considered.

References

Clayton-Smith J, Donnai D (1995) Fetal valproate syndrome. J Med Genet 32(9):724–727

Dean JC, Hailey H, Moore SJ, Lloyd DJ, Turnpenny PD, Little J (2002) Long term health and neurodevelopment in children exposed to antiepileptic drugs before birth. J Med Genet 39(4):251–259

Genton P, Semah F, Trinka E (2006) Valproic acid in epilepsy: pregnancy-related issues. Drug Saf 29:1–21

Kozma C (2001) Valproic acid embryopathy: report of two siblings with further expansion of the phenotypic abnormalities and a review of the literature. Am J Med Genet 98:168–175

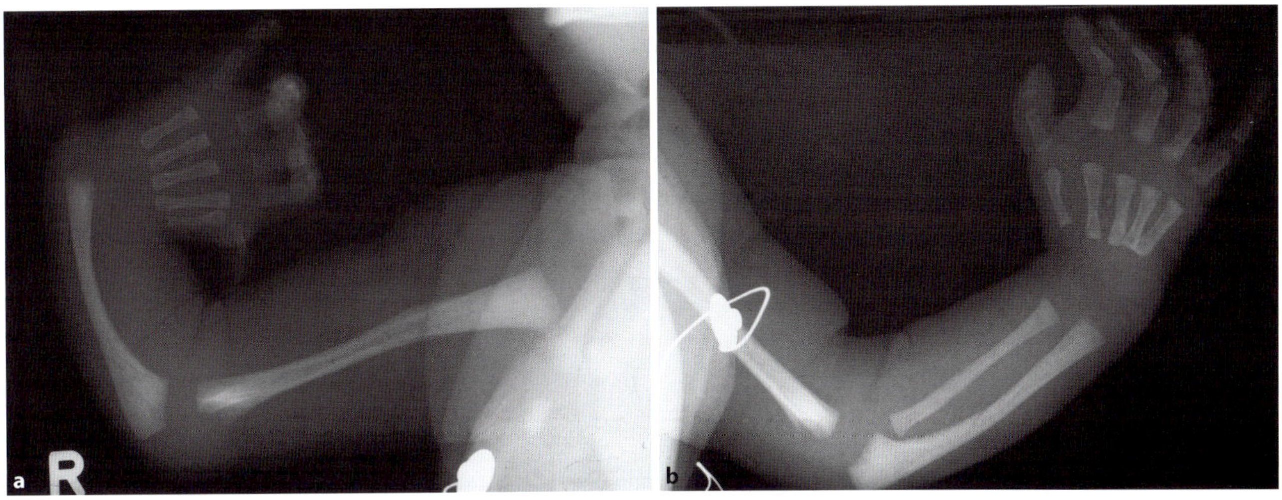

Fig. 88.1 **a** Radial ray deficiency with absent radius and small thumb on the right. **b** Small radius and radial deviation of the hand on the left

S. Mundlos, D. Horn, *Limb Malformations*,
DOI 10.1007/978-3-540-95928-1_88, © Springer-Verlag Berlin Heidelberg 2014

Part XVI

Reduction Anomalies: Split Hand/Foot Malformation

89 Split Hand/Foot Malformation (SHFM)

MIM 246560, MIM 220600, MIM 605289, MIM 119100

Synonyms

Split-hand deformity

Ectrodactyly

Major Clinical Findings

Split-hand/foot malformation (SHFM) typically affects the central rays of the hands/feet, resulting in an extremely variable phenotype consisting of missing digits; aplasia and/or hypoplasia of the phalanges, metacarpals, and metatarsals; and syndactyly of the remaining digits. Two major anatomic types have been discerned. In the first, the hand is split into two by a cone-shaped cleft tapering proximally consisting of fused remnants of radial and ulnar ray fingers. Similar deformities can occur in the feet. In the even more severe type, only a single digit remains (monodactyly). As a general rule, the radial rays are usually absent, with only the 5th digit remaining. Besides these typical findings, a vast variety of less severe phenotypes can be observed that sometimes need close inspection, including radiographs, to not be overlooked. Other less frequent findings include preaxial involvement consisting of absent, proximally placed, and/or triphalangeal thumbs, as well as preaxial polydactyly. Nonpenetrance is another characteristic of SHFM. Many pedigrees have been described that indicate skipping of generations and extreme variability of phenotypes.

Genetic Transmission

Autosomal dominant with variable expressivity. Rarely, families with recessive inheritance have been described.

Differential Diagnosis

SHFM is genetically heterogenous and thus a phenotypic diagnosis. Overlap with other syndromic forms exists, and, based on the limb phenotype, they cannot be differentiated. Thus, it is important to search for other signs such as ectodermal dysplasia.

Molecular Pathology

Several loci have been associated with nonsyndromic SHFM. Mutations in *p63* may result in isolated SHFM (MIM 605289), but this gene is also involved in a variety of conditions with SHFM and ectodermal dysplasia. Duplications of 10q24-q25 involving parts of the *FBXW4* (dactylin) gene, as well as the entire *LBX1*, *BTRC*, and *POLL* genes, are a relatively common cause of SHFM (MIM 246560). This locus is syntenic to mouse chromosome 19 where the mouse dactylaplasia (Dac) gene was mapped. Dactylaplasia closely resembles SHFM. Interestingly, the expression of Dac is regulated by a modifier locus (mdac) as demonstrated by the existence of permissive and nonpermissive strains of mice. The molecular pathology of these duplications remains unclear, but a regulatory effect on the neighboring fibroblast growth factor 8 (FGF8) gene expressed by the apical ectodermal ridge (AER) is likely. The distal-less homeobox 5 and 6 (DLX5/6) genes are expressed in the AER, and disruption of both DLX5 and Dlx6 in mice leads to a SHFM phenocopy. In humans, chromosomal aberrations in the *DLX5/6* region, some of which do not encompass the coding sequences of *DLX5/6*, cause SHFM (MIM 220600). A further locus exists on chromosome 17p13.3, consisting of duplications that harbor the *BHLHA9* gene (MIM 119100). This locus is also associated with a more severe form of SHFM that also involves the lower limbs (SHFM with long bone deficiency). The latter locus appears to be the most frequent one. A cohort study identified 17p13.3 duplications in 30 %, 10q24 duplications in 20 %, and TP63 duplications in 9 % of the affected families.

References

Everman DB, Morgan CT, Lyle R, Laughridge ME, Bamshad MJ, Clarkson KB et al (2006) Frequency of genomic rearrangements involving the SHFM3 locus at chromosome 10q24 in syndromic and non-syndromic split-hand/foot malformation. Am J Med Genet 140A:1375–1383

Gurrieri F, Everman DB (2013) Clinical, genetic, and molecular aspects of split-hand/foot malformation: an update. Am J Med Genet A 161A(11):2860–2872

Ianakiev P, Kilpatrick MW, Toudjarska I, Basel D, Beighton P, Tsipouras P (2000) Split-hand/split-foot malformation is caused by mutations in the p63 gene on 3q27. Am J Hum Genet 67:59–66

Klopocki E, Lohan S, Doelken SC, Stricker S, Ockeloen CW, Thiele de Aguiar RS et al (2012) Duplications of BHLHA9 are associated with ectrodactyly and tibia hemimelia inherited in non-Mendelian fashion. J Med Genet 49:119–125

Lango AH, Caswell R, Xie W, Xu X, Wragg C, Turnpenny PD et al (2014) Next generation sequencing of chromosomal rearrangements in patients with split-hand/split-foot malformation provides evidence for DYNC1I1 exonic enhancers of DLX5/6 expression in humans. J Med Genet 51(4):264–267

Merlo GR, Paleari L, Mantero S, Genova F, Beverdam A, Palmisano GL et al (2002) Mouse model of split hand/foot malformation type I. Genesis 33(2):97–101

S. Mundlos, D. Horn, *Limb Malformations*,
DOI 10.1007/978-3-540-95928-1_89, © Springer-Verlag Berlin Heidelberg 2014

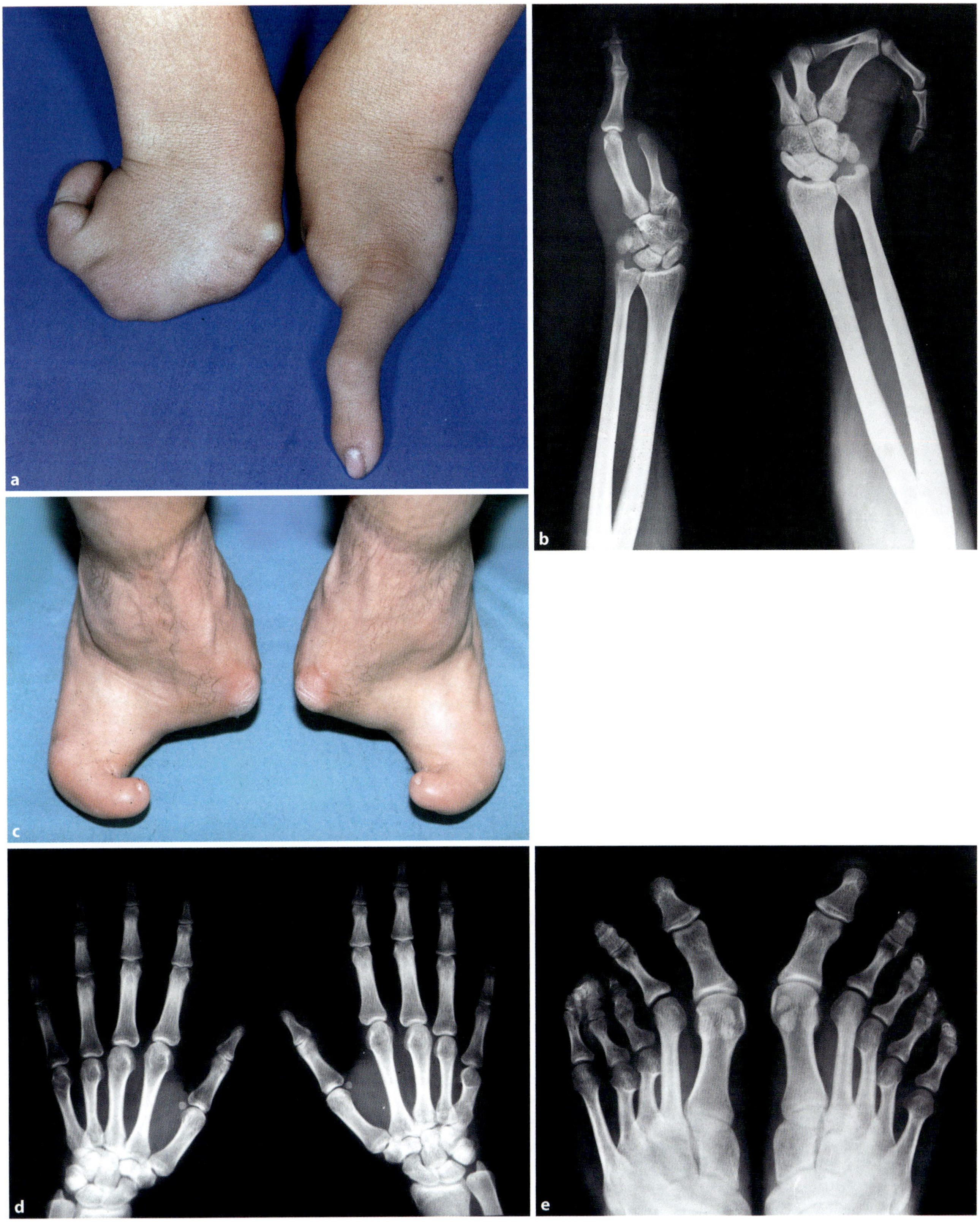

Fig. 89.1 Split-hand/foot malformation (SHFM) caused by duplication on 10q. **a** Severe SHFM with monodactyly. **b** Corresponding radiograph shows two metacarpals and monodactyly on the left and rudimentary metacarpals with remnants of phalanges on the right. **c** Feet of the same individual. Note amputation-like phenotype that is more severe on the medial side. **d, e** Intrafamiliar variability: radiographs of hands (**d**) and feet (**e**) of sister of the patient shown in **a**. Note relatively mild changes, short metacarpal V on the right hand, short metatarsals III/IV and IV/V, and hypoplastic phalanges

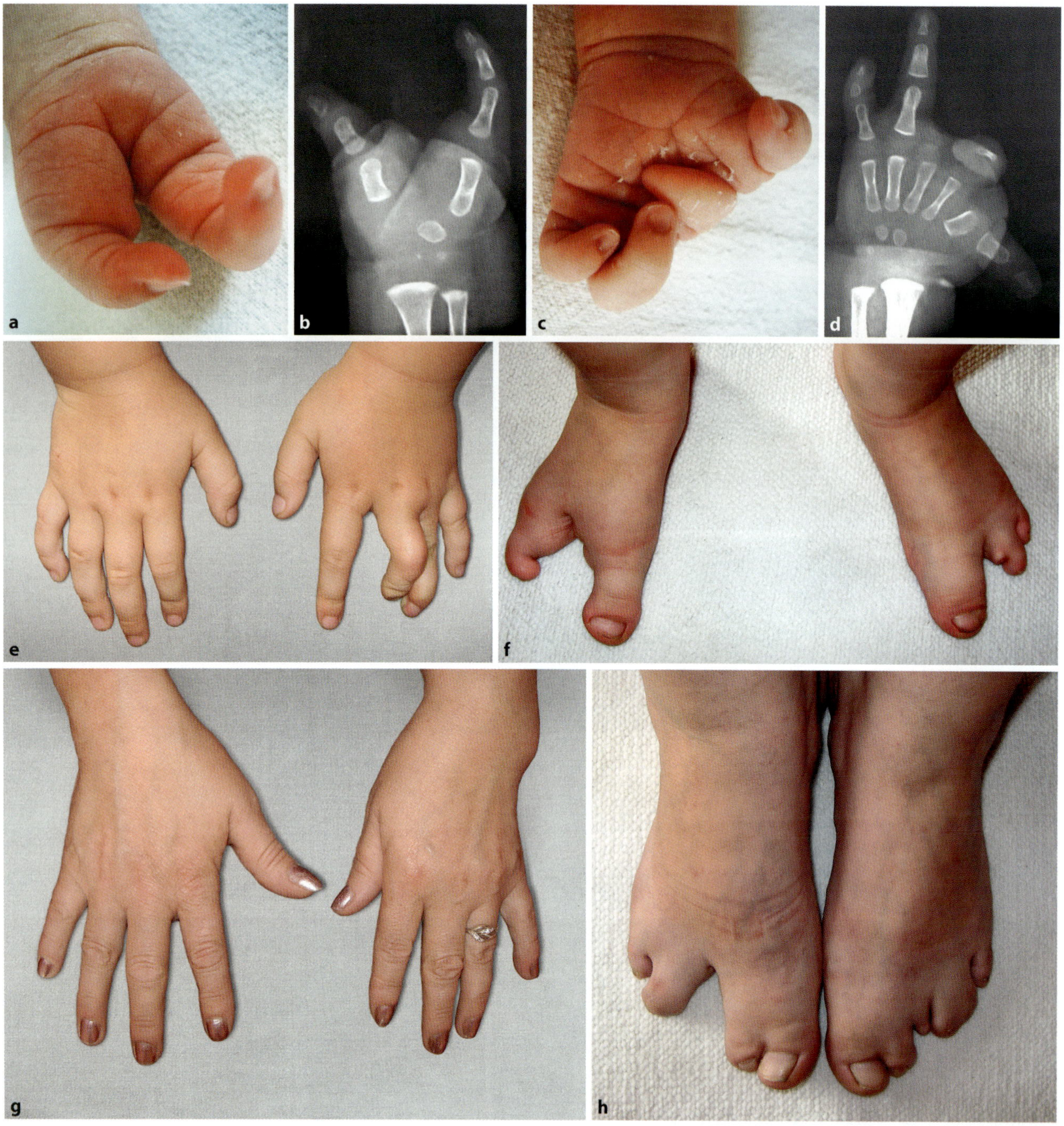

Fig. 89.2 Split-hand/foot malformation (SHFM) associated with mutations in *p63*. **a** Split hand with two digits and corresponding radiograph (**b**) of right hand: fairly normal-size 1st and 5th digits, probable os centralis. **c, d** Hitchhiker thumb with delta phalanx of the 1st metacarpal and absent/partially absent phalanges II and III on the left. **e–h** Intrafamiliar variability: **e, f** and **g, h** show the hands and feet of two siblings. The feet are more severely affected than the hands, and the right hands are normal in both cases

90 Split Hand/Foot Malformation with Long Bone Deficiency (SHFLD)

MIM 612576

Synonyms
Ectrodactyly with tibial hemimelia

Major Clinical Findings
Split-hand/foot malformation (SHFM) occurs as an isolated trait, as a sporadic condition, or as part of a more complex syndromic condition. In most cases the malformation is confined to the hands/feet, but a subtype with more severe involvement exists, featuring variable degrees of lower limb involvement mainly affecting the tibia and fibula. In the latter cases, the condition is referred to as SHFM with long bone deficiency (SHFLD). The hand/foot phenotype in SHFLD is indistinguishable from other forms of SHFM and is extremely variable in its presentation. Affected individuals characteristically have only two digits, which are divided by a large, deep central cleft, with cutaneous syndactyly and/or osseous synostosis in the digits adjacent of the cleft. There may be unilateral involvement, and the individual extremities may be affected to a variable extent, from mild digital changes such as clinodactyly or shortening of individual elements to monodactyly with only the 5th finger remaining. Lower limb involvement ranges from shortening of the tibia to tibial hypoplasia, tibial aplasia, and hypoplasia of the fibula.

Extreme clinical variability and nonpenetrance are characteristic of this condition. Interestingly, females appear to be less frequently affected than males, with approximately 30 % of females being unaffected carriers (versus 12 % in males). This sex bias may result in pedigrees that simulate X-linked inheritance.

Genetic Transmission
Autosomal dominant with reduced penetrance.

Differential Diagnosis
The diagnosis of typical SHFLD is straightforward if ectrodactyly is combined with tibial hemimelia. Without lower limb involvement, however, the phenotype cannot be distinguished from other types of SHFM. The extreme variability with high rates of nonpenetrance, particularly in females, makes SHFLD a differential diagnosis in all SHFM cases.

Molecular Pathology
SHFLD has been shown to be associated with genomic duplications on chromosome 17p that involve the gene *BHLHA9*. The gene is expressed in the developing limb beneath the apical ectodermal ridge in the progress zone. Knockdown experiments in zebrafish have shown that *BHLHA9* is essential for normal limb development, at least in the fish. The duplication has been shown to be the most common cause of nonsyndromic SHFM.

References

Klopocki E, Lohan S, Doelken SC, Stricker S, Ockeloen CW, de Soares Thiele Aguiar R et al (2012) Duplications of BHLHA9 are associated with ectrodactyly and tibia hemimelia inherited in non-Mendelian fashion. J Med Genet 49(2):119–125

S. Mundlos, D. Horn, *Limb Malformations*,
DOI 10.1007/978-3-540-95928-1_90, © Springer-Verlag Berlin Heidelberg 2014

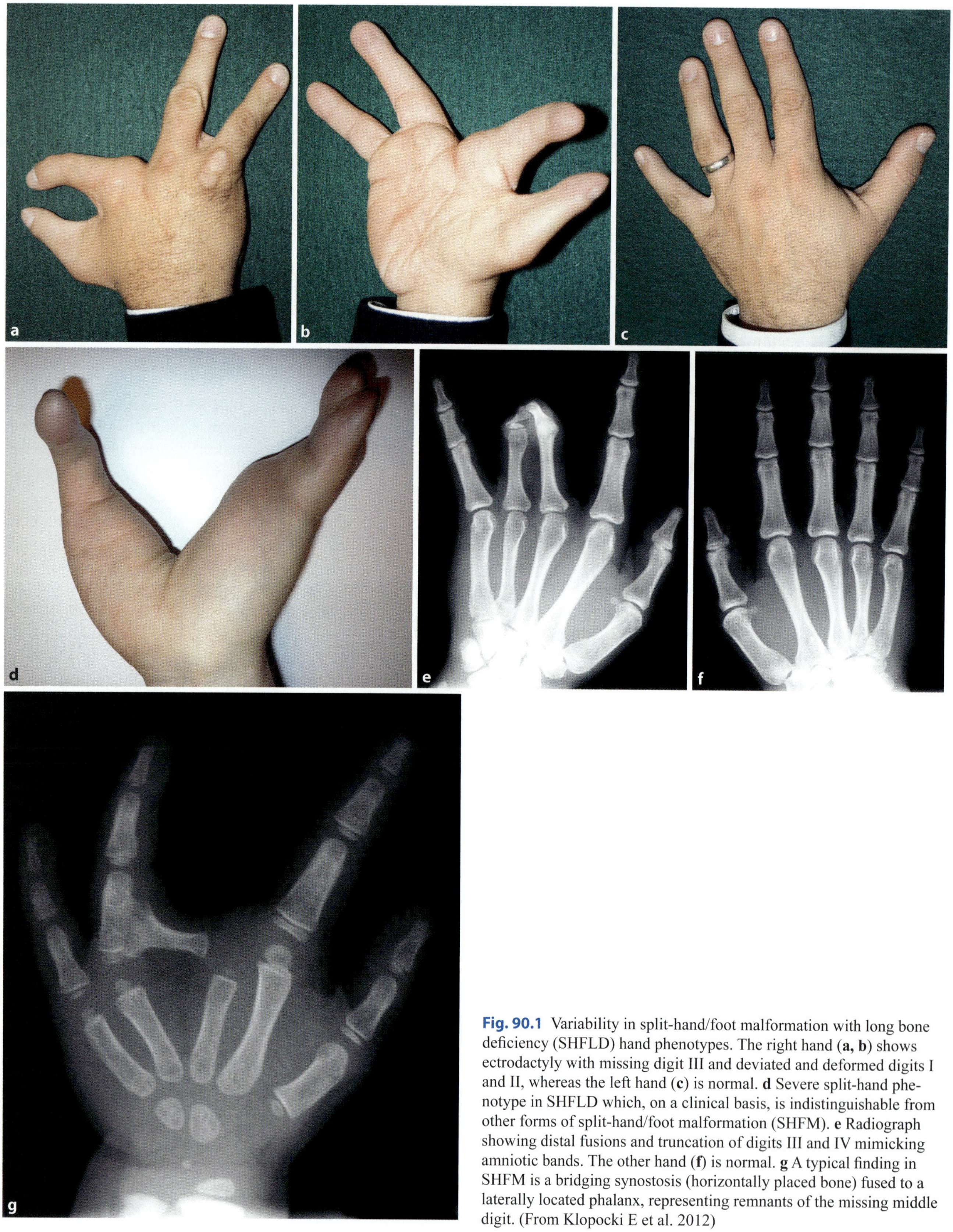

Fig. 90.1 Variability in split-hand/foot malformation with long bone deficiency (SHFLD) hand phenotypes. The right hand (**a, b**) shows ectrodactyly with missing digit III and deviated and deformed digits I and II, whereas the left hand (**c**) is normal. **d** Severe split-hand phenotype in SHFLD which, on a clinical basis, is indistinguishable from other forms of split-hand/foot malformation (SHFM). **e** Radiograph showing distal fusions and truncation of digits III and IV mimicking amniotic bands. The other hand (**f**) is normal. **g** A typical finding in SHFM is a bridging synostosis (horizontally placed bone) fused to a laterally located phalanx, representing remnants of the missing middle digit. (From Klopocki E et al. 2012)

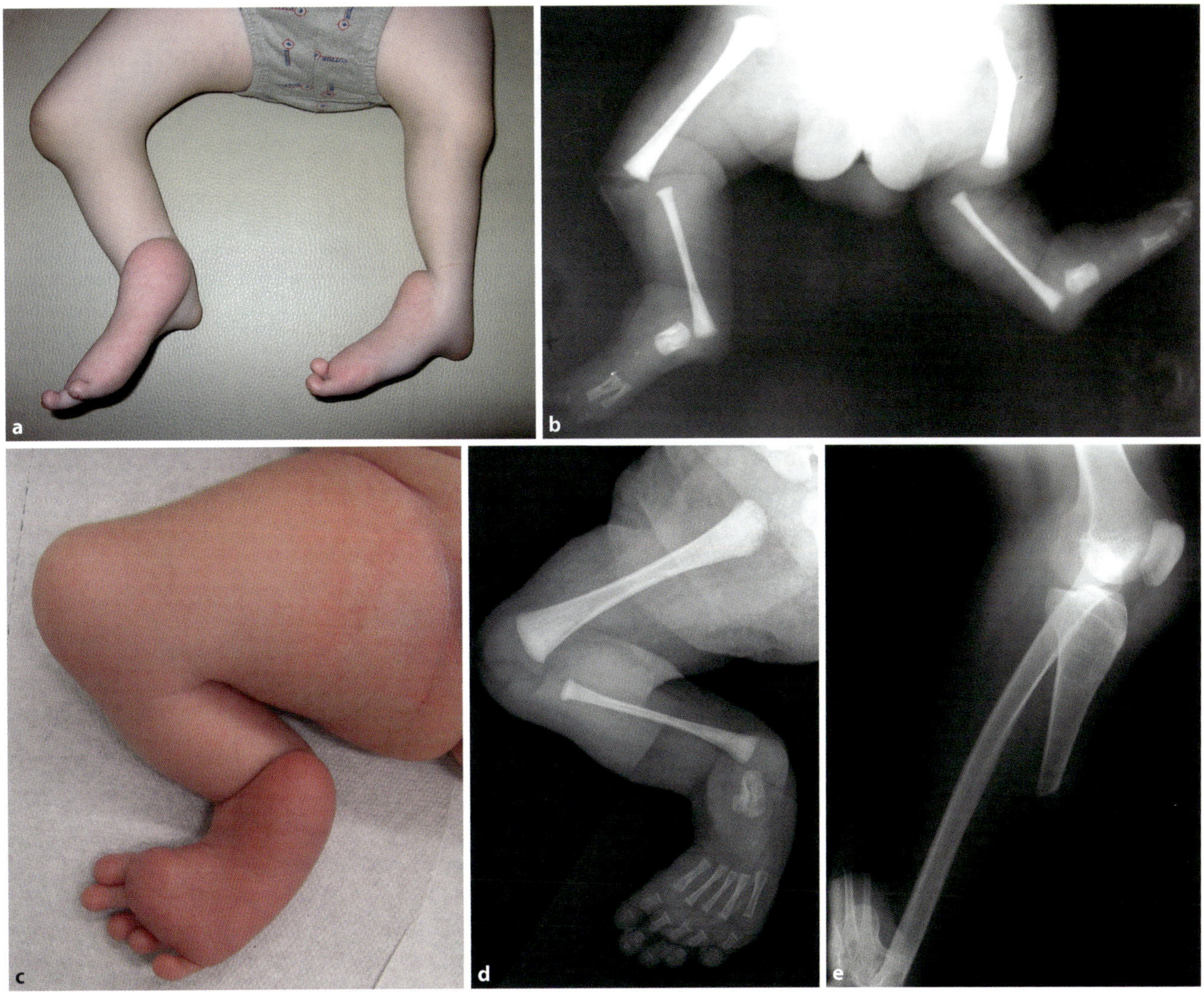

Fig. 90.2 Leg phenotypes in split-hand/foot malformation with long bone deficiency (SHFLD). **a** Bilateral hypoplasia of the tibia with dorsiflexion of the feet. **b** Corresponding radiograph reveals absent tibias. Note unilateral bending of the femur. **c** Newborn with SHFLD and aplasia of the tibia. **d** Corresponding radiograph shows absent tibia. **e** Absent distal tibia with proximal truncation of tibia. (From Klopocki E et al. 2012)

91 Split Hand/Foot Malformation (SHFM), Syndromic, p63 Associated

Synonyms
Ectrodactyly with ectodermal dysplasia, various forms

Includes
Ectrodactyly, ectodermal dysplasia, and cleft lip/palate syndrome 3
MIM 604292
Limb–mammary syndrome
MIM 603543
ADULT syndrome
MIM 103285
Ankyloblepharon–ectodermal defects–cleft lip/palate; Hay–Wells syndrome
MIM 106260
Rapp–Hodgkin syndrome
MIM 129400

Major Clinical Findings
Split-hand/foot malformation (SHFM), typically characterized by defects of the central rays affecting the hands and/or feet, may occur as an isolated condition or in combination with other findings. One group of these conditions shows variable combination of the triad SHFM with ectodermal dysplasia and orofacial clefting. Because these conditions show overlapping features and are caused by mutations in the same gene, *p63*, they are presented together. Besides SHFM, ectodermal dysplasia is a main feature of this group, manifesting as abnormal growth in the development of tissue derived from embryonic ectoderm. This includes skin, teeth, hair, nails, and exocrine glands such as sweat glands and sebaceous glands of the skin. The skin can be very dry, itchy, and hypopigmented. Congenital skin erosions are often observed, which may be life threatening. However, the defects frequently recover after the first year of life. Abnormalities of the hair include alopecia; curly, wiry hair; and absence of the eyelashes, eyebrows, or both. The teeth are often malformed, conical, or missing. The diminished number of sweat glands can result in life-threatening hyperthermia. Lacrimal duct defects of obstruction are another typical feature. Another hallmark of *p63*-associated conditions is clefting consisting of cleft lip and/or cleft palate.

Five different conditions have been delineated clinically.

Ectrodactyly, ectodermal dysplasia, and cleft lip/palate (EEC) syndrome is the prototype of these conditions, characterized by one or more features of SHFM, ectodermal dysplasia, and clefting. The degree and type of ectodermal dysplasia are highly variable, mainly consisting of nail dysplasia, teeth defects, mammary gland/nipple hypoplasia, and hypohidrosis. Cleft lip/palate is present in about 40 %, and SHFM featuring ectrodactyly or syndactyly in approximately 40 %.

Limb–mammary syndrome (LMS) is similar to EEC, but the ectodermal changes are milder. All affected individuals have mammary gland/nipple hypoplasia. Other ectodermal features include nail hypoplasia, lacrimal duct obstruction, hypohidrosis, and teeth defects, whereas abnormalities of the hair and skin are not typically part of this condition. Orofacial clefting in the form of cleft palate occurs in 30 %.

Acro-dermato-ungual-lacrimal-tooth (ADULT) syndrome is very similar to LMS, and clear differences are apparent only when studying larger pedigrees. In ADULT syndrome, orofacial clefting is absent, and teeth, skin, and nail defects are constantly present.

Ankyloblepharon–ectodermal defects–cleft lip/palate (AEC) syndrome, also called Hay–Wells syndrome, is characterized by the severity of the skin lesions, the presence of eyelid fusion at birth, and the absence of limb abnormalities. The eyelid fusion, ankyloblepharon, is present in approximately 45 % of patients but is rarely a feature of other *p63*-associated syndromes. Other ectodermal defects are common. Cleft lip is observed in 40 % and cleft palate in 80 %.

Rapp–Hodgkin syndrome is very similar to AEC but with the absence of ankyloblepharon. A clinical separation between the two conditions is probably not indicated.

Genetic Transmission
Autosomal dominant with variable expressivity.

Differential Diagnosis
Overlap with other isolated SHFM conditions exists, and separation may be difficult based on the limb phenotype. There is general overlap with other ectodermal dysplasia syndromes.

Molecular Pathology
p63 is a transcription factor involved in ectodermal development. It is important for maintaining proliferative activity in specialized ectodermal cells. Accordingly, mice in which p63 is inactive show severe ectodermal abnormalities, including the absence of skin and its derivatives. In the limb it appears to be essential for maintaining the apical ectodermal ridge (AER), which is also ectodermal in origin. Lack

S. Mundlos, D. Horn, *Limb Malformations*,
DOI 10.1007/978-3-540-95928-1_91, © Springer-Verlag Berlin Heidelberg 2014

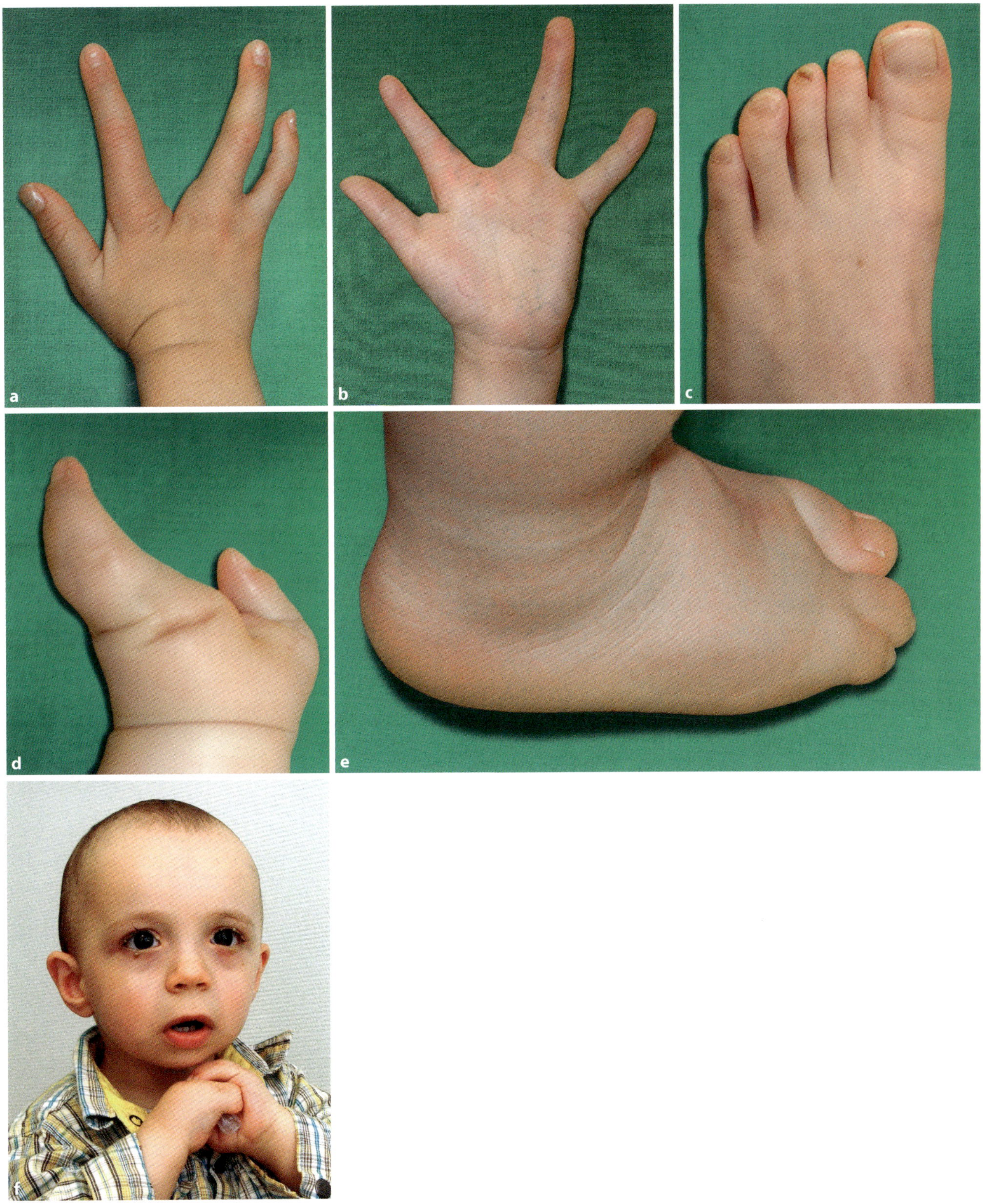

Fig. 91.1 ADULT syndrome. **a, b** Dorsal and palmar views of typical split-hand/foot malformation hand with missing middle digit. **c** Foot of same individual. Note cutaneous syndactyly of toes I and II. **d–f** Son of the individual in **a**. **d** Synmonodactyly of the hand, sparing the thumb. **e** Oligosyndactyly of the foot. **f** Lacrimal duct stenosis and conjunctivitis; thin scalp hair. (Courtesy of Lionel van Maldergem, University de Franche-Comté, Besançon, France)

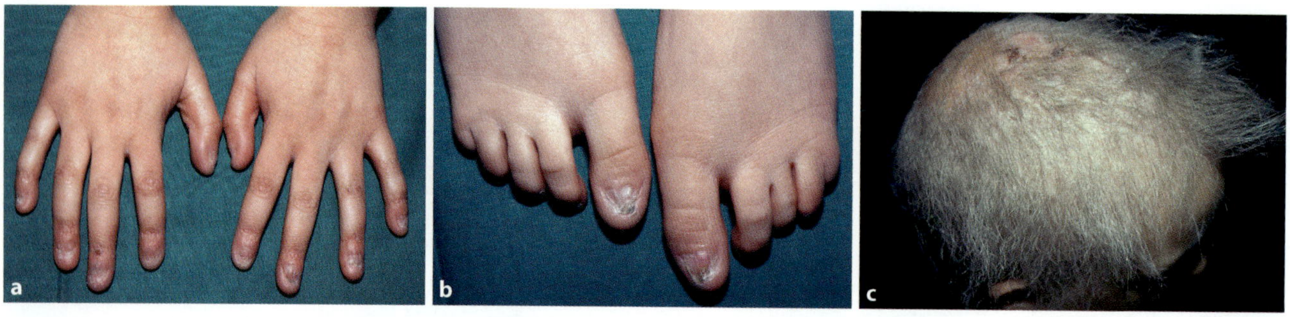

Fig. 91.2 Hay–Wells (AEC) syndrome. Nail dysplasia of the hands (**a**) and feet (**b**). **c** Wiry, sparse hair with patchy alopecia; hyperkeratosis

of AER signaling results in a loss of proliferative activity in the underlying progress zone, which in turn results in the SHFM phenotype. Phenotype–genotype correlations exist to a certain degree. Mutations in the DNA binding domain of p63 result in EEC syndrome. AEC syndrome is characteristically associated with mutations in the SAM and TI domains. The SAM domain binds a member of the RNA processing machinery that is known to regulate alternative splicing, such as FGFR2. As shown in a mouse model, the mutations exert a selective dominant-negative function on wild-type p63 by affecting progenitor cell expansion during ectodermal development, leading to a defective epidermal stem cell compartment via reduced expression of Fgfr2 and Fgfr3. Loss of function mutations in FGFR2 results in lacrimo-auriculo-dento-digital syndrome (LADD), a condition showing several overlapping features with *p63*-associated conditions.

References

Celli J, Duijf P, Hamel BC, Bamshad M, Kramer B, Smits AP et al (1999) Heterozygous germline mutations in the p53 homolog p63 are the cause of EEC syndrome. Cell 99(2):143–153

Ferone G, Thomason HA, Antonini D, De Rosa L, Hu B, Gemei M et al (2012) Mutant p63 causes defective expansion of ectodermal progenitor cells and impaired FGF signalling in AEC syndrome. EMBO Mol Med 4(3):192–205

Rinne T, Brunner HG, van Bokhoven H (2007) p63-associated disorders. Cell Cycle 6(3):262–268

92 Hartsfield Syndrome

MIM 615465

Major Clinical Findings

Hartsfield syndrome refers to the triad of holoprosencephaly, ectrodactyly, and cleft lip/palate. Most affected individuals have semilobar or lobar holoprosencephaly; only a few show mild expression of holoprosencephaly. Depending on the brain anomalies, the condition is lethal. Survivors show developmental delay and intellectual disability. Ectrodactyly is variable, ranging from syndactyly with hypoplastic central digits to monodactyly. Abnormalities of the genitalia in males include small penis, hypospadias, and cryptorchidism. Vertebral segmentation defects may occur.

Genetic Transmission

Autosomal dominant and recessive inheritance.

Differential Diagnosis

A phenotypic overlap exists between this condition and the ectrodactyly, ectodermal dysplasia, and cleft lip/palate (EEC) syndrome because of the presence of ectrodactyly and cleft lip/palate in both.

Molecular Pathology

Dominant or recessive mutations in *FGFR1* cause Hartsfield syndrome.

References

Hartsfield JK Jr., Bixler D, DeMyer WE (1984) Hypertelorism associated with holoprosencephaly and ectrodactyly. J Clin Dysmorph 2:27–31

Konig R, Beeg T, Tariverdian G, Scheffer H, Bitter K (2003) Holoprosencephaly, bilateral cleft lip and palate and ectrodactyly: another case and follow up. Clin Dysmorph 12:221–225

Simonis N, Migeotte I, Lambert N, Perazzolo C, de Silva DC, Dimitrov B et al (2013) FGFR1 mutations cause Hartsfield syndrome, the unique association of holoprosencephaly and ectrodactyly. J Med Genet 50:585–592

Vilain C, Mortier G, Van Vliet G, Dubourg C, Heinrichs C, de Silva D et al (2009) Hartsfield holoprosencephaly-ectrodactyly syndrome in five male patients: further delineation and review. Am J Med Genet 149A:1476–1481

S. Mundlos, D. Horn, *Limb Malformations*,
DOI 10.1007/978-3-540-95928-1_92, © Springer-Verlag Berlin Heidelberg 2014

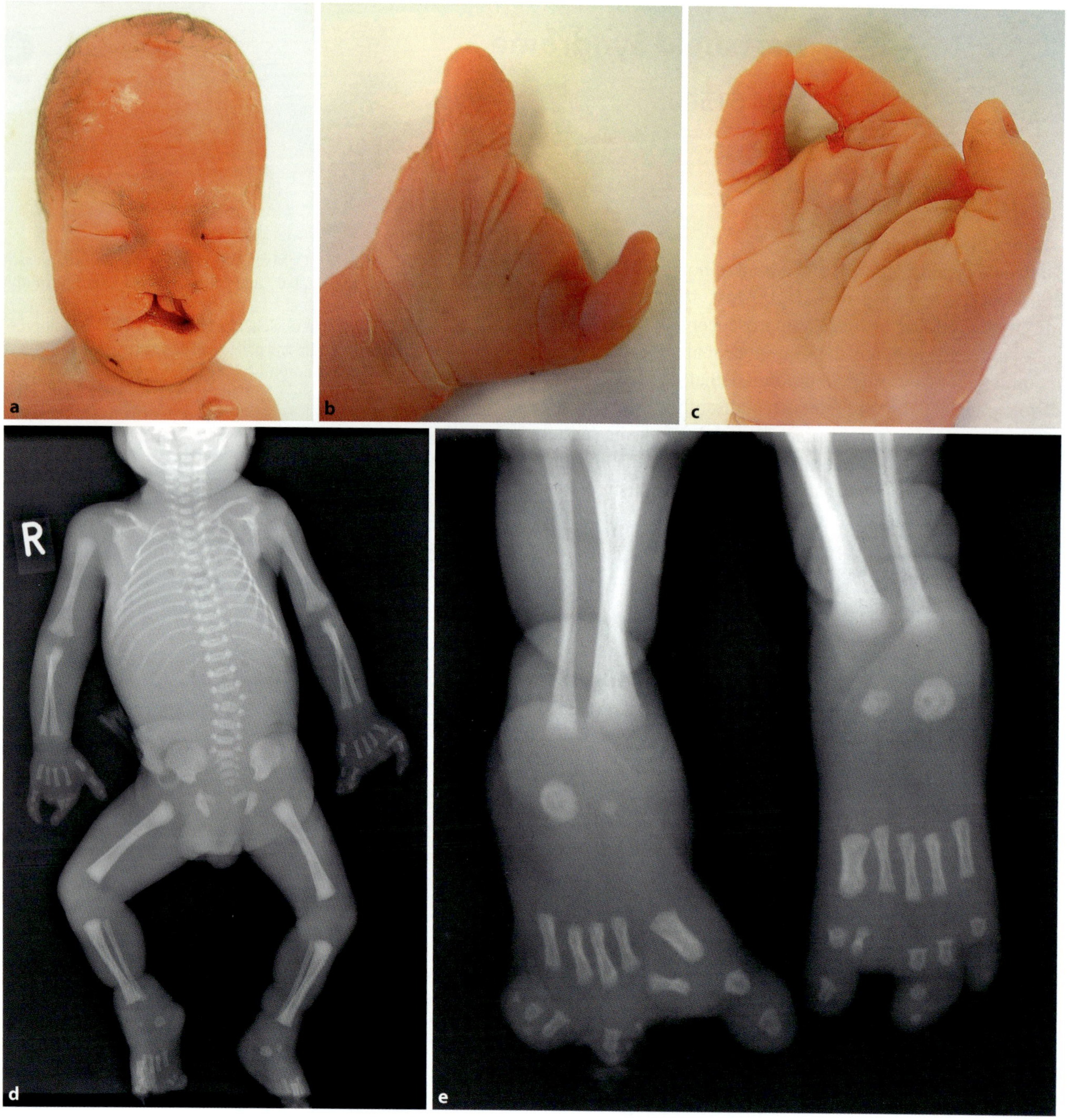

Fig. 92.1 **a** Fetus with Hartsfield syndrome. Note cleft lip/palate. Ultrasound and autopsy showed holoprosencephaly. **b, c** Cleft hand bilaterally. **d** Whole body radiograph. Note asymmetric clefting of the hands and feet and abnormality of the lumbar spine. **e** Anteroposterior view of feet and ankles: asymmetric foot deformities with fusion of toes and centrally missing phalanges

Part XVII
Acromesomelic Dysplasia

93 Acromesomelic Dysplasia, Maroteaux Type

MIM 602875

Major Clinical Findings

The term acromesomelic refers to disproportionate shortening of skeletal elements, predominantly affecting the middle segments (forearms and forelegs) and distal segments (hands and feet) of the appendicular skeleton. Patients with this condition show small to normal birth length, but skeletal growth falls off sharply after birth, resulting in severe short stature from early childhood on. In the limbs there are short tubular bones, bowed forearms, very short and broad fingers, short toes, and large halluces. Also seen are redundant skin on the fingers, short nails, and ligamentous laxity, especially of the finger joints. Disproportionately short limbs are often noted at birth but become more apparent during the first year of life. There is midface hypoplasia with a depressed nasal bridge and a small nose. There are no distinctive radiological signs at birth, but later changes include shortening and bowing of the radius; radial head subluxation or dislocation; very short and broad metacarpals, metatarsals, and phalanges; and cone-shaped epiphyses. The axial skeletal is also involved, characterized by increased lumbar lordosis, lower thoracic kyphosis, and gibbus deformity. Also seen are oval vertebral bodies in early infancy, then relative posterior hypoplasia and anterior central protrusion. Intellectual development is normal.

Genetic Transmission

Autosomal recessive.

Differential Diagnosis

Acrodysostosis and sometimes pseudohypoparathyroidism have similar hand changes but are distinguished by the absence of abnormalities of the forearms and vertebrae.

Molecular Pathology

Acromesomelic dysplasia type Maroteaux is caused by mutations in the gene coding for natriuretic peptide receptor b/guanylate cyclase b (NPR2), a homodimeric transmembrane receptor that produces cytoplasmic cyclic guanosine monophosphate (GMP) from guanosine-5'-triphosphate (GTP) on binding its extracellular ligand, C-type natriuretic peptide (CNP). Npr2 null mice show impaired endochondral ossification, resulting in dwarfism that becomes more prominent as the mice grow older. Thus, NPR2 is involved in the regulation of skeletal growth. Mice lacking the ligand for NPR2, CNP, are dwarfed, and mice overexpressing CNP have longer bones, suggesting that CNP signaling via its receptor NPR2 is important for growth plate function.

References

Bartels CF, Bukulmez H, Padayatti P, Rhee DK, van Ravenswaaij-Arts C, Pauli RM et al (2004) Mutations in the transmembrane natriuretic peptide receptor NPR-B impair skeletal growth and cause acromesomelic dysplasia, type Maroteaux. Am J Hum Genet 75:27–34

Langer LO, Garrett RT (1980) Acromesomelic dysplasia. Radiology 137:349–355

Tsuji T, Kunieda T (2005) A loss-of-function mutation in natriuretic peptide receptor 2 (Npr2) gene is responsible for disproportionate dwarfism in cn/cn mouse. J Biol Chem 280(14):14288–14292

S. Mundlos, D. Horn, *Limb Malformations*,
DOI 10.1007/978-3-540-95928-1_93,

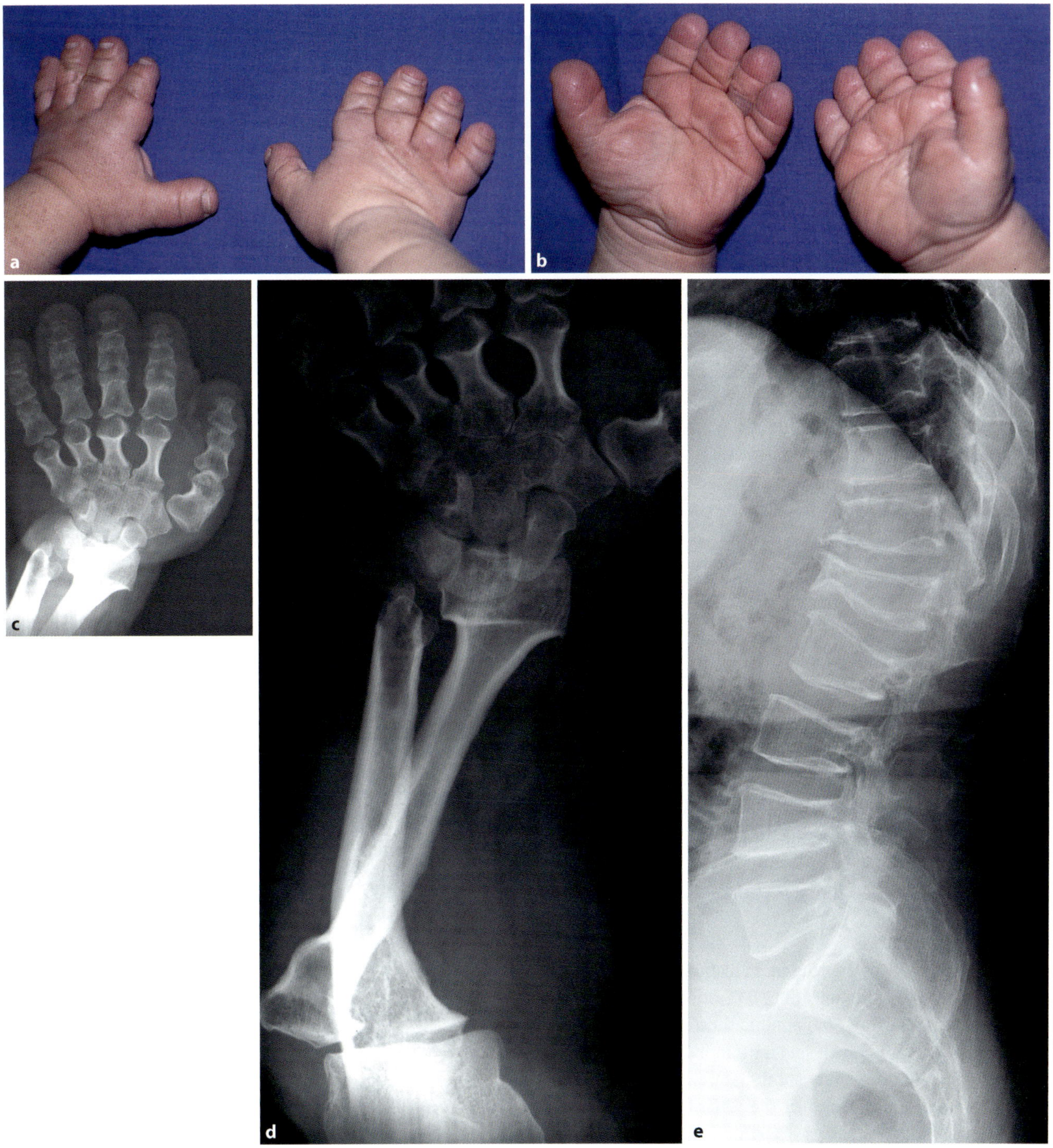

Fig. 93.1 Dorsal (**a**) and palmar (**b**) views of hands in acromesomelic dysplasia Maroteaux type. All elements are very short. **c** Radiograph of hand showing very short and broad phalanges as well as short and distally broad metacarpals and carpal fusions. These hand changes are similar to those in acrodysostosis. **d** Frontal view of forearm shows mesomelia with proportional shortening of the radius and ulna, dislocation of the proximal radius, and multiple carpal fusions. **e** Radiograph of lateral lumbar spine. Note residual anterior wedging of several lumbar vertebrae with generalized osteoporosis

94 Léri–Weill Dyschondrosteosis; Mesomelic Dysplasia, Langer Type

OMIM 127300; OMIM 249700

Major Clinical Findings

Léri–Weill dyschondrosteosis is characterized by short forearms (mesomelia), short stature, and Madelung deformity of the wrist. Madelung deformity is a reducible dorsal subluxation of the distal end of the ulna. It is caused by a growth disturbance in the volar-ulnar distal radial physis, resulting in a volar and ulnar tilt of the distal radial articular surface. The carpal bones show triangulation with the lunate at the proximal apex. The tibias are short, with a prominent medial portion of the proximal tibia. Although the disorder occurs in both sexes, it is usually more severe in females, perhaps due to sex differences in estrogen levels.

Langer mesomelic dysplasia, the homozygous form of Léri–Weill dyschondrosteosis, is a severe mesomelic limb dysplasia affecting the ulna and fibula. The radius and tibia are thickened and curved. These changes can result in displacement deformities of the hands and feet. Hypoplasia of the mandible has been reported.

Genetic Transmission

The mutated genes, *SHOX* or *SHOXY*, are located on the pseudoautosomal region of the X and Y chromosomes, respectively. Accordingly, the inheritance is autosomal dominant in Léri–Weill dyschondrosteosis and recessive in Langer mesomelic dysplasia.

Differential Diagnosis

Together with short stature, the same features can be found in Turner syndrome. Mutations in *SHOX* or *SHOXY* have also been reported as a cause of idiopathic short stature. However, this appears to be infrequent, and most individuals show some degree of disproportionately short stature and at least some (radiological) abnormalities of the wrist (triangularization of the distal radial epiphysis, triangularization of the distal carpal row).

The forearms in Langer mesomelic dysplasia patients show features similar to those of mesomelic dysplasia Kantaputra type.

Molecular Pathology

Dyschondrosteosis is caused by heterozygous deletions or mutations in *SHOX* or *SHOXY*. Regulatory mutations (deletions upstream of *SHOX*) have been shown to be a frequent cause of the condition. Langer mesomelic dysplasia is the homozygous expression of dyschondrosteosis. *SHOX* appears to function as a repressor of growth plate fusion and skeletal maturation in the distal limbs, counteracting the effects of estrogens. Accordingly, *SHOX* overdosage leads to long limbs and tall stature resulting from continued growth into the late teens.

References

Belin V, Cusin V, Viot G, Girlich D, Toutain A, Moncla A et al (1998) SHOX mutations in dyschondrosteosis (Léri–Weill syndrome). Nature Genet 19:67–69

Kunze J, Klemm T (1980) Mesomelic dysplasia, type Langer—a homozygous state for dyschondrosteosis. Europ J Pediat 134:269–272

Ogata T, Matsuo N, Nishimura G (2001) SHOX haploinsufficiency and overdosage: impact of gonadal function status. J Med Genet 38:1–6

Sabherwal N, Bangs F, Roth R, Weiss B, Jantz K, Tiecke E et al (2007) Long-range conserved non-coding SHOX sequences regulate expression in developing chicken limb and are associated with short stature phenotypes in human patients. Hum Molec Genet 16:210–222

S. Mundlos, D. Horn, *Limb Malformations*,
DOI 10.1007/978-3-540-95928-1_94, © Springer-Verlag Berlin Heidelberg 2014

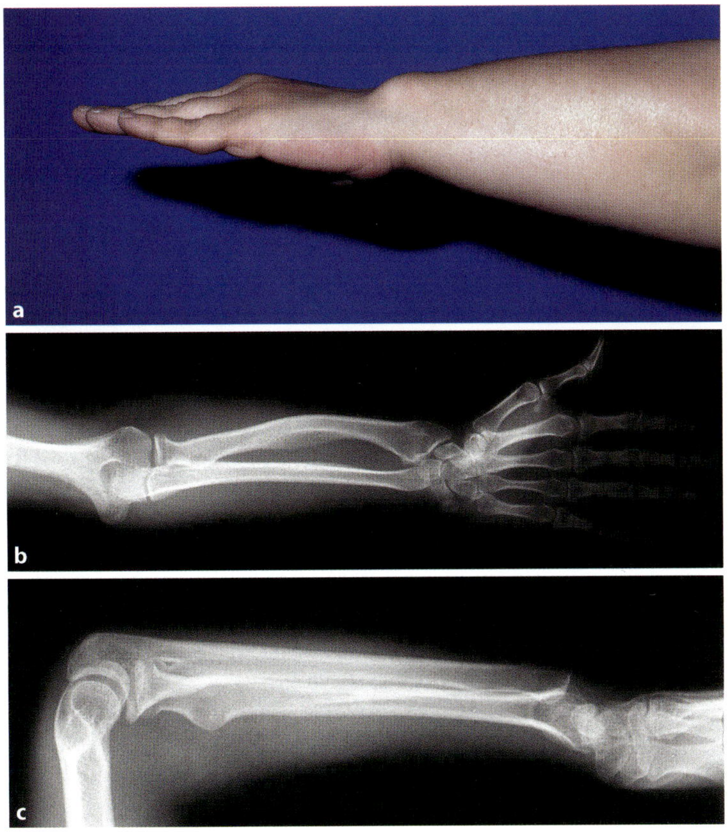

Fig. 94.1 Léri–Weill dyschondrosteosis. **a** Madelung deformity of the wrist. **b, c** Radiographs of the forearm and hand (**b** true anteroposterior view, **c** lateral view) reveal a medial distal slope of the radius with posterior dislocation of the ulna and herniation of the carpal bones, producing a wedge-shaped deformity (Madelung deformity). The radius is bowed

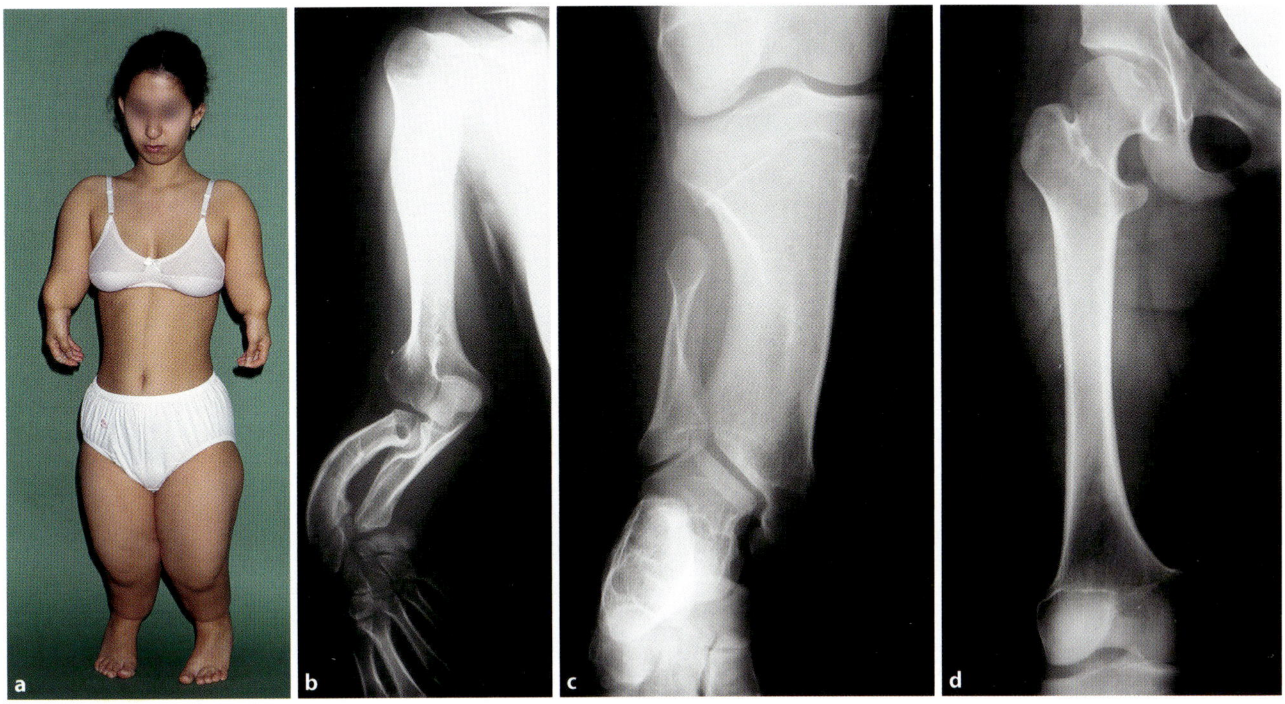

Fig. 94.2 Mesomelic dysplasia, Langer type. **a** Langer mesomelic dysplasia with shortening of the limbs. Note bulging of the distal forearm, which corresponds to a bowed radius. **b** Anteroposterior (AP) view of the right arm. Mildly short humerus, very short radius and ulna, bowed radius. **c** AP view of the lower limb. The tibia is very short and broad; the fibula is small and hypoplastic. **d** Somewhat short, otherwise normally formed femur

95 Robinow Syndrome

MIM 268310

Synonyms
Costovertebral segmentation defect with mesomelia
COVESDEM syndrome

Major Clinical Findings
Robinow syndrome is a complex malformation disorder with mesomelic limb shortening that tends to be more severe in the upper limbs. The digit anomalies are variable but usually comprise brachydactyly with small hands for age, nail dysplasia, broad thumbs, and 5th-finger clinodactyly. In some patients, cutaneous syndactyly and a split-hand phenotype have been described, indicating some overlap with other forms of syndactyly, brachydactyly type B (BDB), and split-hand/foot malformation. Radiographs show short and deformed radius and ulna, radioulnar dislocation, and bifid terminal phalanges of the thumb and occasionally of other digits. Robinow syndrome is characterized by a distinct dysmorphic facies ("fetal face") with macrocephaly; frontal bossing; hypertelorism; wide, downward slanting palpebral fissures; prominent eyes; large anterior fontanel; broad nose with anteverted nostrils; micrognathia; triangular mouth; clefts; ankyloglossia; and a bifid tongue. There is moderate shortness of stature. Scoliosis, hemivertebrae and other vertebral anomalies, rib fusions, and absent ribs indicate a general defect in vertebral segmentation. Genital hypoplasia, renal duplication, hydronephrosis, and cryptorchidism are other common features. Developmental retardation and developmental delay occur in a minority of patients. A second form of Robinow syndrome with autosomal dominant mode of inheritance exists, and there is considerable overlap between the two forms.

Occasional Findings
Madelung deformity, dislocation of the hip, seizures, inguinal hernia, nevus flammeus, and cardiac defects, especially right ventricular outlet obstruction.

Genetic Transmission
Two forms of Robinow syndrome exist, an autosomal recessive variant and an autosomal dominant variant.

Differential Diagnosis
The dominant form of Robinow syndrome is less severe than the recessive. In particular, the vertebral malformations, severe mesomelic shortening, radioulnar dislocation, and triangular-shaped mouth are less pronounced. Aarskog syndrome has a somewhat similar appearance but can be differentiated by the abnormal scrotum and absence of other typical signs such as vertebral malformations. Nail hypoplasia and the cleft in the distal phalanx of the thumb are also seen in brachydactyly type B (BDB); however, in this condition there are usually no abnormalities outside of the hand.

Molecular Pathology
Autosomal recessive Robinow syndrome is caused by homozygous missense, nonsense, and frameshift mutations in *ROR2*, leading to loss of function. Inactivation of ROR2 in the mouse results in shortening of all long bones, spinal malformations, craniofacial malformations, and small external genitals, thus resembling human Robinow syndrome. Truncating mutations in *ROR2* with a dominant negative effect cause BDB.

References

Afzal AR, Rajab A, Fenske CD, Oldridge M, Elanko N, Ternes-Pereira E et al (2000) Recessive Robinow syndrome, allelic to dominant brachydactyly type B, is caused by mutation of ROR2. Nature Genet 25:419–422

Mazzeu JF, Pardono E, Vianna-Morgante AM, Richieri-Costa A, Kim CA, Brunoni D et al (2007) Clinical characterization of autosomal dominant and recessive variants of Robinow syndrome. Am J Med Genet 143A:320–325

Schwabe GC, Trepczik B, Suring K, Brieske N, Tucker AS, Sharpe PT et al (2004) Ror2 knockout mouse as a model for the developmental pathology of autosomal recessive Robinow syndrome. Dev Dyn 229:400–410

Tufan F, Cefle K, Turkmen S, Turkmen A, Zorba U, Dursun M et al (2005) Clinical and molecular characterization of two adults with autosomal recessive Robinow syndrome. Am J Med Genet 136A:185–189

S. Mundlos, D. Horn, *Limb Malformations*,
DOI 10.1007/978-3-540-95928-1_95,

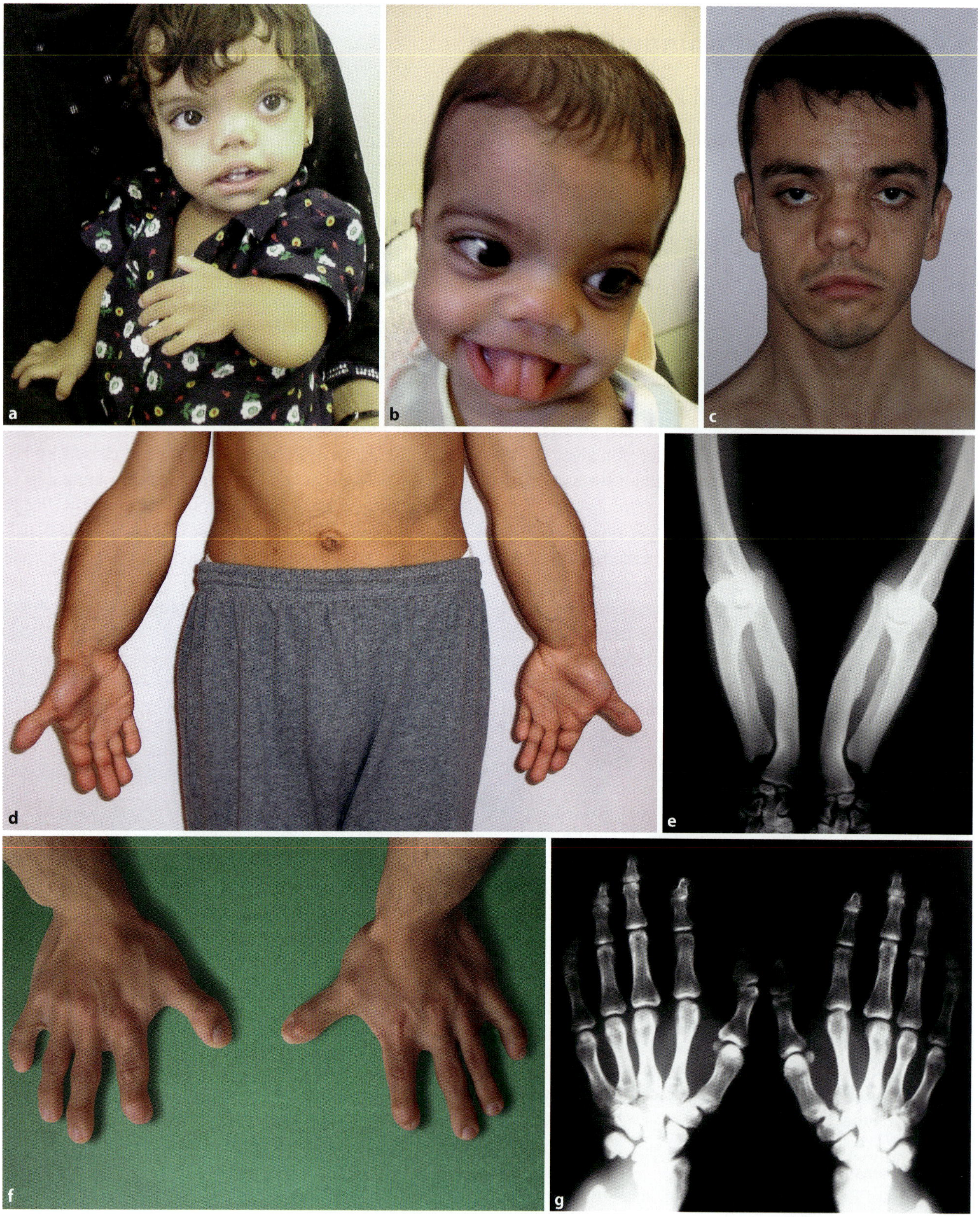

Fig. 95.1 **a, b** Typical Robinow facies with hypertelorism, short upturned nose, and triangular mouth. The limbs show mesomelic shortening. **c** Mild expression of Robinow syndrome in a young adult **d** Mesomelic shortening of the limbs in Robinow syndrome. **e** Corresponding radiograph shows short forearms, broad hypoplastic ulna, and broad radius with distal bending. **f** Hands of individual shown in **d**, with corresponding radiograph in **g**. Note the small hands, short digits, and distal hypoplasia (most severe in digit II) with nail hypoplasia. (**b, d–g** from Tufan et al. 2005)

Mesomelic Dysplasia, Kantaputra Type

OMIM 156232

96

Synonyms

Mesomelic dysplasia with ankle, carpal, and tarsal synostosis
Mesomelic dysplasia, Thai type

Major Clinical Findings

Originally described in a large Thai family, mesomelic dysplasia Kantaputra type (MDK) is characterized by bilateral, symmetrical marked shortening of the forearm. The hands show no major involvement. Radiographs show a very short ulna with a cuboidal shape and a short and bowed radius. The feet are very abnormal in an extended position. Affected individuals walk on the tips of their toes with the dorsal foot deviated laterally. Radiographs of the lower limbs show a shortening of the proximal fibula and synostoses between the tibia and fibula and between the small, malformed calcaneus and talus. A prominent calcaneus on the ventral surface of the distal fibula is a characteristic feature. In this family the average height of affected male adults was 152 cm.

Genetic Transmission

Autosomal dominant.

Differential Diagnosis

The clinical features are very characteristic, in particular those of the feet. A similar type of mesomelic shortening of the forearm also occurs in Langer dysplasia.

Molecular Pathology

MDK is associated with rearrangements at the *HOXD* locus. A very similar MDK-like phenotype exists in the mouse, the mutant ulnaless (Ul). Ul mice have very short ulnas, the radius is short and bowed, and the autopod is normal. Ul is caused by an inversion of the entire HOXD cluster. The original Thai family with MDK was shown to harbor a duplication of the HOXD cluster and a second duplication nearby. The similarity in phenotypes suggests similar pathogenic mechanisms. In Ul the inversion results in a disconnection of the 5' and 3' Hoxd genes from their respective regulatory sequences, moving the 5' genes, Hoxd10–13, in the vicinity of the 3' regulator, and vice versa. This results in an aberrant expression of Hoxd13 in the domain of Hoxd11, causing a functional inactivation of the latter. The MDK duplication is likely to have a similar effect by placing 5' genes next to the 3' regulators.

References

Kantaputra PN, Gorlin RJ, Langer LO Jr. (1992) Dominant mesomelic dysplasia, ankle, carpal, and tarsal synostosis type: a new autosomal dominant bone disorder. Am J Med Genet 44:730–737

Kantaputra PN, Klopocki E, Hennig BP, Praphanphoj V, Le Caignec C, Isidor B et al (2010) Mesomelic dysplasia Kantaputra type is associated with duplications of the HOXD locus on chromosome 2q. Europ J Hum Genet 18:1310–1314

Peichel CL, Prabhakaran B, Vogt TF (1997) The mouse Ulnaless mutation deregulates posterior HoxD gene expression and alters appendicular patterning. Development 124(18):3481–3492

Spielmann M, Mundlos S (2013) Structural variations, the regulatory landscape of the genome and their alteration in human disease. Bioessays 35(6):533–543

Spitz F, Gonzalez F, Duboule D (2003) A global control region defines a chromosomal regulatory landscape containing the HoxD cluster. Cell 113(3):405–417

S. Mundlos, D. Horn, *Limb Malformations*,
DOI 10.1007/978-3-540-95928-1_96, © Springer-Verlag Berlin Heidelberg 2014

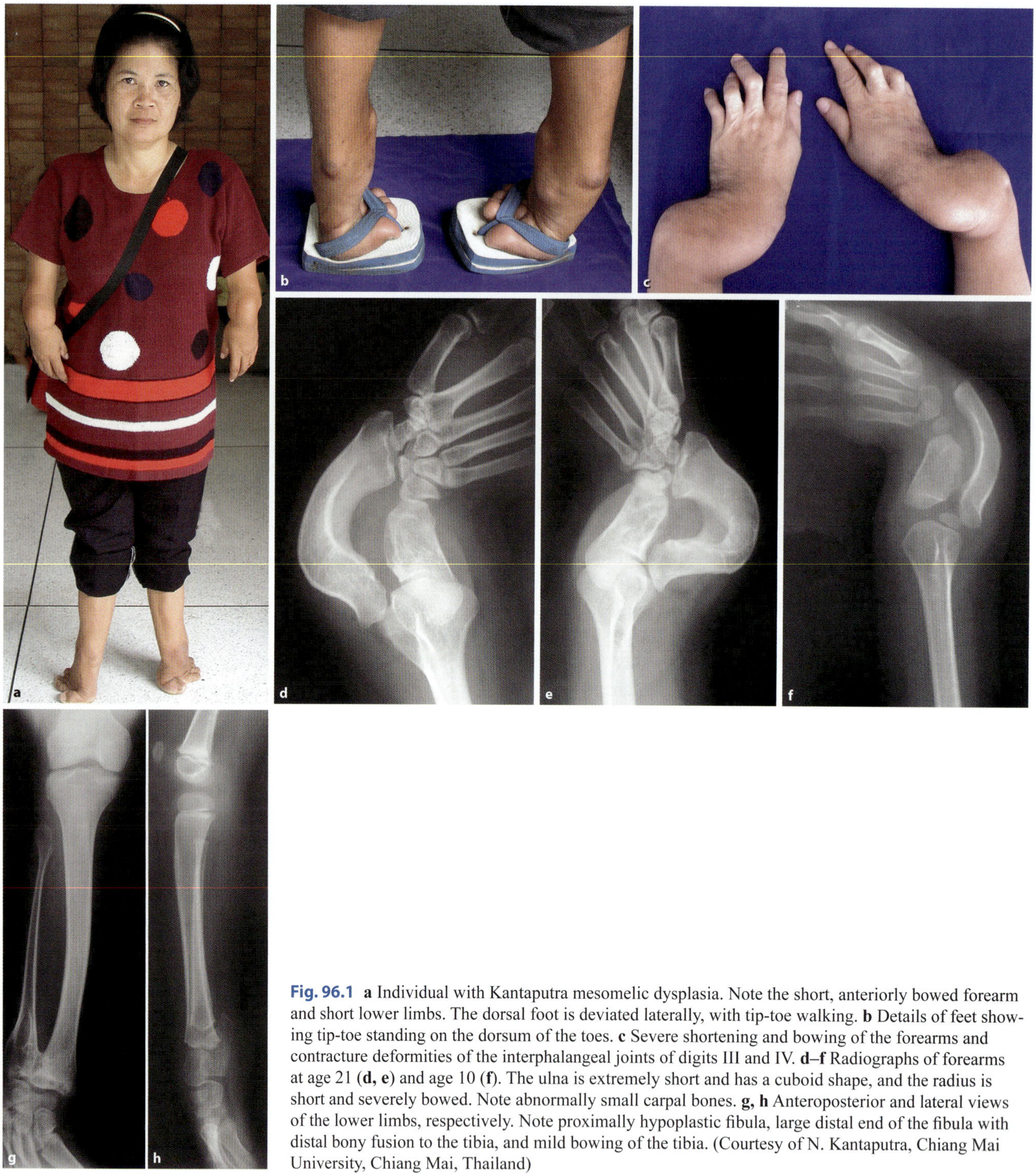

Fig. 96.1 **a** Individual with Kantaputra mesomelic dysplasia. Note the short, anteriorly bowed forearm and short lower limbs. The dorsal foot is deviated laterally, with tip-toe walking. **b** Details of feet showing tip-toe standing on the dorsum of the toes. **c** Severe shortening and bowing of the forearms and contracture deformities of the interphalangeal joints of digits III and IV. **d–f** Radiographs of forearms at age 21 (**d, e**) and age 10 (**f**). The ulna is extremely short and has a cuboid shape, and the radius is short and severely bowed. Note abnormally small carpal bones. **g, h** Anteroposterior and lateral views of the lower limbs, respectively. Note proximally hypoplastic fibula, large distal end of the fibula with distal bony fusion to the tibia, and mild bowing of the tibia. (Courtesy of N. Kantaputra, Chiang Mai University, Chiang Mai, Thailand)

Grebe Dysplasia; Hunter–Thompson Dysplasia; Du Pan Dysplasia; Chondrodysplasia, Acromesomelic, BMPR1B Type

97

Grebe Dysplasia

MIM 200700

Synonyms

Acromesomelic dysplasia, Grebe type

Hunter–Thompson Dysplasia

MIM 201250

Synonyms

Acromesomelic dwarfism

Du Pan Dysplasia

MIM 228900

Synonyms

Fibular hypoplasia and complex brachydactyly

Chondrodysplasia, Acromesomelic, BMPR1B Type

MIM 609441

Synonyms

Chondrodysplasia, acromesomelic, with genital anomalies

Major Clinical Findings

Acromesomelic chondrodysplasias of the Grebe type, Hunter–Thompson type, Du Pan type, and BMPR1B type are a group of conditions predominantly affecting the limbs with increasing severity in a proximodistal fashion. Grebe type dysplasia is the most severe form, characterized by shortening of the upper and lower limbs, bowing of the forearms, and very short, stumplike digits/toes. Affected individuals are of very short stature, with an adult height of approximately 100 cm. The nails are short but otherwise normal. There is limited extension, pronation, and supination of the elbows and normal shoulder movement. The lower extremities are very short, with limited extension and flexion of the knee and very short, overriding toes. Radiographs of the upper limbs show a short humerus and a short, bowed radius and ulna. The ulna is much shorter than the radius. Carpal bones show fusions, and metacarpals are rudimentary. Individual phalanges may appear to be absent due to missing ossification. Radiographs of the lower limb show a mildly short femur, a missing fibula, and a very short cuboid-shaped tibia. The patellae are small or absent. There is fusion of the tarsal bones, which are difficult to identify, and missing proximal and/or middle phalanges. The spine is normal. Heterozygous carriers of the mutation may show reduced penetrance and a mild phenotype consisting of clinodactyly and shortening of the middle phalanges, and thus show features overlapping brachydactyly types A1, A2, and C.

Patients with Hunter–Thompson type dysplasia show a similar picture but are not as severely affected. The radius and ulna are short but not as deformed as in Grebe dysplasia. The ulna may be shorter than or the same size as the radius, and radioulnar dislocation may be present. The digits are longer and partially functional. The metacarpals are very short, and two or three cuboid-shaped phalanges are present per digit. The tibia is relatively short, and the fibula is very short.

Du Pan dysplasia is characterized by mildly short stature, fibular hypoplasia or aplasia, complex brachydactyly, mild shortness of the hands, and short, knoblike toes. Radiographs show very short 1st metacarpals, short metacarpals II–V, relatively long proximal phalanges II–V, and hypoplastic or aplastic middle phalanges. The radius and ulna are of normal length. Tarsal bones are present but deformed, and metatarsals are short and malaligned.

Acromesomelic chondrodysplasia BMPR1B type shows skeletal features are similar to those in Du Pan and Hunter–Thompson dysplasias: aplasia of the fibula, hypoplasia or dysplasia of the tibia, severe brachydactyly with short metacarpals, hypoplastic or aplastic phalanges, and fusion of carpal/tarsal bones. In addition, females with this condition may have genitourinary abnormalities including hypoplasia of the uterus, as well as ovarian dysfunction with consecutive hypergonadotropic hypogonadism.

Genetic Transmission

Autosomal recessive.

Differential Diagnosis

The four conditions overlap in their clinical features and are part of a phenotypic spectrum. In some cases it may be difficult to differentiate among them.

Molecular Pathology

Grebe, Hunter–Thompson, and Du Pan dysplasias are caused by homozygous mutations in *GDF5*. The phenotypic spectrum appears to be due to partial residual function in the less severe conditions. Mutations in Du Pan dysplasia have been

S. Mundlos, D. Horn, *Limb Malformations*,
DOI 10.1007/978-3-540-95928-1_97, © Springer-Verlag Berlin Heidelberg 2014

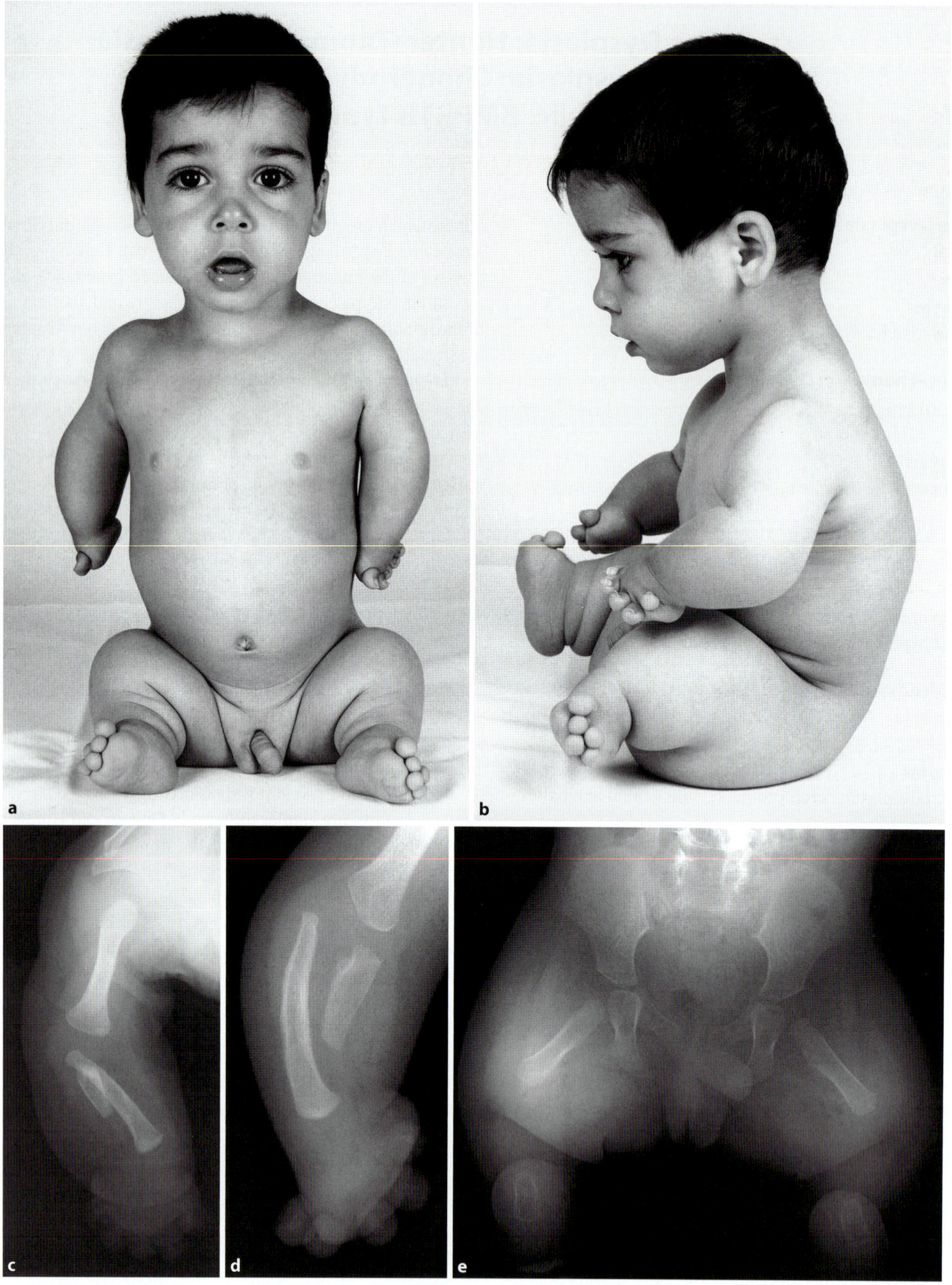

Fig. 97.1 **a, b** Individual with homozygous mutation in *GDF5* (insG206) and Grebe syndrome. Note very short limbs with acromesomelic shortening, which is more severe in the lower limbs, and knoblike digits. **c, d** Radiographs of right arm show short humerus, hypoplastic ulna, short and bowed radius, and absent or very few visible distal ossification centers in the hands. **e** Radiograph of pelvis and lower limbs. Note mildly hypoplastic femurs, absent ossification of fibula, and very short tibia. Calcaneal ossification is present. Normal pelvic bones. (Courtesy of J. Spranger, Sinzheim, Germany)

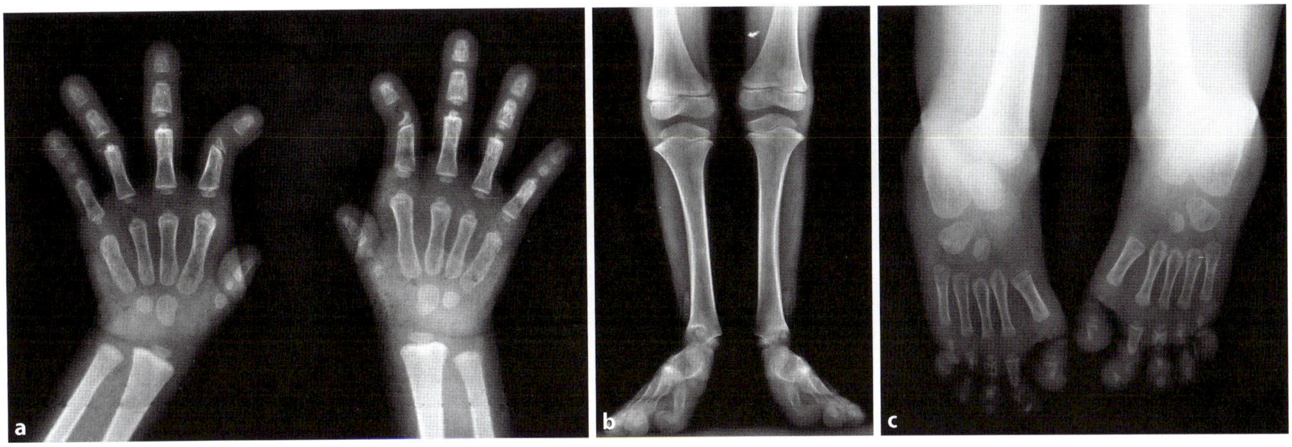

Fig. 97.2 **a** Radiograph of hands of 4-year-old patient with Du Pan syndrome. Note hypoplastic metacarpal I and middle phalanx, well-formed distal phalanx of the thumb, short metacarpals II–V, distal pseudoepiphyses of proximal phalanges II–V, absent middle phalanx of digit II with abnormal distal epiphyses of proximal phalanges of digits II resulting in medial deviation of digits II, and hypoplastic middle phalanx of digit V. **b** Lower limb radiograph of same individual showing almost absent fibula (rudimentary ossification can be seen at distal lateral side of tibia), short tibia with irregular distal tibial epiphyseal ossification, and normal distal femur. **c** Radiograph of feet and ankle region showing mildly short metatarsals, hypoplastic proximal phalanx of great toe, and very small ossification centers of phalanges, which are more pronounced distally and of which some have an angel-like appearance. (Courtesy of J. Spranger, Sinzheim, Germany)

described to be caused by BDA2 in the heterozygous state. The mouse mutant brachypodism (bp), caused by a loss of function mutation of Gdf5, exhibits similar cartilage and joint formation and serves as a model for these conditions. Acromesomelic chondrodysplasia BMPR1B type is caused by loss of function mutations in the BMP receptor 1B (BMPR1B). GDF5 is the high-affinity ligand for BMPR1B, thus explaining the overlapping phenotype with Du Pan syndrome. In the ovaries, however, BMPR1B is the receptor for other BMPs, including the ovary-specific BMP15.

References

Costa T, Ramsby G, Cassia F, Peters K-R, Soares J, Correa J et al (1998) Grebe syndrome: clinical and radiographic findings in affected individuals and heterozygous carriers. Am J Med Genet 75:523–529

Demirhan O, Turkmen S, Schwabe GC, Soyupak S, Akgul E, Tastemir D et al (2005) A homozygous BMPR1B mutation causes a new subtype of acromesomelic chondrodysplasia with genital anomalies. J Med Genet 42:314–317

Douzgou S, Lehmann K, Mingarelli R, Mundlos S, Dallapiccola B (2008) Compound heterozygosity for GDF5 in Du Pan type chondrodysplasia. Am J Med Genet 146A:2116–2121

Faiyaz-Ul-Haque M, Ahmad W, Zaidi SHE, Haque S, Teebi AS, Ahmad M et al (2002) Mutation in the cartilage-derived morphogenetic protein-1 (CDMP1) gene in a kindred affected with fibular hypoplasia and complex brachydactyly (DuPan syndrome). Clin Genet 61:454–458

Graul-Neumann LM, Deichsel A, Wille U, Kakar N, Koll R, Bassir C et al (2014) Homozygous missense and nonsense mutations in BMPR1B cause acromesomelic chondrodysplasia-type Grebe. Eur J Hum Genet 22(6):726–733

Hunter AGW, Thompson MW (1976) Acromesomelic dwarfism: description of a patient and comparison with previously reported cases. Hum Genet 34:107–113

Langer LO, Cervenka J, Camargo M (1989) A severe autosomal recessive acromesomelic dysplasia, the Hunter–Thompson type, and comparison with the Grebe type. Hum Genet 81:323–328

Thomas JT, Kilpatrick MW, Lin K, Erlacher L, Lembessis P, Costa T et al (1997) Disruption of human limb morphogenesis by a dominant negative mutation in CDMP1. Nature Genet 17:58–64

Thomas JT, Lin K, Nandekar M, Camargo M, Cervenka J, Luyten FP (1996) A human chondrodysplasia due to a mutation in a TGF-beta superfamily member. Nature Genet 12:315–317

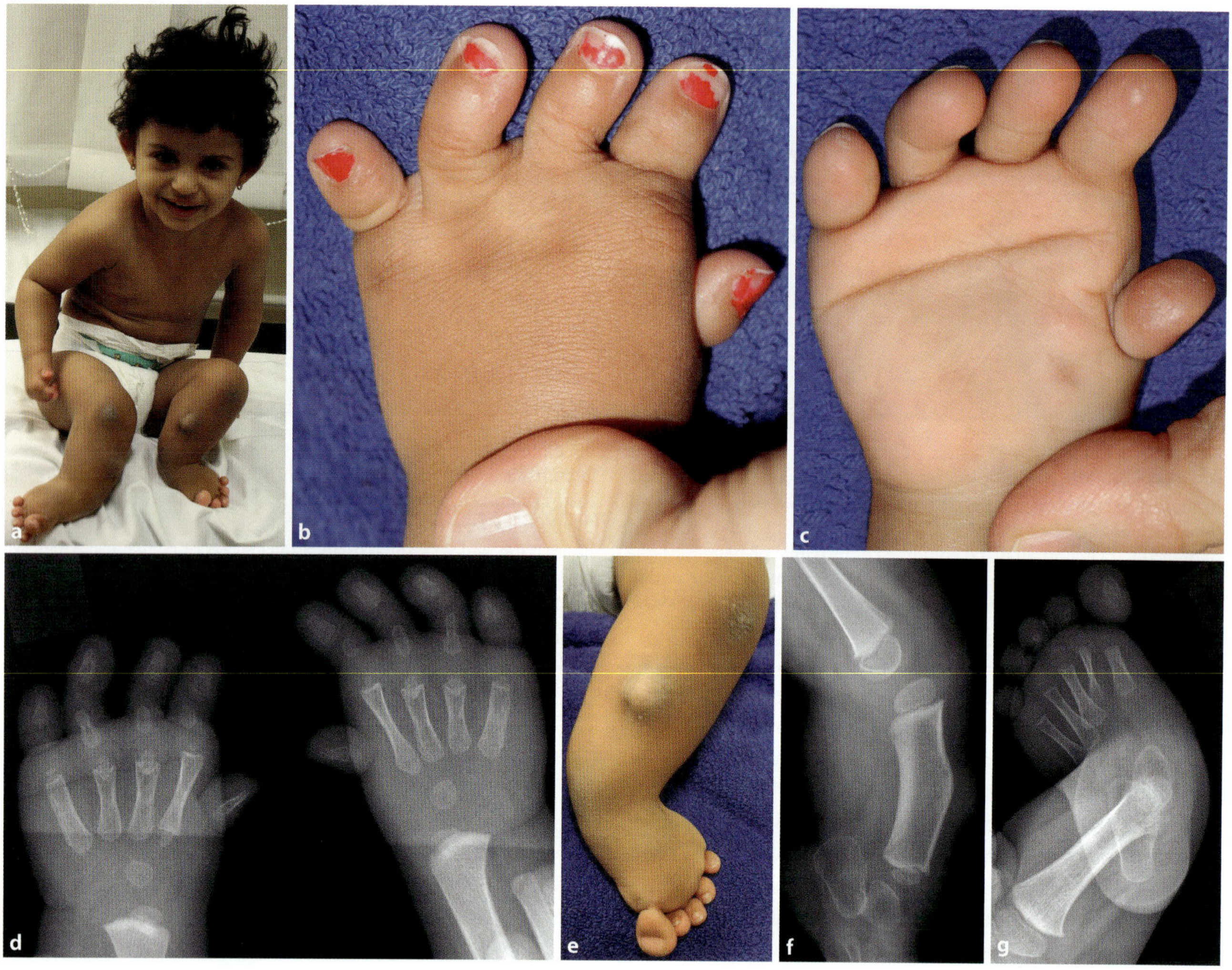

Fig. 97.3 **a** Two-year-old child with mutation in BMPR1B. Note short lower limbs with protrusion at the lateral medial tibia and knoblike toes. **b, c** Left hand dorsal (**b**) and palmar (**c**) views show very short fingers and missing interdigital creases. **d** Radiograph of hands and wrist showing short ulna, normal distal radius, single carpal ossification center, absent ossification middle phalanges III–V, hypoplastic/absent proximal phalanges II–V, cone-shaped epiphyses of metacarpals II and IV, absent ossification of metacarpal and proximal phalanx of thumb, and a single enlarged ossified carpal bone. **e** Protuberance at midshaft of lower leg and bulbous distal phalanges of toes. **f** Radiograph showing lateral view of distal femur to ankle. Note very short tibia with relatively normal epiphyseal ossification, anterior protrusion of the diaphysis, and absence of fibula. **g** Radiograph of foot shows thin/hypoplastic 2nd metatarsal, absent/hypoplastic ossification of multiple/all phalanges, and relatively normal talus/calcaneus. (From Graul-Neumann et al. 2014)

Mesomelic Dysplasia, Werner Type

MIM 188770

98

Synonyms

Tibial hemimelia-polydactyly-triphalangeal thumb syndrome

Major Clinical Findings

Mesomelic dysplasia Werner type is characterized by hypoplasia of the tibia with polydactyly of the feet and hands. Polydactyly of the hands is often of the triphalangeal type, featuring a thumb that is partially or completely duplicated and has three phalanges. The thumbs may also be hypoplastic, and fusion with the index finger may occur. Severe shortening of the legs is present due to the absence or severe hypoplasia of the tibia, with bowing and/or dislocation of the fibula. The fibula may be thickened or even duplicated. The lower limb findings can be asymmetric. Preaxial polydactyly and central polydactyly of the feet are seen. There is extended clinical variability in this condition.

Genetic Transmission

Autosomal dominant.

Differential Diagnosis

Mesomelic dysplasia Werner type is allelic with triphalangeal thumb polydactyly syndrome (TPT), Haas-type syndactyly, and Laurin–Sandrow syndrome. All conditions can be considered part of a phenotypic spectrum. Tibial hemimelia together with polydactyly has been described as being caused by deletions of the *PITX1* gene.

Molecular Pathology

Mesomelic dysplasia Werner type belongs to a group of conditions that are caused by alterations within the zone of polarizing activity regulatory sequence (ZRS), the regulatory region that controls *Sonic hedgehog* (*SHH*) expression in the limb bud. Mutations in the ZRS have been shown to result in misexpression of Shh in the anterior part of the limb bud, resulting in an ectopic, additional Shh signal.

References

Girisha KM, Bidchol AM, Kamath PS, Shah KH, Mortier GR, Mundlos S et al (2014) A novel mutation (g.106737G>T) in zone of polarizing activity regulatory sequence (ZRS) causes variable limb phenotypes in Werner mesomelia. Am J Med Genet A 164A(4):898–906

Kantaputra PN, Chalidapong P (2000) Are triphalangeal thumb-polysyndactyly syndrome (TPTPS) and tibial hemimelia-polysyndactyly-triphalangeal thumb syndrome (THPTTS) identical? A father with TPTPS and his daughter with THPTTS in a Thai family. Am J Med Genet 93(2):126–131

Wieczorek D, Pawlik B, Li Y, Akarsu NA, Caliebe A, May KJ et al (2010) A specific mutation in the distant sonic hedgehog (SHH) cis-regulator (ZRS) causes Werner mesomelic syndrome (WMS) while complete ZRS duplications underlie Haas type polysyndactyly and preaxial polydactyly (PPD) with or without triphalangeal thumb. Hum Mutat 31(1):81–89

S. Mundlos, D. Horn, *Limb Malformations*,
DOI 10.1007/978-3-540-95928-1_98, © Springer-Verlag Berlin Heidelberg 2014

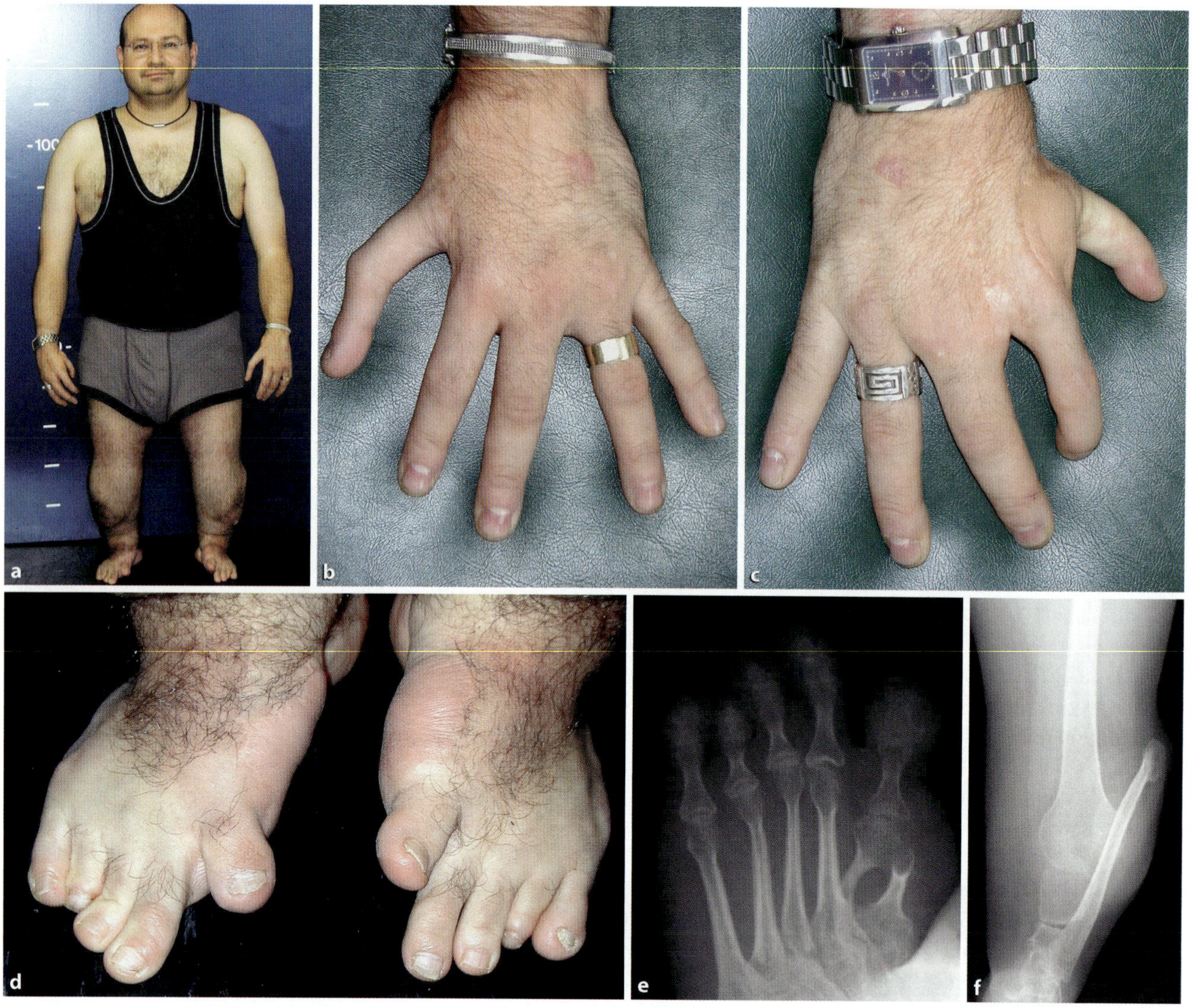

Fig. 98.1 **a** Patient 1. Short stature, shortening of forearms, triphalangeal thumb on the right side. The femurs are mildly shortened, with severely short lower legs due to very short tibia. **b, c** Close-up of hands showing five fingers with a triphalangeal first ray on the left and surgical correction on the right. **d** Small feet and short 1st toes. **e** Radiographically visible duplication of hypoplastic metatarsal I with shortening. **f** Radiograph of lower limb showing hypoplastic cuboid-shaped tibia with marked overgrowth of almost normal fibula with proximal dislocation. (From Wieczorek et al. 2010)

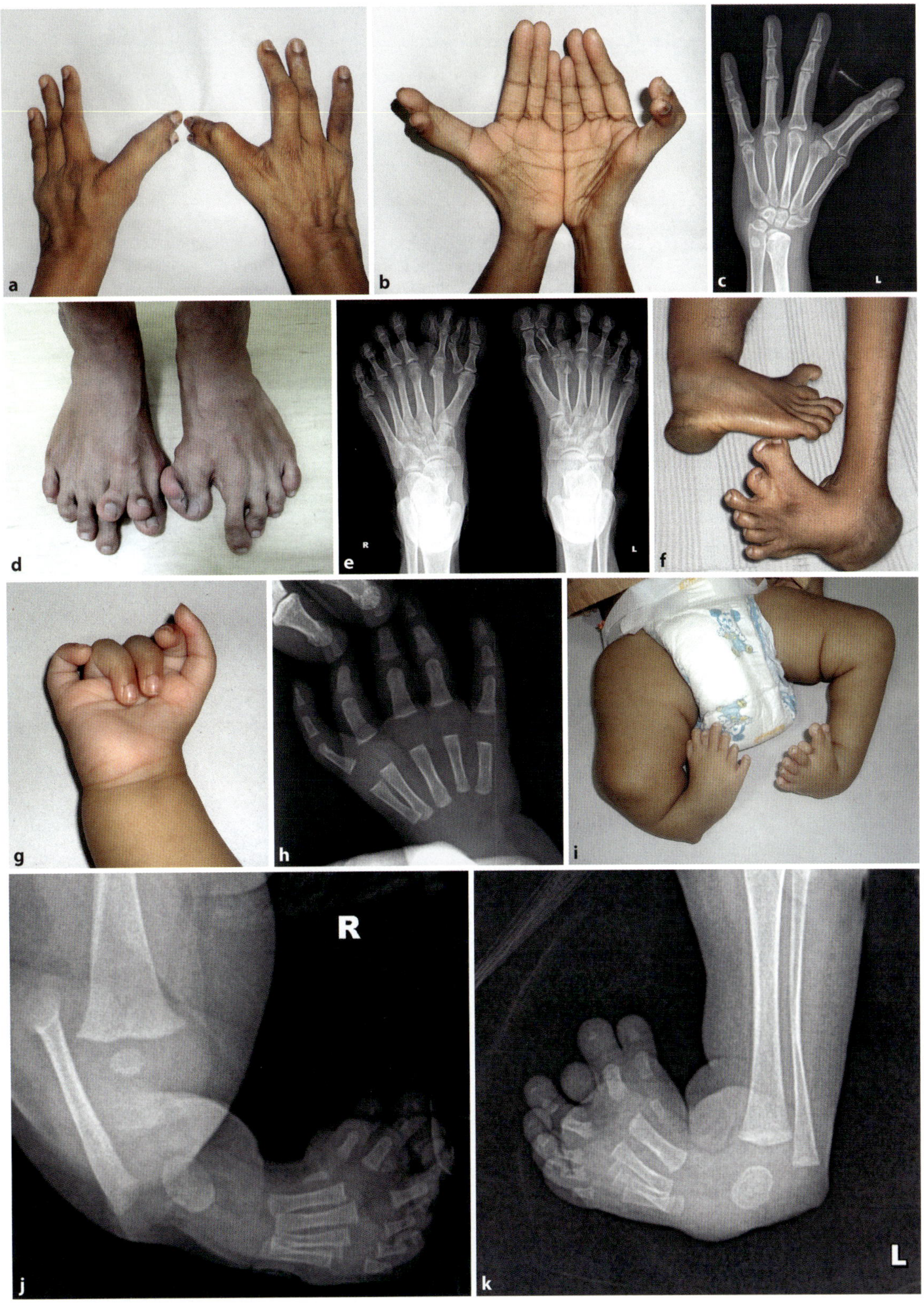

Fig. 98.2 Variability in a family with Werner syndrome. Dorsal (**a**) and palmar (**b**) views of hands show complete syndactyly of digits I and II. Radiograph (**c**) shows normal digits III–V but fusion (soft tissue) of a normal digit II with a small, digit-like triphalangeal thumb. The carpal bones are crowded and displaced. **d** Feet of the same individual with extensive polydactyly. **e** Radiograph shows seven digits, with an additional full digit bilaterally between toes I and II that originates from the tarsal bones. Additional toes branch from the metatarsals (interaxial polydactyly). **f** Mesomelic dysplasia with bilateral clubfoot due to short or absent (left) tibia; polydactyly. **g–i** Newborn with triphalangeal thumb (**g**) and corresponding radiograph (**h**); lower limb mesomelia (**i**) with clubfeet, absent talus, and seven-digit polydactyly. **j, k** Radiographs show absent (right) and short (left) tibia. (Courtesy of Hitesh Shah, Kasturba Medical College, Manipal, India)

99 Nievergelt Syndrome

MIM 163400

Synonyms

Mesomelic dysplasia, Nievergelt type

Major Clinical Findings

Nievergelt syndrome refers to a rather ill-defined group of conditions with specific deformities of the tibia. The tibia is severely hypoplastic and of rhomboid shape due to an abnormal position of the epiphysis, which is located laterally. The original family described by Nievergelt showed autosomal dominant inheritance of radioulnar synostosis as well as triangular tibias and fibulas. Subsequent descriptions included cases with triangular tibias, absent fibulas, and mild mesomelic shortening of the arms. In addition, malformations of the brain and internal organs, including horseshoe kidney and ambiguous genitalia, were observed.

Genetic Transmission

Unclear. Autosomal dominant in one family.

Differential Diagnosis

The rhomboid shape of the tibia is characteristic and differentiates this condition from other types of mesomelic dysplasia. Mesomelic dysplasia Savarirayan type (MIM 605274) is a related disorder.

References

Savarirayan R, Cormier-Daire V, Curry CJ, Nashelsky MB, Rappaport V, Rimoin DL et al (2000) New mesomelic dysplasia with absent fibulae and triangular tibiae. Am J Med Genet 94:59–63

Steichen-Gersdorf E, Gassner I, Superti-Furga A, Ullmann R, Stricker S, Klopocki E et al (2008) Triangular tibia with fibular aplasia associated with a microdeletion on 2q11.2 encompassing LAF4. Clin Genet 74:560–565

Tuysuz B, Zeybek C, Zorer G, Sipahi O, Ungur S (2002) Patient with the mesomelic dysplasia, Nievergelt syndrome, and cerebellovermian agenesis and cataracts. Am J Med Genet 109:206–210

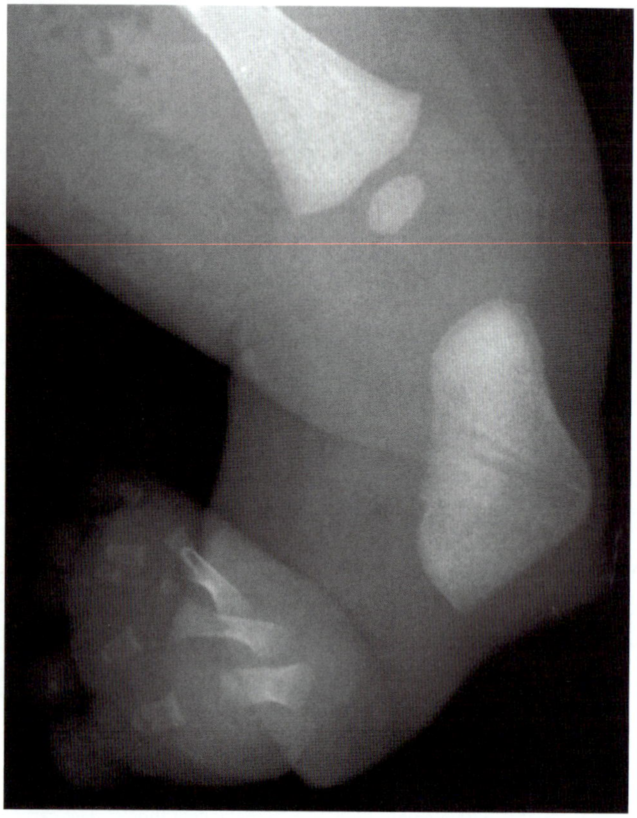

Fig. 99.1 Radiograph of lower limb showing triangular tibia and absence of fibula. There is abnormal ossification of the metatarsal and phalangeal bones of the feet

S. Mundlos, D. Horn, *Limb Malformations*,
DOI 10.1007/978-3-540-95928-1_99, © Springer-Verlag Berlin Heidelberg 2014

Part XVIII

Macrodactyly/Overgrowth

100 Hemihyperplasia, Isolated

MIM 235000

Synonyms
Hemihypertrophy, isolated

Major Clinical Findings
Isolated hemihyperplasia is characterized by asymmetric overgrowth of one or more regions of the body. The affected area may be a single digit, a single limb, unilateral facial involvement, or involvement of half the body. Hemihyperplasia may be crossed in a few cases and most frequently involves multiple tissues, such as muscle, bone, and the vascular system. Asymmetry is usually evident at birth and becomes more prominent with growth. Cutaneous anomalies include nevus flammeus and telangiectasia. Different neoplasms have been reported in association with hemihyperplasia. Most commonly, Wilms tumor, adrenal cortical carcinoma, and hepatoblastoma have been documented during childhood.

Occasional Findings
Enlarged tongue on affected side, hemimegalencephaly, unilateral nephromegaly, increased birth weight, scoliosis.

Genetic Transmission
Most of the cases are sporadic. Familial instances have been reported in some cases.

Differential Diagnosis
A distinct subtype has been delineated with static or mildly progressive hemihyperplasia and multiple lipomata, named hemihyperplasia–multiple lipomatosis syndrome. Hemihyperplasia can occur as a feature of Beckwith–Wiedemann syndrome. Asymmetry of limbs may also occur in Klippel–Trénaunay syndrome, Proteus syndrome, Silver–Russell syndrome, and CLOVE syndrome (congenital lipomatous overgrowth, vascular malformations, and epidermal nevi). Hemihyperplasia may be part of the epidermal nevus syndrome and different chromosomal mosaicisms, such as mosaic trisomy 8.

Molecular pathology
Patients with isolated hemihyperplasia were found to have paternal uniparental disomy of 11p15 or hypomethylation at KCNQ10T1 (LIT1) or H19. Patients with paternal uniparental disomy of 11p15 seem to have a higher tumor risk compared with patients without molecular alterations of these regions. The results suggest that isolated hemihyperplasia can be part of the spectrum of Beckwith–Wiedemann syndrome.

References

Hoyme HE, Seaver LH, Jones KL, Procopio F, Crooks W, Feingold M (1998) Isolated hemihyperplasia (hemihypertrophy): report of a prospective multicenter study of the incidence of neoplasia and review. Am J Med Genet 79:274–278

Shuman C, Smith AC, Steele L, Ray PN, Clericuzio C, Zackai E et al (2006) Constitutional UPD for chromosome 11p15 in individuals with isolated hemihyperplasia is associated with high tumor risk and occurs following assisted reproductive technologies. Am J Med Genet 140A:1497–1503

Viljoen D, Pearn J, Beighton P (1984) Manifestations and natural history of idiopathic hemihypertrophy: a review of eleven cases. Clin Genet 26:81–86

West PMH, Love DR, Stapleton PM, Winship IM (2003) Paternal uniparental disomy in monozygotic twins discordant for hemihypertrophy. J Med Genet 40:223–226

S. Mundlos, D. Horn, *Limb Malformations*,
DOI 10.1007/978-3-540-95928-1_100, © Springer-Verlag Berlin Heidelberg 2014

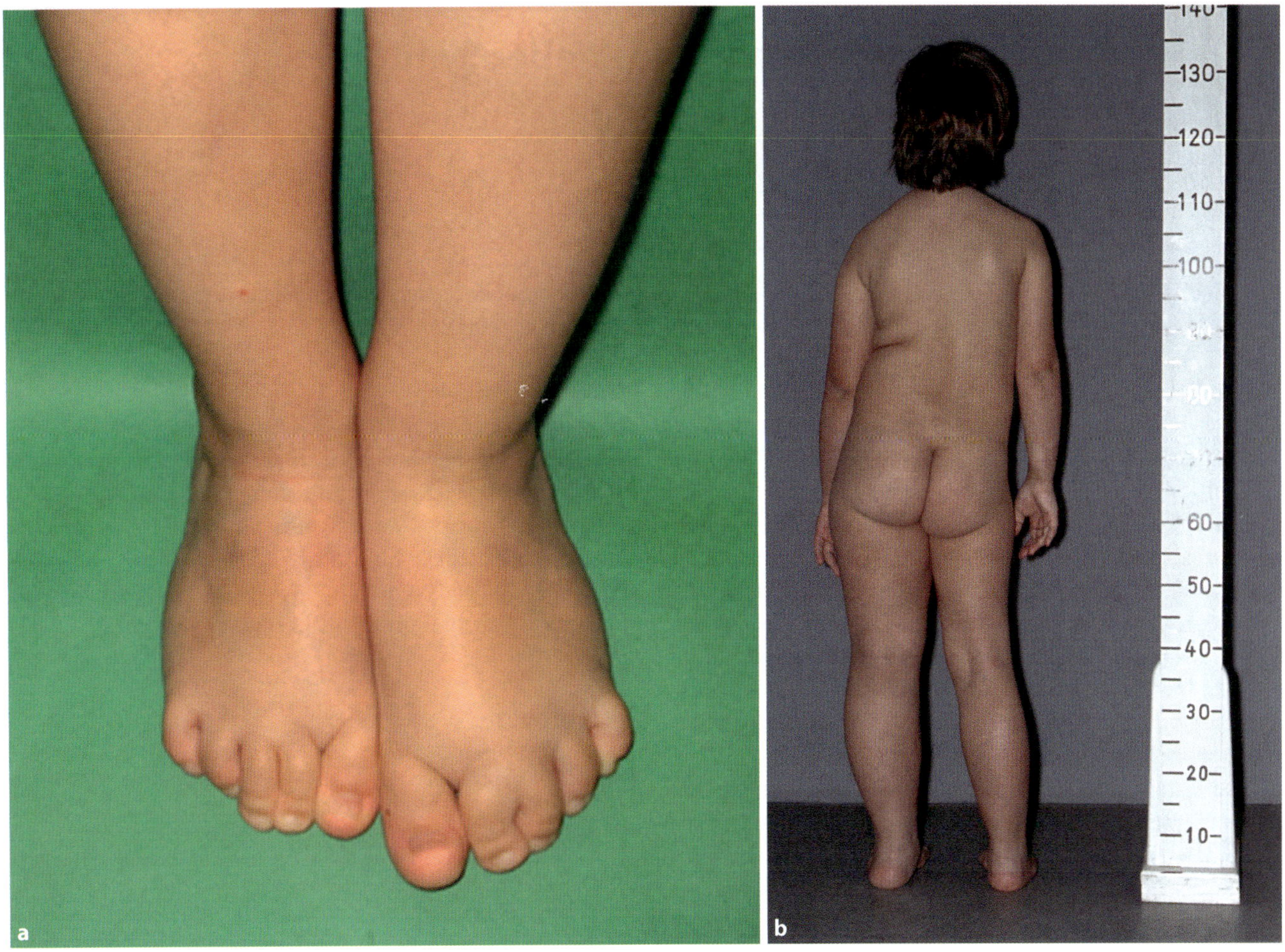

Fig. 100.1 **a** Enlargement of the left foot and lower leg. **b** Hemihyperplasia of the left leg with consecutive scoliosis

101 Klippel–Trénaunay–Weber Syndrome

MIM 149000

Synonyms
Angioosteohypertrophy syndrome

Major Clinical Findings
Klippel–Trénaunay–Weber syndrome consists of cutaneous angiomatosis, varicose veins, and enlargement of the bone and soft tissue of the limbs presenting as asymmetric limb hypertrophy. Hemodynamically, significant arteriovenous communications have been reported. The most frequent finding is unilateral leg hypertrophy, which may occur at any age and progressively increase. In some cases, only the proximal or the distal limb segment is affected. Radiographs of the affected limb show enlargement of underlying subcutaneous tissues, muscle, and bones. Very rarely, limb hypotrophy has been reported.

The visible vascular abnormalities are usually present in the body parts in which the hypertrophy is located. Hemangiomatous lesions include nevus flammeus, varicosities, phlebectasia, cutaneous and subcutaneous hemangiomas, and arteriovenous fistula. Hemangiomatous lesions may also affect the viscera, including the gastrointestinal tract, urinary system, and visceral organs. Macrodactyly and cutaneous syndactyly may be present. In some cases, craniofacial involvement similar to that seen in Sturge–Weber syndrome is present. These patients have a higher risk for neurologic complications, especially intellectual disability. Patients without craniofacial involvement show normal psychomotor development. In some instances, intracranial vascular malformations have been described, including arteriovenous malformations and infarction of the brain and spinal cord.

Occasional Findings
Polydactyly, oligodactyly, hyperpigmented areas, eye abnormalities, macrocephaly, visceromegaly, pulmonary vein varicosity.

Genetic Transmission
Almost all cases are sporadic. Occasional familial aggregation has been reported.

Differential Diagnosis
Isolated hemihyperplasia should be excluded. Other syndromes with hemangiomatous involvement such as Proteus syndrome and CLOVES syndrome must be differentiated. Neurofibromatosis may be associated with limb hypertrophy and skin hemangiomas.

Molecular Pathology
Somatic mosaicism for a missense mutation in the *PIK3CA* gene has been shown in patients with CLOVES syndrome, an overgrowth syndrome with features overlapping those of Klippel–Trénaunay–Weber syndrome. Analysis of affected tissue from patients who had been diagnosed with Klippel–Trénaunay–Weber syndrome showed somatic mosaicism for a missense mutation in PIK3C in some individuals.

References

Berry SA, Peterson C, Mize W, Bloom K, Zachary C, Blasco P et al (1998) Klippel–Trenaunay syndrome. Am J Med Genet 79:319–326

Hall BD, Cadle RG, Morrill-Cornelius SM, Bay CA (2007) Phakomatosis pigmentovascularis: implications for severity with special reference to mongolian spots associated with Sturge–Weber and Klippel–Trenaunay syndromes. Am J Med Genet 143A:3047–3053

Kurek KC, Luks VL, Ayturk UM, Alomari AI, Fishman SJ, Spencer SA et al (2012) Somatic mosaic activating mutations in PIK3CA cause CLOVES syndrome. Am J Hum Genet 90:1108–1115

S. Mundlos, D. Horn, *Limb Malformations*,
DOI 10.1007/978-3-540-95928-1_101, © Springer-Verlag Berlin Heidelberg 2014

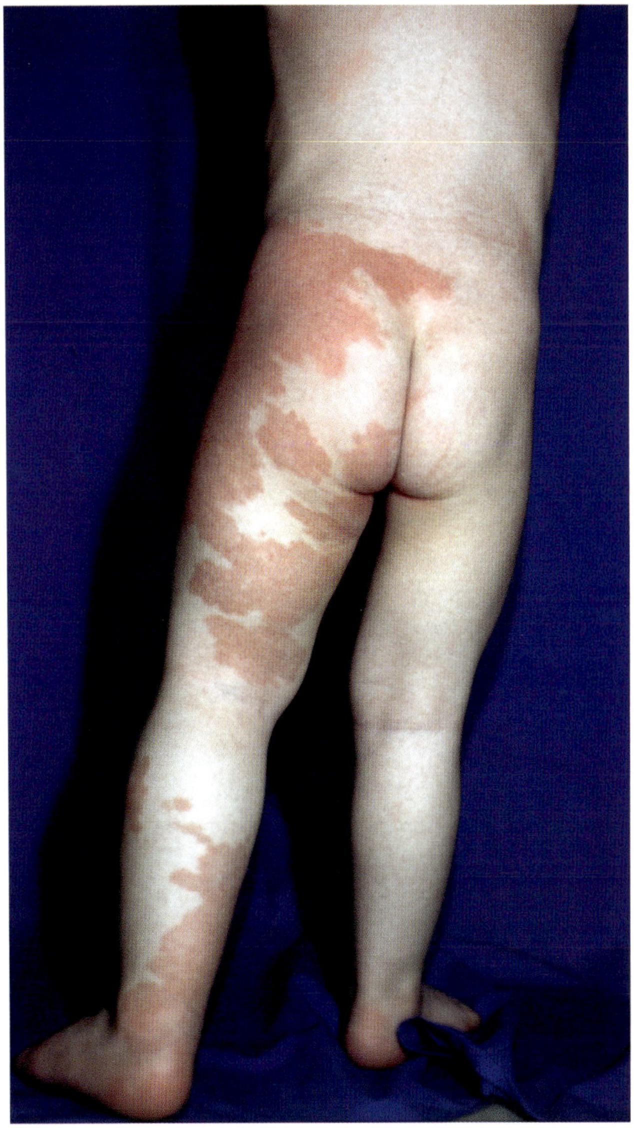

Fig. 101.1 Hemihypertrophy on left side with large cutaneous hemangiomata

102 Proteus Syndrome

MIM 176920

Major Clinical Findings

Proteus syndrome is, as the name implies, a remarkably variable disorder characterized by asymmetric and disproportionate overgrowth of body parts, connective tissue nevi, epidermal nevi, and vascular malformations. Manifestations include partial gigantism of the hands, feet, or both; growth asymmetry of the limbs; macrocephaly; and cranial hyperostosis. Birth weight is often increased. Increased growth tendency persists during the first years of life. Gyriform hyperplasia of the palms and soles is a specific sign. Rounded hyperostosis of the skull can develop, leading to enlargement and asymmetry of the skull. Subcutaneous hamartomas, hemangiomas, lipomas, and lymphangiomas may be noted, which are located on the thorax and upper abdomen in most cases. Abdominal and pelvic lipomatosis has been seen. Skin abnormalities such as pigmented intradermal nevi, hyperpigmented and hypopigmented areas, and linear verrucous epidermal nevi have been described. Moderate psychomotor delay and intellectual disability have been documented in more than half of the affected individuals. General diagnostic criteria suggested as mandatory are mosaic distribution of lesions, a progressive course, and sporadic occurrence. Connective tissue nevi are pathognomonic for the syndrome, although they are not present in all cases. Other combinations of manifestations (epidermal nevus, disproportionate overgrowth, specific tumors) are suggested to meet the diagnostic criteria, too.

Occasional Findings

Frontal bossing, scoliosis, hip dislocation, bony protuberances, central nervous system abnormalities, seizures, goiter, eye abnormalities such as strabismus and heterochromia, cataract, pulmonary embolism, deep venous thrombosis, tumors (ovarian cystadenoma, parotid monomorphic adenoma).

Genetic Transmission

Sporadic.

Differential Diagnosis

A Proteus-like syndrome is associated with germline and somatic mutations of the *PTEN* gene. Klippel–Trénaunay syndrome, CLOVES syndrome, and neurofibromatosis should be clinically excluded.

Molecular Pathology

Proteus syndrome is caused by mosaicism for a somatic activating mutation (E17K) in the *AKT1* gene on chromosome 14q32.3. No association between the proportion of mutant alleles and the clinical severity or specific manifestations of the phenotype has been observed. AKT, also called protein kinase B, is a target of the phosphoinositide 3-kinases, which generate specific inositol lipids that are implicated in the regulation of cell growth, proliferation, survival, and differentiation. The specific AKT mutation was shown to be present in the affected body part only with a fraction of mutant DNA ranging from 1 % to 50 %. This finding supports the hypothesis that Proteus syndrome, like other sporadically occurring syndromes with an irregular distribution of skin involvement, is due to mosaic mutations that are likely to be lethal in the germline.

References

Biesecker LG, Happle R, Mulliken JB, Weksberg R, Graham JM Jr., Viljoen DL et al (1999) Proteus syndrome: diagnostic criteria, differential diagnosis, and patient evaluation. Am J Med Genet 84:389–395

Happle R (1987) Lethal genes surviving by mosaicism: a possible explanation for sporadic birth defects involving the skin. Am Acad Derm 16:899–906

Lindhurst MJ, Sapp JC, Teer JK, Johnston JJ, Finn EM, Peters K et al (2011) A mosaic activating mutation in AKT1 associated with the Proteus syndrome. New Eng J Med 365:611–619

Wiedemann H-R, Burgio GR, Aldenhoff P, Kunze J, Kaufmann HJ, Schirg E (1983) The Proteus syndrome: partial gigantism of the hands and/or feet, nevi, hemihypertrophy, subcutaneous tumors, macrocephaly or other skull anomalies and possible accelerated growth and visceral affections. Europ J Pediat 140:5–12

S. Mundlos, D. Horn, *Limb Malformations*,
DOI 10.1007/978-3-540-95928-1_102, © Springer-Verlag Berlin Heidelberg 2014

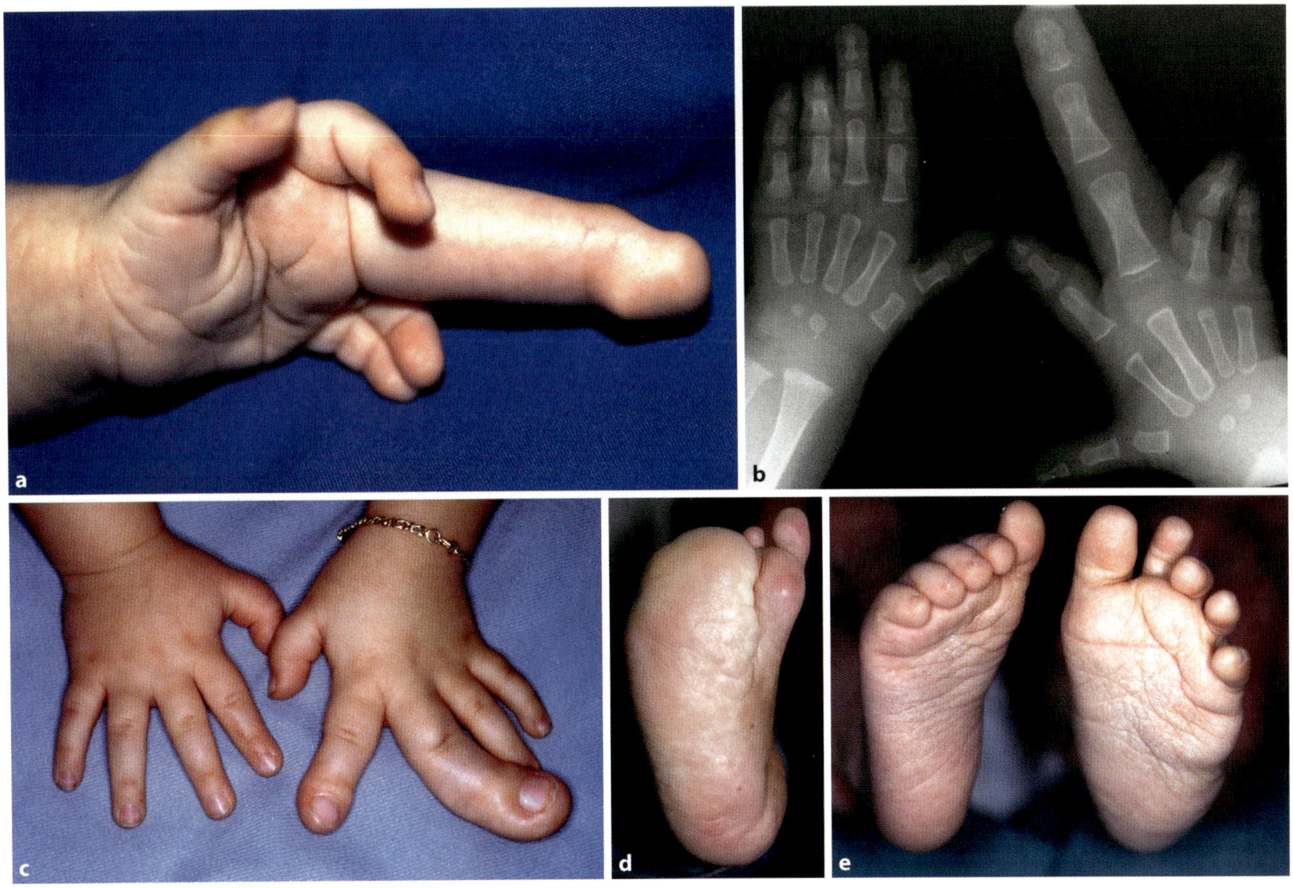

Fig. 102.1 **a** Hypertrophy of the middle finger in Proteus syndrome. **b** Corresponding radiograph shows enormously enlarged phalanges of digit III and enlarged metacarpal III of the right hand (and somewhat reduced size of the other digits). **c** Similar case with enlargement of digits II and III of the left hand. **d** Enlargement and thickening of sole. **e** Broadening of the left foot and thick skin with wrinkling

Subject Index

S. Mundlos, D. Horn, *Limb Malformations*,
DOI 10.1007/978-3-540-95928-1, © Springer-Verlag Berlin Heidelberg 2014

Printing: Ten Brink, Meppel, The Netherlands
Binding: Stürtz, Würzburg, Germany